Novel Drug Delivery Systems for Chinese Medicines

Nianping Feng • Zhijun Yang
Editors

Novel Drug Delivery Systems for Chinese Medicines

Springer

Editors
Nianping Feng
Department of Pharmaceutical Sciences
Shanghai University of Traditional
Chinese Medicine
Shanghai, China

Zhijun Yang
School of Chinese Medicine
Hong Kong Baptist University
Kowloon Tong, Hong kong, China

ISBN 978-981-16-3443-7　ISBN 978-981-16-3444-4 (eBook)
https://doi.org/10.1007/978-981-16-3444-4

This Springer imprint is published by the registered company Springer Nature Singapore Pte Ltd.
The registered company address is: 152 Beach Road, #21-01/04 Gateway East, Singapore 189721, Singapore

Editorial Board

Preface

Traditional Chinese Medicine (TCM) has been around for thousands of years and is enjoying increasing popularity all over the world for its more than ten thousand chemical ingredients with potential effects in healthcare. Even though great progress has been made in novel drug delivery systems for Chinese medicines during the last decades, the most effective chemical ingredients of TCM are still waiting for the reasonable designed novel drug delivery systems to reveal the significant pharmacological actions and to apply in clinical services. This book describes the fundamental concepts based on the frontier of pharmaceutical research in TCM, underlying scientific principles, and current advancements of drug delivery systems for Chinese medicines, including sustained-release drug delivery systems, nasal drug delivery systems, dermal and transdermal drug delivery systems, etc. Novel carriers and emerging technologies (such as pharmaceutical nanotechnologies and 3D printing) are also covered. The book provides readers with an overall picture of drug delivery systems for Chinese medicines and also yields benefits for the pharmaceutical industry with regard to TCM-based drug development.

The successful completion of this book is the result of the cooperation and confidence of many people. First, we thank all the chapter authors for their expertise, patience, and dedication during the frustrating and difficult time of the COVID-19 pandemic. Their contributions have really made this project realizable. We express our gratitude to Professor En Zhou for his help on the translation of professional TCM terms. Thanks also go to Prof. Xisong Ke, Dr. Ying Liu, and Dr. Xuefeng Hou for the review and comments on some chapters. We acknowledge the support of our publisher Springer Nature and thank Miss Xianxian Sun and Dr. Ke Liu for their encouragement, assistance, and guidance during the preparation of the book.

Shanghai, China — Nianping Feng
Kowloon Tong, Hong kong, China — Zhijun Yang

Marketing Text

This book describes the essential and cutting-edge concepts based on the frontier of pharmaceutical research in TCM, underlying scientific principles, and current advancements of drug delivery systems for Chinese medicines, including sustained-release drug delivery systems, trans-nasal drug delivery systems, dermal and transdermal drug delivery systems, etc. Novel carriers and emerging technologies (such as 3D printing) are also covered. The book provides readers with an overall picture of drug delivery systems for Chinese medicines and also yields benefits for the pharmaceutical industry with regard to TCM-based drug development.

Contents

About the Editors

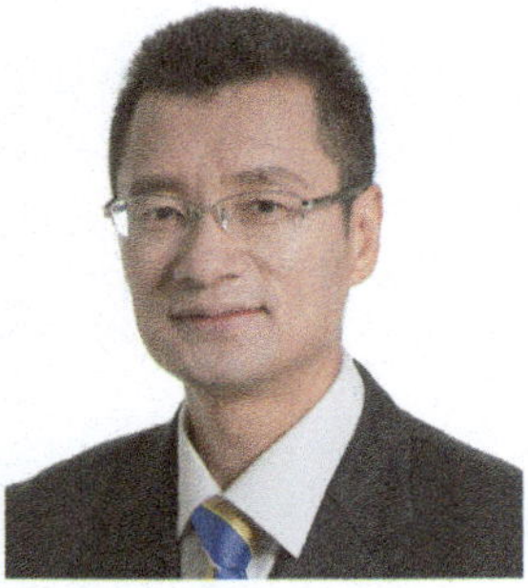

Nianping Feng is a Chair Professor and the Director of the Department of Pharmaceutical Sciences at Shanghai University of Traditional Chinese Medicine, Shanghai, China. He received his Ph.D. degree from China Pharmaceutical University in June 1997 and took up a lectureship at the same university prior to joining the Shanghai University of Traditional Chinese Medicine in October 1998. Dr. Feng worked as a senior research scientist at Purdue University from September 2012 to September 2013. His research interests include novel drug delivery systems, pharmaceutical nanotechnologies, and TCM-based new drug development. Dr. Feng has co-authored more than 200 research papers, reviews, and patents.

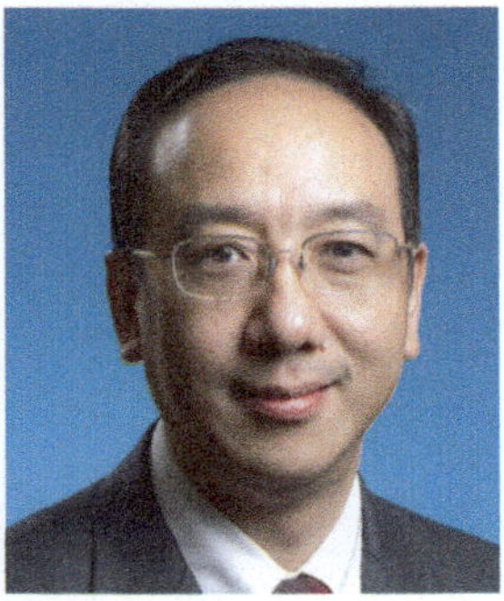

Zhijun Yang is a Professor at the School of Chinese Medicine, Hong Kong Baptist University, Hong Kong, China. He graduated from Shenyang College of Pharmacy, received his Ph.D. from Chiba University. He was an AP, a lecturer in China Pharmaceutical University, a researcher in Gifu Pharmaceutical University and TaiYo Pharmaceutical Industry Ltd., a postdoctoral at the University of British Columbia, and a scientist in Northern Lipids Inc. Canada. Dr. Yang attained remarkable results both in publications and pharmaceutical products. Currently, Dr. Yang is focusing on the forefront of the formulation by combining the theories of TCM and DDS.

Chapter 1
A Historical Overview and Concepts of Chinese Medicine Preparations and Novel Delivery Systems

Yongtai Zhang, Zehui He, Yuanzhi He, Xiaolin Hou, and Nianping Feng

Abstract Traditional Chinese medicine (TCM) is widely used in clinic for a long time in China, especially for certain chronic diseases with reliable clinical effects. However, there are challenges in the controllable quality, safety and efficiency, and patient compliance of TCM due to the traditional pharmaceutical approaches in preparation of Chinese medicines. During the past decades, novel drug delivery systems (NDDS) have been developed for Chinese medicines. This chapter presents the historical overview of Chinese medicines regarding the fundamental concepts, sources, characteristics, and preparation approaches. The design principles and current advancements of NDDS for Chinese medicines were also highlighted in this chapter.

Keywords Chinese medicine · Chinese medicinal materials · Active substances · Drug delivery system · Pharmaceutical nanotechnology

1.1 Introduction

Chinese medicines refer to the substances possessing the function of rehabilitation and healthcare and are generally used for the prevention, treatment, and diagnosis of diseases under the guidance of the theory of traditional Chinese medicine (TCM). There are a variety of Chinese medicines, including natural (herbs, animals, minerals) and processed (chemicals, biologics) products, and herbs are the most frequently used resource among these materials. Before being applied to clinical practice, Chinese medicines should be prepared to some dosage forms under the guidance of TCM theory.

The origin of Chinese medicine preparations can be traced back to the *Xia* dynasty (about 2070 BC–1600 BC), when medicinal liquor prepared in infusing

Y. Zhang · Z. He · Y. He · X. Hou · N. Feng (✉)
Department of Pharmaceutical Sciences, Shanghai University of Traditional Chinese Medicine, Shanghai, China
e-mail: npfeng@shutcm.edu.cn

N. Feng, Z. Yang (eds.), *Novel Drug Delivery Systems for Chinese Medicines*,
https://doi.org/10.1007/978-981-16-3444-4_1

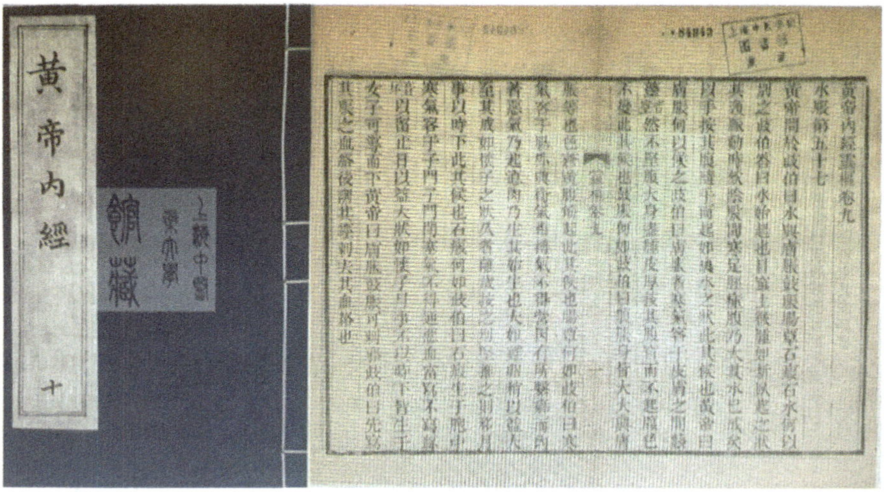

Fig. 1.1 A photocopy of the book *Huang Di Nei Jing* (*Huangdi's Internal Classic, or The Yellow Emperor's Classic of Medicine*), which is hoarded in the library of Shanghai University of Traditional Chinese Medicine

method was developed. In *Shang* dynasty (about 1600 BC–1046 BC), *Yi Yin* (1649 BC–1550 BC) invented the decoction.

Huang Di Nei Jing (*Huangdi's Internal Classic*) (Fig. 1.1) is the earliest medical classic extant in China, in which the "*Jun* (monarch), *Chen* (minister), *Zuo* (assistant), *Shi* (guide)" hierarchy of a prescription was firstly proposed, and various dosage forms including decoction, pill, powder, paste, wine, etc. as well as their preparation methods were recorded. The pharmaceutical theory and technology of Chinese medicines developed rapidly during the *Qin* and *Han* dynasties (221 BC–220). *Wu Shi Er Bing Fang* (*Prescriptions for Fifty-two Diseases*; written before 168 BC) unearthed from *Mawangdui Han* Tombs (Changsha city, Hunan province) recorded not only conventional external application and oral administration but also diverse application methods of Chinese medicines like medicated bath, fumigation, steam fumigation, and hot medicinal compress. *Shang Han Za Bing Lun* (*Treatise on Cold Damage and Miscellaneous Diseases*) and *Jin Gui Yao Lue* (*Synopsis of Prescriptions of the Golden Chamber*) were written by *Zhang Zhongjing* (150–154 to 215–219) in the *Donghan* (*Eastern Han*) dynasty (25–220). In these two books, more than 60 species of Chinese medicinal herbs were recorded, and gelatin, refined honey, and gooey starch were first used as excipients for pills, which are still adopted nowadays. During the *Dongjin* (Eastern *Jin*) dynasty (317–420), *Ge Hong* (283–363) compiled *Zhou Hou Bei Ji Fang* (*Handbook of Prescriptions for Emergencies*), which documented black plaster (lead soap), dry extract, waxed pill, concentrated pill, pastille, medicated roll, moxibustion formula, medicinal cake, and other dosage forms. *Xin Xiu Ben Cao* (*Newly Revised Materia Medica*) is the earliest pharmacopeia in the world, and it was promulgated officially in the *Tang* dynasty in 659.

The Chinese traditional patent medicines witnessed great development from the Song dynasty to the *Yuan* dynasty (960–1368). The *Song* dynasty government established the *He Ji JU* (the *Imperial Medical Bureau*) to sell Chinese medicine preparations in 1076, and a government-operated pharmaceutical factory named *Xiu He* was set up. In 1080, the Imperial Medical Bureau issued the earliest Good Preparation Practice of TCM, entitled *Tai Ping Hui Min He Ji Ju Fang* (*Prescriptions of Peaceful Benevolent Dispensary*), which recorded a total of 788 preparations. *Ben Cao Gang Mu* (*Compendium of Materia Medica*), written by *Li Shizhen* (1518–1593), recorded 1892 medicines, over 13,000 prescriptions, and almost 40 kinds of dosage forms. This book is recognized as a comprehensive summary of Chinese pharmacy before the sixteenth century. In the *Qing* dynasty (1636–1912), *Wu Shiji* (1806–1886) compiled *Li Yue Pian Wen* (*Rhymed Discourse for Topical Remedies*), which was the first monograph on the external application of Chinese medicines. This book expounds the theory of external therapies and recorded the preparation methods, usage, and therapeutic effects of various plasters. Unfortunately, in the huge number of TCM prescriptions or formulas, few herb-drug were indicated the role as the "*Jun*, *Chen*, *Zuo*, *Shi*" in its formula, while the "*Shi* (guide)" may be considered to hold the most similar function of drug delivery system (DDS).

From the beginning of the nineteenth century to the middle of the twentieth century, dosage forms of Chinese medicines such as tablets and injectable formulations were developed. Chinese medicine preparations marched forward to modern dosage forms from old ones, which is of great significance for the improvement of the therapeutic efficacy and patient compliance. More than 20 kinds of dosage forms for Chinese medicines such as injections, granules, tablets, capsules, dripping pills, suppositories, ointments, and aerosols have been available on the market. Since the 1990s, as the advances in the research on pharmacodynamic material basis and effect mechanism of Chinese medicines, the development of Chinese medicine preparations has entered the stage of novel drug delivery systems (NDDS). However, there are still many concerns in the design of NDDS for Chinese medicines, such as unclarified mechanism and effective ingredients of Chinese medicines, extraction and purification of active substances, and unknown in vivo fate and biopharmaceutical characteristics [1].

1.2 Characteristics of Chinese Medicines

*1.2.1 Medicinal Materials' Growing Areas and Geo-Authentic Medicinal Materials (*Daodi Yaocai*)*

The geographical distribution and production of crude medicinal materials are closely related to certain natural conditions. The species, yield, and quality of various medicinal materials are determined by their growing areas [2–4]. Geo-authentic medicinal materials refer to medicinal materials with a long historical standing, suitable origin, superior breed, high yield, particular processing, outstanding therapeutic effect, and special local feature [5]. There are a large number of representative geo-authentic medicinal materials, such as *Danggui* (*Angelicae Sinensis Radix*) from Gansu province; *Gouqizi* (*Lycii Fructus*) from Ningxia province; *Dahuang* (*Rhei Radix et Rhizoma*) from Qinghai province; *Huangqi* (*Astragali Radix*) from Inner Mongolia; *Dangshen* (*Codonopsis Radix*) from Shanxi province; *Renshen* (*Ginseng Radix et Rhizoma*), *Dengzhanxixin* (*Erigerontis Herba*), and *Wuweizi* (*Schisandrae Chinensis Fructus*) from the northeast provinces; and *Dihuang* (*Rehmanniae Radix*) from Henan province.

1.2.2 Harvesting of Chinese Medicinal Materials

The time and method of harvesting medicinal materials are closely related to quality. The active ingredients and toxic constituents in medicinal parts are different at various growth stages of plants and animals, and the therapeutic efficacy and side effects are consequently different. For example, the total flavonoids content was reduced at the fruiting stage and then raised at the fruit ripening stage of *Astragalus membranaceus* (Fisch.) Bge.var. *mongholicus* (Bge.) Hsiao [6]. Therefore, Chinese medicinal materials must be harvested at the appropriate season.

1.2.3 Processing of Medicinal Materials

Processing of medicinal materials refers to a necessary process of crude medicinal materials according to the needs of medical treatment and formulation before application. Conventional processing methods include processing of net and cut, water processing, fire processing, water and fire co-processing, etc. The purpose of processing is to cleanse the medicinal materials, sort different medical parts, and distinguish commercial grades. Decoction pieces (also known as prepared slices of Chinese medicinal materials) bearing processing reduces toxicity and side effects, enhances therapeutic efficacy, changes the performance of medicinal materials, and expands their application fields [7]. It has been reported that herbal-processing technology can significantly impair hepatotoxicity and nephrotoxicity evoked by *Tripterygium wilfordii* Hook. f. [8]. *Pinellia pedatisecta* has proinflammatory toxicity related to the *Pinellia pedatisecta* lectin, and the alum and quicklime solution processing reduces the toxicity by inducing protein denaturation [9]. The dried gizzard membrane of *Gallus gallus domesticus* with fire processing enhances the effect on urolithiasis [10].

1.2.4 Compatibility of Chinese Medicines

According to the requirement for the indications, the characteristic of Chinese medicines, and the theory of TCM, the combination of two or more Chinese medicines is called compatibility. There are seven features of compatibility of Chinese medicines, including using a single drug (or going alone) and six kinds of compatibility in TCM clinic. Mutual promotion (or mutual reinforcement) and mutual assistance can increase the therapeutic effectiveness of Chinese medicines, which are generally applied in clinical use, such as compatibility of *Mahuang* (*Ephedrae Herba*) and *Rougui* (*Cinnamomi Cortex*), *Huangqi* (*Astragali Radix*), and *Fuling* (*Poria*). Mutual restraint (or incompatibility between two drugs) and mutual detoxication can alleviate toxicity or side effects, which can be utilized in the processing and clinical application of Chinese medicines with strong toxicity, e.g., *Banxia* (*Pinelliae Rhizoma*) is incompatible with *Shengjiang* (*Zingiberis Rhizoma Recens*) [11]. Mutual inhibition may weaken each other's therapeutic actions, and antagonism will induce toxic reactions or severe side effects, e.g., *Shengjiang* has mutual inhibition with *Huangqin* (*Scutellariae Radix*), and *Chuanbeimu* (*Fritillariae Cirrhosae Bulbus*) is antagonism with *Chuanwu* (*Aconiti Radix*). Reports have shown that the synergistic mechanism of the *Baishao* (*Paeoniae Radix Alba*) and *Gancao* (*Glycyrrhizae Radix et Rhizoma*) herbal pair is associated with their coregulation of bile secretion and ATP-binding cassette transporter pathways [12]. The root of *Gansui* (*Kansui Radix*) has an effect on treating malignant pleural effusion, but could be weakened by the co-use of *Gancao*, even causing serious toxicity [13]. The toxicity is related to the selenoamino acid, nicotinate, and nicotinamide metabolism [14], and impacting the gut microbiota diversity and related metabolic functions [15]. Therefore, mutual antagonism and mutual suppression should be avoided in the compatibility of Chinese medicines.

1.3 Active Substances of Chinese Medicine Preparations

1.3.1 Diversity of the Active Substances of Chinese Medicine Preparations

Diversity is the main characteristic of active substances of Chinese medicine preparations, covering the following aspects.

1.3.1.1 Diversity of Source

The decoction pieces and extracts are obtained from processed medicinal materials. Diversity of the source of medicinal herbs generally affects the quality of active substances of Chinese medicines, e.g., the chemicals of *Chishao* (*Paeoniae Radix*

Rubra) and *Baishao* in *Huangqin* Decoction differ from that in single herbs, especially in terms of monoterpenoids and hydrolyzable tannins [16]. Therefore, the source of materials should be controlled according to the botanical origin, specific species, and medicinal part.

1.3.1.2 Diversity of Ingredients and Effects

Chinese medicines generally contain multitudinous active ingredients, for example, *Renshen* contains polysaccharides, organic acids, esters, and more than 30 kinds of ginsenosides [17]; gintonin contains lysophosphatidic acids that are the intracellular lipid mitogenic mediator, and gintonin activates the G protein-coupled receptors for lysophosphatidic acids, which can be associated with *Yin* and *Yang* components [18]. Moreover, Chinese medicine preparations are generally made of two or more ingredients, combinations of medicinal multi-components, and exert multi-targeting and multi-actions.

1.3.1.3 Diversity of Factors Affecting the Quality

Many factors affect the quality of raw active substances of Chinese medicines, such as the species, growing areas, harvesting and processing methods, and transport and storage conditions. Some Chinese medicines with the same popular name have differences in quality, while they are of different families or genera. Besides, the quality of herbs in the same family and genera can be affected by the ecological environment, harvest season, and processing technic. For example, there were more than ten kinds of medicinal herbs belonging to Menispermaceae Juss. and Aristolochiaceae Juss. family used as *Fangji*, such as *Stephania tetrandra* S. Moore, *Cocculus orbiculatus* (L.) DC., *Aristolochia fangchi* Y.C.Wu ex L.D. Chou et S.M, and Sichuan *Stephania tetrandra* [19]. *Stephania tetrandra* S. Moore (*Stephaniae Tetrandrae Radix*) contains active constituents with muscle relaxation function, exerting the effect of dispelling pathogenic wind to relieve pain [20]. However, *Aristolochia fangchi* Y.C.Wu ex L.D. Chou et S.M contains aristolochic acid which shows renal toxicity [21]. In Chinese Pharmacopoeia (2020 edition), only *Stephania tetrandra* S. Moore (*Stephaniae Tetrandrae Radix*) has been included as the medicinal herb *Fangji*. The original growing area of *Fangji* is northeast provinces and Inner Mongolia, and after being introduced to southern China, herbs undergo lignification and have different characteristics and ingredients [22]. Moreover, the content of rutin is the highest in the buds of the sophora flower, while it's much lower in the blooming flowers [23, 24]. Besides, there are some Chinese medicines like frankincense, myrrh, and catechu that tend to be sticky in hot or humid storage conditions.

1.3.2 Types of Active Substances of Chinese Medicine Preparations

The active substances of Chinese medicine preparations include the decoction pieces, vegetable oils and fat oils, extracts, and purified active ingredients.

1.3.2.1 Decoction Pieces

The decoction pieces refer to the processed Chinese medicinal materials that can be directly used in TCM clinic as prescription drugs. In general, the components of a TCM compound prescription refer to decoction pieces.

1.3.2.2 Volatile Oil and Fatty Oil

The volatile oil is a type of liquid oil that can be distilled with water vapor and is immiscible with water, and most of them have aromatic odors. Representative volatile oil like clove basil oil, patchouli oil, and perilla leaf oil can be obtained by hydrodistillation or/and steam distillation, and they are important active substances for the preparation of *Fufang Dingxiangluole* Oil and *Huoxiang Zhengqi* Tincture (patchouli oil and perilla leaf oil).

Tea oil, spicebush oil, sesame oil, and castor oil are common fatty oils, which are obtained by pressing or refining process. Tea oil is the material of injectable tea oil and ointment, spicebush oil is used in the preparation of suppository, and sesame oil can be used as a lubricant and excipient.

1.3.2.3 Extracts

Extracts of Chinese medicine generally fall into total extracts and effective fractions.

Total extracts are crude extracts obtained from Chinese medicinal materials by using water, ethanol, or other solvents.

Effective fractions are one or several types of constituents extracted from Chinese medicines. Quantitative determination of representative active ingredients should be carried out, and the upper and lower limits should be specified; for those toxic ingredients, an upper limit is necessary. The effective fractions have a relatively definite pharmacodynamic substance base and specific pharmacological activity and can represent the efficacy of medicinal materials and initial prescription, such as total saponin of *Huangqi* and total flavonoids of *Gegen* (*Puerariae Lobatae Radix*).

1.3.2.4 Active Ingredients

Active ingredients are defined as the substances with the therapeutic effect, which are generally chemical monomeric compounds with high purity above 90%, specific molecular formula or structural formula, and certain physicochemical properties, such as salidroside and baicalin. A single Chinese medicine usually contains a variety of active ingredients, for example, active ingredients of *Wuzhuyu* (*Euodiae Fructus*) include evodiamine, rutecarpine, limonin, and synephrine.

Preparations made with active ingredients have the advantages of a definite foundation and controllable quality. However, a single active ingredient usually cannot represent the comprehensive effect of TCM compound prescription, which results in a limited number of Chinese medicine preparations made from active ingredients.

1.3.3 Preparation of Active Substances of Chinese Medicine Preparations

Active substances of Chinese medicine preparations can be regarded as intermediates of the final products, and the preparation process mainly includes extraction, refining, concentrating, and drying processes of the prepared slices of Chinese medicinal materials.

1.3.3.1 Pretreatment of Chinese Medicinal Materials

According to the properties of crude drugs and the need for extraction method, pretreatment like grinding should be adopted. For a small number of preparations that can be directly used as powder in the production of preparations, the fineness of pulverization should be controlled to obtain appropriate particle size according to the requirements of the preparations. The decoction pieces must be inspected according to mandatory standard, and only those that reach the standard could be used in production.

1.3.3.2 Extraction

The extraction process depends on the physical properties, chemical components, therapeutic efficacy, and clinical requirements of Chinese medicines. The prescription composition is different, and the extraction process varies accordingly. In general, for oral preparations or external preparations, if the effective constituents of medicinal materials are one or several categories of compounds with different therapeutic effects, purified total extract with no toxicity is not necessary to achieve high purity and can be directly applied in preparation in consideration of actual production. It's an economical method to extract all the Chinese medicines in the prescription together, which is the traditional way of decoction preparation under the guidance of TCM theory.

For optimization of the extraction process, an accurate, convenient, representative, and quantifiable comprehensive evaluation index system should be created, and the content of active ingredients and the therapeutic effect of a prescription can be regarded as indicators. To select an appropriate extraction process and design a feasible process route, the active ingredients and pharmacological effect of each Chinese medicine in the prescription need to be analyzed, and factors like clinical requirements, physicochemical properties of the effective constituents, or fractions should be taken into consideration.

Factors related to the process can be optimized by using design of experiments, such as orthogonal test design, uniform test design, composite design, and response surface methodology. At present, some modern extraction technologies such as supercritical fluid extraction, smashing tissue extraction, microwave-assisted extraction, and ultrasonic extraction provide more choices for the extraction of active substances from Chinese medicines. For example, a deep eutectic solvent belongs to green chemistry is reported for extracting flavonoids from *Huaihua* (*Flos Sophorae*) efficiently [25], and the online near-infrared technique has been used for determination of rutin from *Huaihua* in the extraction process of formula particles [26].

1.3.3.3 Separation and Purification

The objective of separation is to obtain pharmacodynamic compositions from the crude extract, and the selection of separation methods and conditions depends on the physicochemical properties of the active ingredients. The role of purification is to eliminate non-active and noxious ingredients, get purified active ingredients or fractions, and provide qualified active ingredients for preparations.

The refining process should be designed according to the dosage form, administration route, prescription dosage, and physicochemical properties of the extracted active ingredients. High-speed centrifugation, membrane separation, macroporous resin adsorption and purification, molecular distillation, and other purification techniques can be used for refining, e.g., flavonoid glycosides in *Huaihua* are extracted by using ultrasonic-assisted extraction and isolated by high-speed countercurrent chromatography [27].

1.3.3.4 Concentration and Drying

The concentration and drying process is utilized to achieve required relative density or water content of the extract and facilitate the shaping of preparations. The design of the concentration and drying process is related to the physicochemical properties of the materials. For those that contain thermolabile and fusible ingredients, special concentration and drying method should be chosen to ensure the quality of the concentrated or dried products.

1.4 NDDS of Chinese Medicines

1.4.1 Design of NDDS for Chinese Medicines

When developing the NDDS for Chinese medicines, the requirements of safety, therapeutic effect, stability, controllability, and patient compliance of the NDDS should be achieved. For example, the total alkaloids extracted from *Aconitum sinomontanum* showed strong anti-inflammatory and analgesic effects but exhibited poor oral bioavailability and short half-life, and microneedle-mediated nanostructured lipid carriers were demonstrated as excellent transdermal system for decreasing cytotoxicity and increasing biocompatibility of those total alkaloids [28, 29]. In general, for active substances of Chinese medicines with strong local irritation, the inclusion or microencapsulation technology can be utilized to reduce irritation, e.g., aconitine is an active ingredient isolated from *Chuanwu* with high toxicity, and by using solid lipid nanoparticles as the sustained-release carrier and administered by transdermal route, the medication safety is improved [30]. Dripping pills are suitable for sublingual administration, and the rapid drug absorption facilitates first aid of angina. Oral tablets and transdermal patches tend to be applied in the prophylactic treatment of angina [31, 32]. Besides, the adaptability of production technology and economic efficiency should be added as evaluation indicators in the processes of extraction and separation, the selection of excipients, and the optimization process of Chinese medicine preparation formulations.

During developing formulations, factors including characteristics of administration routes, the compliance and physiological conditions of treated patients, and the pharmaceutical and biopharmaceutical properties of active substances of Chinese medicines should also be taken into consideration. The dosage forms can play a key role in exerting therapeutic efficacy in certain conditions, which is mainly reflected in the effect on drug release, absorption, and biological distribution. Sustained-release tablets and capsules are suitable for chronic diseases, and a time-controlled drug release system can be applied to diseases with periodic rhythmic changes such as asthma and angina pectoris which often bring an attack in the evening or early morning. Additionally, treatment of local skin diseases usually adopts ointments or gels. In order to enhance the therapeutic efficacy, accelerate or delay the effect, increase the targeting ability and tissues retention, and meet the needs for treatment, the corresponding NDDS can be developed, such as *Subing* Dripping Pills for coronary heart disease and angina pectoris, Vitex Oil Microcapsules for tracheitis, and elastic liposomes made as carriers of cinnamic acid for enhanced transdermal delivery [33]. Furthermore, the antitumor drugs are advisable to be loaded in the targeted drug delivery systems (nanoparticles, liposomes, etc.) to improve the therapeutic efficacy and reduce toxicity and side effects. In another case, oridonin is the main active ingredient in *Donglingcao* (*Rabdosiae Rubescentis Herba*), and its therapeutic antitumor efficacy is improved by loading into atactic poly(D,L-lactic acid) nanoparticles and surface cross-linking with the peptide Arg-Gly-Asp (RGD) for active tumor-targeted therapy [34].

1.4.2 NDDS Technologies Used in Chinese Medicines

NDDS technologies can be employed for improving the efficacy and avoiding the side effects of Chinese medicines. In consideration of Chinese medicines usually containing multitudinous active ingredients, most NDDS designs focused on sustained- or controlled-release systems for oral and transdermal administration, while targeted drug delivery systems were generally developed for specific active ingredients (Fig. 1.2). Besides, NDDS technologies used in Chinese medicines such as transdermal, mucosal, targeted, and smart drug delivery systems also have been developed rapidly.

1.4.2.1 Oral Sustained-Release Systems

Pills and black plasters (Fig. 1.3) are representatives of early sustained-release drug delivery systems for oral and topical routes, respectively. Beeswax is used in waxed pills as a matrix, which can reach the intestinal tract to release the drug continuously after oral administration; lead plaster is used in black plasters as a matrix to improve skin hydration and lessen the stratum corneum to enhance drug permeation into the skin. Sustained- or controlled-release technologies like coating technology, solid dispersion, and inclusion compound have been applied to Chinese medicines. For

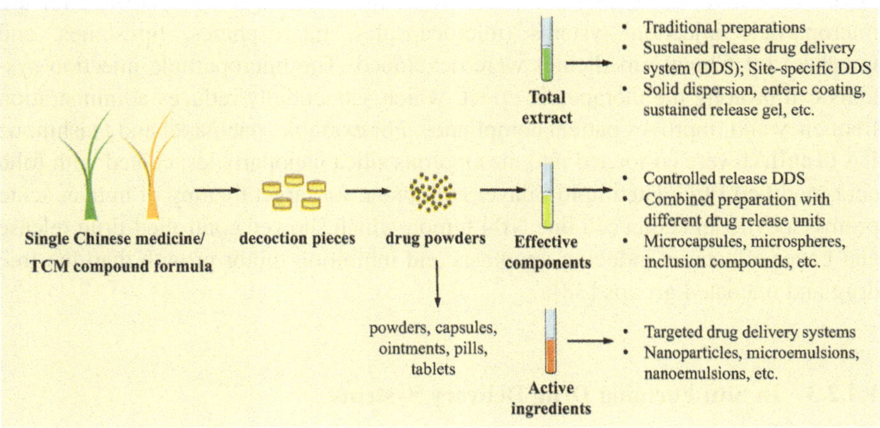

Fig. 1.2 Drug delivery systems and carriers suitable for different types of active substances of Chinese medicines

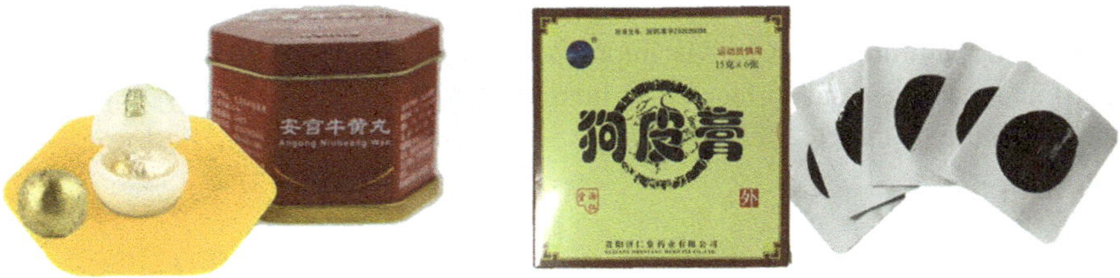

Fig. 1.3 Pills (left, *Angong Niuhuang* Pills) and black plasters (right, *Goupi* Plasters). (Photos by Dr. Yang Lu, Beijing University of Chinese Medicine)

example, paeonol is isolated from *Mudanpi* (*Moutan Cortex*), and the protective effects of sustained-release gastroretention tablets of paeonol are more conducive to the rapid clearance of free paeonol on gastric ulcer and intestinal flora in rats [35]. The poor solubility and permeability across the gastrointestinal mucosa limit the clinical efficacy of glycyrrhizic acid, which has been used for the treatment of acute and chronic hepatitis. By using mixed micelles as a vehicle based on poloxamer 188 and D-α-tocopheryl polyethylene glycol 1000 succinate, its oral bioavailability has been improved via sustained release [36]. Compound *Danshen* consists of *Danshen* (*Salviae Miltiorrhizae Radix et Rhizoma*) extract and *Sanqi* (*Notoginseng Radix et Rhizoma*) extract, and *Tianranbingpian* (*Borneolum*); when the *Borneolum* is designed as a colon-specific osmotic pump capsule by using a semipermeable shell with the core components, of which the relative bioavailability achieved 330.58% and the retention time was greatly prolonged as compared with the commercially available *Fufang Danshen* Tablets [37].

1.4.2.2 Sustained-Release Systems for Intravenous Administration

Based on conventional liquid injection systems, sustained- or controlled-release microparticle injection systems (microcapsules, microspheres, liposomes, and micelles) for Chinese medicines were developed. The microparticle injection systems can prolong the therapeutic effect, which sequentially reduces administration frequency and improves patient compliance. For example, paclitaxel and tanshinone IIA (TanIIA) were co-loaded into mesoporous silica nanoparticles, coated with folic acid-modified PEGylated lipid-bilayer membrane for target therapy of human acute promyelocytic leukemia cell line NB4 tumor, which showed controlled-drug release and better effects on inducing apoptosis and inhibiting tumor growth than the free drug and uncoated groups [38].

1.4.2.3 In Situ Forming Drug Delivery Systems

In situ forming drug delivery systems can be used for local drug delivery which avoids the surgical operation of implantation; decreases administration frequency, dosage, and adverse reactions; and improves patient compliance. Besides, the manufacturing technique is simple and stable. A recent report pronounced that by loading *Chansu* (*Bufonis Venenum*) and *Xionghuang* (*Realgar*) (respectively encapsulated in solid lipid nanoparticles and ground into nano-realgar in advance) into a poloxamer 188/407-based temperature-sensitive in situ gel for the treatment of cervical cancer, and the drug release was improved and local irritation was reduced after vaginal administration [39].

1.4.2.4 Transdermal Drug Delivery Systems

Most drugs can hardly penetrate the skin to acquire desirable therapeutic effects, and a variety of new technologies such as pharmaceutical approaches (nanocarriers, etc.), chemical routes (penetration enhancers, prodrugs, ion pairs, etc.), physical means (iontophoresis, electroporation, ultrasound, laser, microneedles, and heating), and physiological methods (meridian point administration) have been developed to increase the transdermal absorption of drugs, i.e., the distribution of tetramethylpyrazine in the brain is increased by adding borneol and iontophoresis with microneedles assistant via transdermal route, and the effect on preventing middle cerebral artery occlusion was enhanced [40]. Emodin has potent activity against methicillin-resistant *Staphylococcus aureus*, and its effect is improved by encapsulating in the core of hydrophilic poly(vinylpyrrolidone) in the coaxial electrospinning nanofibers with a hygroscopic cellulose acetate sheath for topical administration [41].

1.4.2.5 Mucosal Drug Delivery Systems

Mucosal drug delivery systems aim at delivering the drug to specific areas such as nasal, buccal, ocular, rectal, and vaginal mucosa. In situ gels and buccal adhesive tablets can promote the drug to be absorbed through the mucosa, avoid the first-pass effect, prolong the action time, and improve bioavailability. In general, the appropriate dosage form is required to have the following characteristics: small in size, convenient to use, simple in the preparation process, and suitable for various administration routes. For example, the trimethyl chitosan-coated lipid nanoparticles were chosen as carriers for the ocular delivery of baicalein, to obtain a sustained release, enhanced permeability without ocular irritation, and improved ocular bioavailability [42].

1.4.2.6 Targeted Drug Delivery Systems

The development of targeted drug delivery systems provides a more effective, safe, convenient, and economical drug administration route for drugs with a narrow therapeutic window and requirement of high concentration in specific tissue or organ.

The composition of active substances of Chinese medicines is complex and multi-targeted. Therefore, in the research process of targeted drug delivery systems, based on the acting sites of the effective substances, the corresponding targeted units of each component should be prepared, and the interaction between the drug and the target should be clarified. At present, targeted drug delivery systems of Chinese medicines are mainly designed for monomer active ingredients. For example, in order to improve the efficacy of vincristine sulfate on metastatic tumors and malignant lymphoma, the poly(butylcyanoacrylate) nanoparticles were employed and modified with poloxamer 188, and the modified nanoparticles showed sustained drug release, lower clearance in systemic circulation, and higher lymphatic targeting efficiency when compared with the unmodified nanoparticles and free drug [43]. As another example, biopeptide-lipid hybrid nanoparticles modified with tLyP-1-fused apolipoprotein A-I-mimicking peptides possess long circulation and the ability to penetrate deeply into tumors, which shows potential use as vectors for targeted drug delivery systems of Chinese medicines [44].

1.4.2.7 Smart Drug Delivery Systems

Smart drug delivery systems can realize time-controlled and site-controlled drug release which are based on the information of pathological changes; as a result, the smart drug delivery systems can improve efficacy and reduce damage of the encapsulated drug to normal tissues. The present researches focus on pulsed drug release technology, which utilize external changes (such as magnetic field, light, temperature, electric field, or specific chemical substances) and in vivo environmental factors (such as pH, enzyme, and bacteria) to control the drug release. In order to improve the oxidative stress and anticancer efficacy of melittin, nanocomplexes were fabricated with condensed epigallocatechin gallate and covered with phenylboronic acid derivatized hyaluronic acid [45]. In another case, the TCM compound *Shuxiong* prescription was developed into sustained-release capsules that prepared by multi-particulate time-controlled explosion technology, so as to achieve the synchronous and release of *Panax notoginseng* saponins, hydroxysafflor yellow A, and ferulic acid [46]. Also, some commercially available Chinese patent medicines, e.g., *Tripterygium wilfordii* Bilayer Tablet, which can deliver one part of the drug rapidly release in the stomach and the other part slowly release in the intestine, thus to produce efficacy steadily and continuously.

1.5 Novel Pharmaceutical Technologies for Chinese Medicines

Applying novel pharmaceutical technologies is crucial to the development of new preparations and new dosage forms of Chinese medicines. Hitherto, novel pharmaceutical technologies have performed extensive researches and applications in the field of Chinese medicine preparation, including inclusion compounds, solid dispersion, microcapsules and microspheres, and especially pharmaceutical nanotechnologies. Herein, the above mentioned technologies were concisely introduced.

1.5.1 Inclusion Compounds

Inclusion compounds are that guest molecules enclosed in the cavity of host molecules to form host-guest inclusion compounds, which mostly rely on highly specific host-guest interactions. Materials used for inclusion include cholic acid, starch cellulose, protein, and cyclodextrin and its derivatives.

Inclusion compounds have the following advantages:

1. Increase the solubility and bioavailability of drugs, for instance, the solubility of both peppermint oil and eucalyptus oil is increased by about 50 times by using inclusion technique.
2. Reduce the irritation, objectionable odor, and mucosa irritation of the drug, e.g., the deficiencies of *Bufonis Venenum* and borneol in *Liushen* Pills can be covered up when enclosed in cyclodextrin.
3. Improve the stability of drugs which are susceptible to heat, moisture, and light, e.g., the stability of cinnamon oil is improved by inclusion.
4. Reduce the loss of volatile components; liquid components can be prepared to powder, for example, inclusion compound of garlic essential oil is a white powder with reduced irritation and masked odor.
5. Adjust drug release rate, e.g., inclusion compounds of camphor and menthol with β-cyclodextrin can be made into inhalant to achieve homogeneous drug release.

1.5.2 Solid Dispersion

As an intermediate of preparations, solid dispersion can be made into various dosage forms such as injections, capsules, tablets, pills, suppositories, and ointments. Solid dispersion made from various materials with different properties can meet different medication requirements, and the encapsulation effect of carriers may improve the chemical stability of drugs, change the liquid ingredients into solid forms, and reduce the objectionable odor or irritation of Chinese medicines. For instance, a novel porous silica carrier (AEROPERL® 300 Pharma) formed solid dispersions improved the in vitro release and oral bioavailability of puerarin, which also has excellent flowability and hydrophilic properties [47].

1.5.3 Microcapsules and Microspheres

Typically, the particle diameters of microcapsules and microspheres are in micron size. Microencapsulation technology can improve the stability of drugs such as β-carotene and menthol, shelter drugs from inactivation, reduce irritation and objectionable odor of the drug, and achieve taste masking and controlled drug release. Biological medicines such as enzymes and hemoglobin can also be encapsulated to improve biocompatibility and stability. Besides, embolic microspheres can block tumor vessels, cut off tumor tissue from nutrients, and suppress cancer cell proliferation, and embolic microspheres such as *Bletilla striata* polysaccharide are dual antitumor agents [48]. Shi et al. [49] reported a realgar nanoparticle-based microcapsule prepared by using a solvent evaporation technique, which exhibited higher bioavailability and improved antitumor efficacies than that of realgar nanoparticles and crude realgar.

1.5.4 Pharmaceutical Nanotechnologies

With nano-scale size, nanoparticles in pharmaceutics can enhance biomembrane permeability and promote absorption of active substances, increase the solubility of poorly soluble drugs, and improve bioavailability and target delivery of drugs. Generally, nanoparticles for drug delivery can be divided into three categories: nanosuspension of active ingredients, functionalized drug-loaded nanocarriers, and self-assembly nanoparticles of the ingredients in Chinese medicines [50].

It was found that daidzein nanosuspensions with steric (hydroxypropyl methylcellulose E5) and electrostatic (sodium dodecyl sulfate) stabilizers increased the solubility and dissolution rate of the drug, e.g., the oral bioavailability of nanosuspension in rats was 1.63–2.19 times greater than that of crude daidzein [51].

In recent years, various functionalized nanocarriers have been applied in drug delivery. A biomimetic nanoparticle is one of them, such as cell membrane-coated nanovesicles and natural extracellular vesicles like exosomes [52, 53], and nanocarriers camouflaged with membranes derived from tumor cells or exosomes have the ability to target the homologous tumor [54]. Liposomes are also called "biological membrane," which are easily modified to obtain various functions, such as active targeting, environmentally responsive drug release, and deformability [55]. Recently reported a new liposome that was co-hybridized with hyaluronic acid, ethanol, and the encapsulated volatile oil medicines (clove oil and cinnamon oil), which had excellent deformability and stability, thereby enhanced cargo permeability via transdermal administration [56]. Besides, solid lipid nanoparticles

(SLNs) as drug carriers can also improve the efficacy of the insoluble drug. Shi et al. [57] prepared SLNs for the delivery of frankincense and myrrh essential oils (FMO), and the results demonstrated that the SLN formulation increased the antitumor efficacy of FMO than that of FMO suspension and FMO β-CD inclusion complex.

Additionally, spontaneously formed nanoparticles have been developed to promote oral absorption of active ingredients [58]. For instance, microemulsion and submicroemulsion are formulated by self-emulsifying, which have an excellent performance in improving oral and transdermal absorption of drugs [59, 60]. Further, berberine and flavonoid glycosides can self-assemble to form nanoparticles and nanofibers, which showed significantly enhanced bacteriostatic activity [61]. Berberine and cinnamic acid can also self-assemble into nanoparticles with good bacteriostatic activity [62].

1.6 Multi-Component Drug Delivery System

The multi-component drug delivery system (MCDDS) is designed to achieve targeted delivery, programmed release, and multi-level synergy. According to the medicinal properties and clinical efficacy of Chinese medicines, different effective fractions are combined into prescriptions, and different drug release units are designed according to the physicochemical properties and pharmacological characteristics, to achieve the overall multi-channel and multi-targeted treatment concept. The components of Chinese medicines with similar physicochemical properties and activities are formed into different component units according to a certain ratio and integrated into a multi-unit drug release system with programmed release characteristics to improve the efficacy of Chinese medicines. In this regard, the TCM compound *Niuhuang Xingxiao* Pills was formulated into four units (realgar, frankincense, and myrrh oil, musk, and bezoar) using micro–/nanotechnologies, which obtained higher bioavailability and efficacy [63].

1.7 Conclusions

This chapter highlighted some aspects of the history of the Chinese medicine preparations, and the general information on the DDS of Chinese medicines were also covered.

The development of the DDS of Chinese medicines arose in the 1990s in China. Now several NDDS of Chinese medicines appeared on the market, and the number of patent applications about NDDS of Chinese medicines is growing rapidly. Sustained- and controlled-release formulations are the focus of the research and development of NDDS of Chinese medicines, which are suitable for the multi-component and multi-targeted characteristics of Chinese medicines.

As the chemical components of Chinese medicines are complicated and coexisting ingredients have great differences in physicochemical properties, it brings great difficulty to the pretreatment process, excipient selection, formulation design, quality evaluation, and construction of NDDS. At present, there are a few varieties of industrialized NDDS production based on Chinese medicines, and it remains a big challenge to establish in vivo and in vitro evaluation methods for NDDS which conforms to the features of Chinese medicines.

The following chapters provide more information on current and future design as well as the development of Chinese medicine-based NDDS, including design concepts, evaluation methods, and application prospects.

Acknowledgments This work was financially supported by the National Natural Science Foundation of China [82074279, 82074031] and the Natural Science Foundation of Shanghai [20ZR1458300].

References

1. Liu, Y., & Feng, N. (2015). Nanocarriers for the delivery of active ingredients and fractions extracted from natural products used in traditional Chinese medicine (TCM). *Advances in Colloid and Interface Science, 221*, 60–76.
2. Feng, T., Jia, Q., Meng, X., et al. (2020). Evaluation of genetic diversity and construction of DNA fingerprinting in Polygonatum Mill. based on EST-SSR and SRAP molecular markers. *3 Biotech, 10*(7), 322.
3. Yang, M., Abdalrahman, H., Sonia, U., et al. (2020). The application of DNA molecular markers in the study of Codonopsis species genetic variation, a review. *Cellular and Molecular Biology (Noisy-le-Grand, France), 66*(2), 23–30.
4. Shi, Y., Qiu, L., Guo, L., et al. (2020). K fertilizers reduce the accumulation of Cd in Panax notoginseng (Burk.) F.H. by improving the quality of the microbial community. *Frontiers in Plant Science, 11*, 888.
5. Hu, L., Chen, X., Yang, J., et al. (2019). Geographic authentication of the traditional Chinese medicine Atractylodes macrocephala Koidz. (Baizhu) using stable isotope and multielement analyses. *Rapid Communications in Mass Spectrometry, 33*(22), 1703–1710.
6. Liang, J., Li, W., Jia, X., et al. (2020). Transcriptome sequencing and characterization of Astragalus membranaceus var. mongholicus root reveals key genes involved in flavonoids biosynthesis. *Genes Genomics., 42*(8), 901–914.
7. Chen, Z., Ye, S. Y., & Zhu, R. G. (2020). The extraordinary transformation of traditional Chinese medicine: Processing with liquid excipients. *Pharmaceutical Biology, 58*(1), 561–573.
8. Wang, J. M., Li, J. Y., Cai, H., et al. (2019). Nrf2 participates in mechanisms for reducing the toxicity and enhancing the antitumour effect of Radix Tripterygium wilfordii to S180-bearing mice by herbal-processing technology. *Pharmaceutical Biology, 57*(1), 437–448.
9. Wang, N., Zhang, D., Zhang, Y. T., et al. (2019). Endothelium corneum gigeriaegalli extract inhibits calcium oxalate formation and exerts anti-urolithic effects. *Journal of Ethnopharmacology, 231*, 80–89.
10. Wang, W., Mao, S., Yu, H., et al. (2019). Pinellia pedatisecta lectin exerts a proinflammatory activity correlated with ROS-MAPKs/NF-κB pathways and the NLRP3 inflammasome in RAW264.7 cells accompanied by cell pyroptosis. *International Immunopharmacology, 66*, 1–12.

11. Chen, L., Hu, C., Hood, M., et al. (2020). An integrated approach exploring the synergistic mechanism of herbal pairs in a botanical dietary supplement: A case study of a liver protection health food. *Int J Genomics., 2020*, 9054192.
12. Fueki, T., Tanaka, K., Obara, K., et al. (2020). The acrid raphides in tuberous root of Pinellia ternata have lipophilic character and are specifically denatured by ginger extract. *Journal of Natural Medicines, 74*(4), 722–731.
13. Yu, J., Guo, J., Tao, W., et al. (2018). Gancao-Gansui combination impacts gut microbiota diversity and related metabolic functions. *Journal of Ethnopharmacology, 214*, 71–82.
14. Shen, J., Pu, Z. J., Kai, J., et al. (2017). Comparative metabolomics analysis for the compatibility and incompatibility of kansui and licorice with different ratios by UHPLC-QTOF/MS and multivariate data analysis. *Journal of Chromatography B Analytical Technologies in the Biomedical Life Sciences, 1057*, 40–45.
15. Shen, J., Wang, J., Shang, E. X., et al. (2016). The dosage-toxicity-efficacy relationship of kansui and licorice in malignant pleural effusion rats based on factor analysis. *Journal of Ethnopharmacology, 186*, 251–256.
16. Du, K., Yang, J., Yang, L., et al. (2020). Chemical profiling and marker characterization of Huangqin decoction prepared with three types of peony root by liquid chromatography with electrospray ionization mass spectrometry. *Journal of Separation Science, 43*(13), 2558–2570.
17. Shin, B. K., Kwon, S. W., & Park, J. H. (2015). Chemical diversity of ginseng saponins from Panax ginseng. *Journal of Ginseng Research, 39*(4), 287–298.
18. Im, D. S., & Nah, S. Y. (2013). Yin and Yang of ginseng pharmacology: Ginsenosides vs gintonin. *Acta Pharmacologica Sinica, 34*(11), 1367–1373.
19. Zhang, H. M., Zhao, X. H., Sun, Z. H., et al. (2019). Recognition of the toxicity of aristolochic acid. *Journal of Clinical Pharmacy and Therapeutics, 44*(2), 157–162.
20. Jiang, Y., Liu, M., Liu, H., et al. (2020). A critical review: Traditional uses, phytochemistry, pharmacology and toxicology of Stephania tetrandra S. Moore (Fen Fang Ji). *Phytochemical Review, 19*, 1–41.
21. Zhang, Y., Qi, D., Gao, Y., et al. (2020). History of uses, phytochemistry, pharmacological activities, quality control and toxicity of the root of Stephania tetrandra S. Moore: A review. *Journal of Ethnopharmacology, 260*, 112995.
22. Paniwnyk, L., Beaufoy, E., Lorimer, J. P., et al. (2001). The extraction of rutin from flower buds of Sophora japonica. *Ultrasonics Sonochemistry, 8*(3), 299–301.
23. Violon, C. (1997). Belgian (Chinese herb) nephropathy: Why? *Journal de Pharmacie de Belgique, 52*(1), 7–27.
24. Sim, H. J., Kim, J. H., Lee, K. R., et al. (2013). Simultaneous determination of structurally diverse compounds in different Fangchi species by UHPLC-DAD and UHPLC-ESI-MS/MS. *Molecules, 18*(5), 5235–5250.
25. Li, Y., Shi, X., Wu, Z., et al. (2015). Near-infrared for on-line determination of quality parameter of Sophora japonica L. (formula particles): From lab investigation to pilot-scale extraction process. *Pharmacognosy Magazine, 11*(41), 8–13.
26. Wang, G., Cui, Q., Yin, L. J., et al. (2019). Efficient extraction of flavonoids from Flos Sophorae Immaturus by tailored and sustainable deep eutectic solvent as green extraction media. *Journal of Pharmaceutical and Biomedical Analysis, 170*, 285–294.
27. Xie, Z., Sun, Y., Lam, S., et al. (2014). Extraction and isolation of flavonoid glycosides from Flos Sophorae Immaturus using ultrasonic-assisted extraction followed by high-speed counter-current chromatography. *Journal of Separation Science, 37*(8), 957–965.
28. Guo, T., Zhang, Y. T., Zhao, J. H., et al. (2015). Nanostructured lipid carriers for percutaneous administration of alkaloids isolated from Aconitum sinomontanum. *Journal of Nanbiotechnology, 13*, 47.
29. Guo, T., Zhang, Y. T., Li, Z., et al. (2018). Microneedle-mediated transdermal delivery of nanostructured lipid carriers for alkaloids from Aconitum sinomontanum. *Artificial Cells, Nanomedicine and Biotechnology, 46*(8), 1541–1551.

30. Zhang, Y. T., Han, M. Q., Shen, L. N., et al. (2015). Solid lipid nanoparticles formulated for transdermal aconitine administration and evaluated in vitro and in vivo. *Journal of Biomedical Nanotechnology, 11*(2), 351–361.
31. Yao, H., Huang, X., Li, S., et al. (2017). Simultaneous determination of eight phenolic acids, five saponins and four tanshinones for quality control of compound preparations containing Danshen-Sanqi Herb-pair by HPLC-DAD. *Pharmacognosy Magazine, 13*(49), 64–75.
32. Liu, J. H., Han, Y. L., Zhang, S. Y., et al. (2019). Efficacy and safety of low dose sublingual nifedipine dripping pills (5 mg) in the acute treatment of moderate and severe hypertension: A randomized, double-blind, positive-drug parallel-controlled, multi-center clinical study. *Zhonghua Xin Xue Guan Bing Za Zhi, 47*(5), 374–380.
33. Zhang, Y. T., Xu, Y. M., Zhang, S. J., et al. (2014). In vivo microdialysis for the evaluation of transfersomes as a novel transdermal delivery vehicle for cinnamic acid. *Drug Development and Industrial Pharmacy, 40*(3), 301–307.
34. Xu, J., Zhao, J. H., Liu, Y., et al. (2012). RGD-modified poly (D,L-lactic acid) nanoparticles enhance tumor targeting of oridonin. *International Journal of Nanomedicine, 7*, 211–219.
35. Guo, Y., Du, Y., Xie, L., et al. (2020). Effects of paeonol and gastroretention tablets of paeonol on experimental gastric ulcers and intestinal flora in rats. *Inflammation, 43*(6), 2178–2190.
36. Shen, C., Zhu, J., Song, J., et al. (2020). Formulation of pluronic F127/TPGS mixed micelles to improve the oral absorption of glycyrrhizic acid. *Drug Development and Industrial Pharmacy, 46*(7), 1100–1107.
37. Nie, X., Wang, B., Hu, R., et al. (2020). Development and evaluation of controlled and simultaneous release of compound Danshen based on a novel colon-specific osmotic pump capsule. *AAPS PharmSciTech, 21*(2), 38.
38. Li, Z., Zhang, Y., Zhu, C., et al. (2020). Folic acid modified lipid-bilayer coated mesoporous silica nanoparticles co-loading paclitaxel and tanshinone IIA for the treatment of acute promyelocytic leukemia. *International Journal of Pharmaceutics, 586*, 119576.
39. Zhang, S., Zhang, Y., Wang, Z., et al. (2020). Temperature-sensitive gel-loaded composite nanomedicines for the treatment of cervical cancer by vaginal delivery. *International Journal of Pharmaceutics, 586*, 119616.
40. Ye, P., Wei, S., Luo, C., et al. (2020). Long-term effect against methicillin-resistant Staphylococcus aureus of emodin released from coaxial electrospinning nanofiber membranes with a biphasic profile. *Biomolecules, 10*(3), 362.
41. Xiao, S., Yan, Y., Zhao, J., et al. (2020). Increased microneedle-mediated transdermal delivery of tetramethylpyrazine to the brain, combined with borneol and iontophoresis, for MCAO prevention. *International Journal of Pharmaceutics, 575*, 118962.
42. Li, J., Jin, X., Yang, Y., et al. (2020). Trimethyl chitosan nanoparticles for ocular baicalein delivery: Preparation, optimization, in vitro evaluation, in vivo pharmacokinetic study and molecular dynamics simulation. *International Journal of Biological Macromolecules, 156*, 749–761.
43. Wang, R., Zhang, C., Li, J., et al. (2019). Laser-triggered polymeric lipoproteins for precision tumor penetrating theranostics. *Biomaterials, 221*, 119413.
44. Tan, R., Niu, M., Zhao, J., et al. (2014). Preparation of vincristine sulfate-loaded poly (butyl cyanoacrylate) nanoparticles modified with pluronic F127 and evaluation of their lymphatic tissue targeting. *Journal of Drug Targeting, 22*(6), 509–517.
45. Xu, Y., Liu, L. S., Wang, H., et al. (2020). High order self-assembly of dextran nanogels induced by Con A. *Journal of Functional Polymer, 33*(1), 30–38.
46. Song, H. T., Zhang, Q., Wang, H. J., et al. (2007). Preparation of the traditional Chinese medicine compound recipe Shuxiong sustained-release capsules by multiparticulate time-controlled explosion technology. *Pharmazie, 62*(5), 372–377.
47. Wang, Z., Ye, B. N., Zhang, Y. T., et al. (2019). Exploring the potential of mesoporous silica as a carrier for Puerarin: Characterization, physical stability, and in vivo pharmacokinetics. *AAPS PharmSciTech., 20*(7), 289.

48. Chen, Z., Cheng, L., He, Y., et al. (2018). Extraction, characterization, utilization as wound dressing and drug delivery of Bletilla striata polysaccharide: A review. *International Journal of Biological Macromolecules, 120*(Pt B), 2076–2085.
49. Feng, S., Feng, N., & Emmanuel, O. S. (2015). Realgar nanoparticle-based microcapsules: Preparation and in-vitro/in-vivo characterizations. *Journal of Pharmacy and Pharmacology, 67*(1), 35–42.
50. Bonifácio, B. V., Silva, P. B. D., Negri, K. M. S., et al. (2014). Nanotechnology-based drug delivery systems and herbal medicines: A review. *International Journal of Nanomedicine, 9*(1), 1–15.
51. Wang, H., Xiao, Y., Wang, H., et al. (2019). Development of daidzein nanosuspensions: Preparation, characterization, in vitro evaluation, and pharmacokinetic analysis. *International Journal of Pharmaceutics, 566*, 67–76.
52. Amith, K. B., Habbu, P., Thimmasetty, T., et al. (2017). Phytosomes as novel drug delivery system for herbal medicine-a review. *Systamatic Reviews in Pharmacy, 8*(1), 5–7.
53. Liu, Y., Huang, P., Hou, X., et al. (2019). Hybrid curcumin-phospholipid complex-near-infrared dye oral drug delivery system to inhibit lung metastasis of breast cancer. *International Journal of Nanomedicine, 14*, 3311–3330.
54. He, Z., Zhang, Y., & Feng, N. (2020). Cell membrane-coated nanosized active targeted drug delivery systems homing to tumor cells: A review. *Materials Science & Engineering. C, Materials for Biological Applications, 106*, 110298.
55. Zhang, Y., Zhang, H., Zhang, K., et al. (2020). Co-hybridized composite nanovesicles for enhanced transdermal eugenol and cinnamaldehyde delivery and their potential efficacy in ulcerative colitis. *Nanomedicine, 28*, 102212.
56. Liu, Y., Xie, X., Chen, H., et al. (2020). Advances in next-generation lipid-polymer hybrid nanocarriers with emphasis on polymer-modified functional liposomes and cell-based-biomimetic nanocarriers for active ingredients and fractions from Chinese medicine delivery. *Nanomedicine, 29*, 102237.
57. Feng, S., Zhao, J. H., Liu, Y., et al. (2012). Preparation and characterization of solid lipid nanoparticles loaded with frankincense and myrrh oil. *International Journal of Nanomedicine, 7*, 2033–2043.
58. Huang, X., Wang, P., Li, T., et al. (2020). Self-assemblies based on traditional medicine berberine and cinnamic acid for adhesion-induced inhibition multidrug-resistant Staphylococcus aureus. *ACS Applied Materials & Interfaces, 12*(1), 227–237.
59. Liu, Y., Zhang, P., Feng, N., et al. (2009). Optimization and in situ intestinal absorption of self-microemulsifying drug delivery system of oridonin. *International Journal of Pharmaceutics, 365*(1–2), 136–142.
60. Zhang, Y. T., Zhao, J. H., Zhang, S. J., et al. (2011). Enhanced transdermal delivery of evodiamine and rutaecarpine using microemulsion. *International Journal of Nanomedicine, 6*, 2469–2482.
61. Li, T., Wang, P., Guo, W., et al. (2019). Natural berberine-based chinese herb medicine assembled nanostructures with modified antibacterial application. *ACS Nano, 13*(6), 6770–6781.
62. Zhao, Q., Luan, X., Zheng, M., et al. (2020). Synergistic mechanisms of constituents in herbal extracts during intestinal absorption: Focus on natural occurring nanoparticles. *Pharmaceutics, 12*(2), 128.
63. Shi, F., Zhang, Y., Yang, G., et al. (2015). Preparation of a micro/nanotechnology based multi-unit drug delivery system for a Chinese medicine Niuhuang Xingxiao Wan and assessment of its antitumor efficacy. *International Journal of Pharmaceutics, 492*(1–2), 244–247.

Chapter 2
Multi-Component Drug Delivery Systems for Chinese Medicines Based on the TCM Theory

Xiaobin Jia, Zhiwei Xiong, Liang Feng, and Bei Wang

Abstract Multi-component preparation of traditional Chinese medicine (TCM) is an important direction of TCM preparation in the future. The technology to make component unit preparation based on component physical properties can effectively overcome various biological barriers and help to deliver the components to the action sites for improving the bioavailability and curative effects. However, the advantages of overall view of TCM could not be presented only by a component preparation unit. Therefore, developing the multi-component drug delivery system (MCDDS) based on the TCM theory, which is designed according to the component's medicine properties and disease priority, rhythm, and so on, could take the advantages of improving the accuracy of drug using. Besides, establishing an evaluation system of the MCDDS can improve not only the effectiveness but also the safety of the MCDDS. In the future, the design and evaluation of MCDDS will be more scientific by using multidisciplinary knowledge, combined with computer science and mathematics. It is also hoped that our review will be helpful for the further development of complex MCDDS of TCM.

Keywords Multi-component · Drug delivery system · Chinese medicine · Medicine properties · Physical properties · Evaluation system

2.1 Introduction

In the middle of the twentieth century, most of the traditional Chinese medicine (TCM) preparations stayed in the molding research. The development of physical pharmacy helped to solve the molding problem of the TCM preparation. However, there are still problems such as unclear active components, poor solubility, poor permeability, multiple barriers in vivo [1], and difficult to find the right targets. With

X. Jia (✉) · Z. Xiong · L. Feng · B. Wang
School of Traditional Chinese Pharmacy, China Pharmaceutical University, Nanjing, China
e-mail: 1020182571@cpu.edu.cn

N. Feng, Z. Yang (eds.), *Novel Drug Delivery Systems for Chinese Medicines*,
https://doi.org/10.1007/978-981-16-3444-4_2

the development of TCM extraction, separation, and preparation technologies, the second-generation TCM preparations, such as tablets, granules, capsules, and injections, have been formed, but they still have the shortcomings of extensive extraction, unclear material basis, the disorderly release of drugs, and large oral dosage. Based on previous studies on the related components of TCM, our research creatively put forward the theory of "component structure." We believed that the bioavailability, accuracy, and efficacy of drug can be improved through scientific dosage form design and preparation technologies.

The components of TCM are composed of a group of ingredients with similar activities and properties, which are integrated organically according to a certain proportion. The chemical structure and pharmacological activities of each component are completely clear. The components with different activities and action sites have a specific "component structure" in a certain proportion. The components can be divided into two groups, which are called the active components and the functional components. The latter usually have the abilities of solubilizing, promoting absorption, and forming carrier, which could assist the active components to pass through the biological barrier smoothly [2]. Inspired by the thought of "theory, method, formula, and herb" and "syndrome differentiation treatment" of TCM, we studied the "component structure" in-depth and found that the design of MCDDS guided by the traditional TCM theory is highly consistent with the modern precision medicine.

The MCDDS takes a component as the unit and has the characteristics of targeted delivery, programmed release, and multi-level synergy. To develop the MCDDS, we should take into account the factors, such as medicine properties, physical properties, disease status, and individual differences, to control the distribution and drug release accurately. Then it will take advantages of multi-component to meet the needs of clinical precise drug use, and get better curative effects (Fig. 2.1). However, there is still a gap between the dosage form design and preparation technical level of MCDDS. It is also hard to get the goals of "rapid and long effect, small dose and safety, high efficiency, and convenience." Therefore, it is urgent to develop preparation technologies of Chinese medicine with clear ingredients, controllable quality, and steady effects for improving human health [3] and taking advantage of the synergy of multi-unit and multi-target [4]. In addition, with the cross-fusion of multidisciplinary knowledge such as molecular pharmacy and computer science, the evaluation system of MCDDS is being perfected.

2.2 Properties of Components

Based on analyzing the composition structure of multi-component, it is the general trend to realize the modern component of Chinese medicine preparation guided by the TCM theory. Therefore, the component preparation and dosage form design should fully reflect the thinking characteristics of TCM. Taking medicine properties and physical properties as the core content of the component property system can

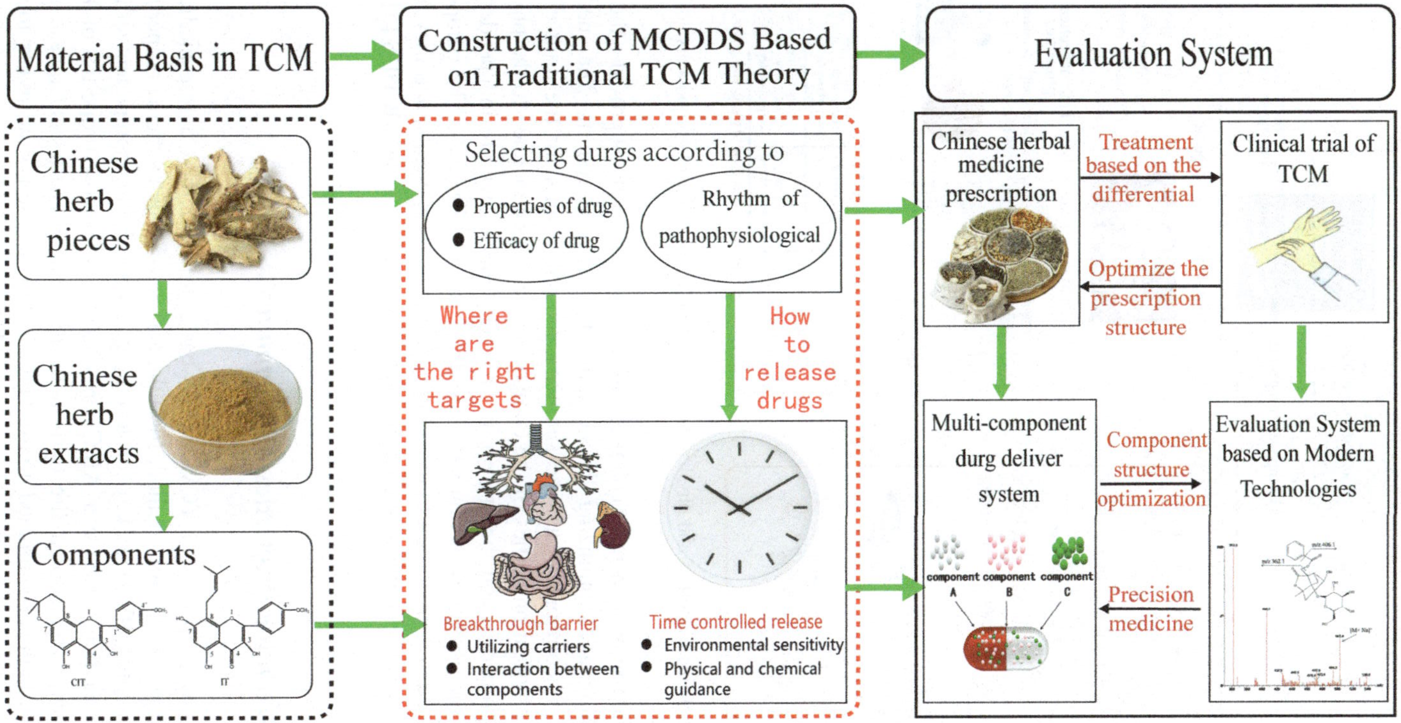

Fig. 2.1 Construction of multi-component delivery system and evaluation system based on TCM theory

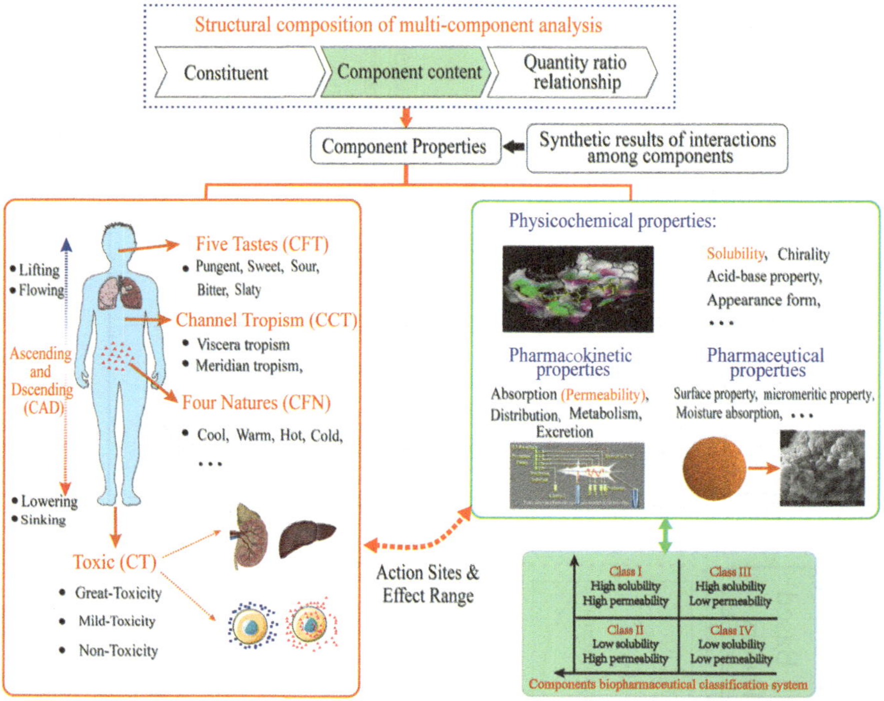

Fig. 2.2 Medicine properties and physical properties evaluation system of components

describe the components more comprehensively and accurately. It provides the basis for designing and optimizing the components' delivery system. The medicine properties of components are the summary and sublimation of the drug effects, while the physical properties of the components are more inclined to the physicochemical properties and the process in vivo. Generally, they are independent but related in the aspects of action sites and effect range (Fig. 2.2). The component property system is important to the "druggability" of components, and they are an important basis for component unit preparation technologies and MCDDS [5].

2.2.1 Medicine Properties of Components

The medicine properties of TCM are the basic principle for Chinese medicine's thinking mode of "theory, method, formula, and herb." The medicine properties of the components (MPCs) are key for designing and developing component structure of Chinese medicine. However, MPCs are different from those properties of TCM, and they cannot be inherited directly from the medicine properties of Chinese herbal pieces, nor can they be summed up from clinical practice, so it is necessary to study MPCs by modern research methods. The MPCs are highly summarized to the biological effects in the human body, and the pharmacological activities, action sites, and trends of the components can be reflected. The core theories of MPCs include four natures, five tastes, channel tropism (meridian and viscera), ascending and descending, toxic. In recent years, the prediction platform of MPCs has adopted data mining technology [6], which is mainly based on the medicinal properties and pharmacological effects of Chinese herbal medicines. In a word, using modern research techniques to elucidate the scientific connotation of MPCs is fundamental to guide the design of MCDDS and accurate drug use.

2.2.1.1 Four Natures of Components

The four natures of components (CFN) include cold, cool, warm, and hot. The cold and cool, warm and hot are essentially the same but different in degree. They are also called cold-heat nature of components which were opposite to heat or cold syndromes. The modern researches on CFN usually have the observations of animal tendency behavior, changes of heat production in the body, and biological effects such as metabolomics, enzyme activity, cold-heat-sensing channel, etc. [7, 8]. Besides, modern research on the mechanism of fever caused by bacteria, viruses, and other factors showed that this kind of fever will appear to leukocyte adhesion and release inflammatory mediators, body fluid exudation, and other inflammatory reactions, showing red, swollen, hot, pain, and other symptoms. This kind of febrile disease has a common pathological mechanism, while the cold components have the effects of scavenging inflammatory factors in varying degrees and repairing the vascular injury, which reflects the thought of "same treatment for different diseases" in the TCM theory.

2.2.1.2 Five Tastes of Components

The five tastes of components (CFT) mainly include pungent, sweet, sour, bitter, and salty. The tastes of TCM according to the sense of taste and smell belong to sensory taste and later evolved to divide the five flavors according to the similarity of efficacy, which belongs to functional taste. Modern studies on taste receptor expression and molecular docking indicate that CFT is highly correlated with its real tastes [9]. The pungent components generally have antipyretic, analgesic, anti-inflammatory, and improve microcirculation effects, such as volatile oil. The sweet components are related to the expression of T1R and T2R receptors, such as polysaccharide components, which could probably improve immunity and reduce blood sugar. The sour components are related to the activation of PKD1L3-PKD2L1 receptors, such as organic acids and tannins, which generally have hemostatic, antidiarrheal, and other effects. The bitter components are related to the expression of T2R receptors, such as alkaloids, which generally have the effect of scavenging oxidative free radicals and inflammatory factors. The salty components are related to

TRPV1 receptors, such as inorganic salt, which generally have the effects of "softening hard masses" (including tumor) and relieving diarrhea.

2.2.1.3 Channel Tropism of Components

The channel tropism of components (CCT) is the reflection of the trends of components and detail action sites. Using modern research methods such as pharmacokinetics of TCM to clarify the connotation of CCT is helpful to achieve the clinical accurate administration of component preparations. The CCT includes the viscera tropism and meridian tropism. The distribution of 23 kinds of ingredients of TCM in human organs was compared with their channel tropism. The results indicate that the organs where the active components distributed and the name of viscera tropism were matched 87% [10]. The viscera tropism is not only related to the exposure of the components to the corresponding viscera but also may be related to the strong biological affinity to it. The meridian tropism may have a situation that the distribution of components is not consistent with the sites of final bioeffects. For example, the lesions of allergic conjunctivitis are in the eyes, but the use of mulberry leaves and chrysanthemum components belonging to the liver meridian has better therapeutic effects.

2.2.1.4 Ascending and Descending of Components

The syndromes of a disease often show a certain movement tendency, and the ascending and descending of components (CAD) can resist it. The CAD embraced lifting, lowing, sinking, and floating, and they are all opposite to disease tendency. The lowing or lifting components, such as the antidiarrheal or antiasthmatic components, can resist the downward or upward trend of the diseases, while the sinking or floating components can resist the internal and external movement tendency of the diseases. Some TCM has the mechanism of bidirectional regulation. For instance, *Ephedra intermedia* can not only perspire but also relieve cough, asthma, and diuresis. Astragalus can not only tonify "Qi" and "Yang" but also has the effects of diuretic detumescence, perspiration, and so on. However, the components may also trend both ascending and descending, and the properties of TCM are not the simple superposition of each ingredient, so the characterization of the CAD should also be based on modern pharmacological researches.

2.2.1.5 Toxic of Components

The broad concept of toxic components (CT) refers to the "deviation" of drugs to correct the imbalance of the body, and the narrow concept is in line with modern toxicological research. According to the toxicity intensity, CT is generally divided into great toxicity, mild toxicity, and non-toxicity. Toxicological studies show that the toxicity of components is closely related to their dosage and it should be strictly controlled. Some toxic components also have pharmacological activities such as aconitine, which has the effects of strengthening the heart and anticancer, etc. [11]. When both components are used, it is possible to reduce the toxicity, called "mutual decreasing toxicity," but also to produce stronger toxicity, called "mutual opposite." Therefore, when characterizing the CT by modern methods, we should not only pay attention to the relationship between toxicity and dosage but also investigate the effect of interaction between components on toxicity.

2.2.2 *Physical Properties of Components*

The state of materials before the preparation of TCM has been an important limiting factor in the development of TCM preparation [12, 13]. As the basic unit of the novel delivery system in the future, the components have different physical properties from the raw powder and extraction of TCM. Due to the removal of a large number of irrelevant ingredients in the refining process, the physical properties of TCM are changed significantly. The core content of the physical property system includes physicochemical properties, pharmaceutical properties, and ADME properties, and it will be a powerful tool for designing dosage forms and optimizing the preparation unit.

2.2.2.1 Physicochemical Properties and Structure Characteristics of Components

The physicochemical properties of the components are the embodiment of intrinsic characteristics of each component, and they are important content of physical property system, including appearance form, acidity and basicity, solubility, stability, and so on. A component is a unit containing chemicals of the same or similar core structure after the purification of the Chinese herb extracts. The components with more chromophores in the core structure can show a certain color, and as the number of chromophores increases, the color becomes more obvious. The appearance form of the components is the result of the physical and chemical interaction of chemicals, such as low eutectic, glassy, gluey, and liquid.

Acidity and basicity are inherent properties of components. The alkaloid is mainly composed of a series of nitrogen compounds, which has alkalinity and can bind to acid to form salts, while the quinone consists of a series of compounds with quinoid structure, with phenolic hydroxyl groups and certain acidity. Under different pH conditions, components with different acids and bases have a different degree of dissociation [14], and its absorption, distribution, metabolism, and excretion processes in the body are also different. For example, the distribution of components in vivo is influenced by acid-base scale. Acid components are often highly bound to plasma proteins, while lipophilic basic components tend to be stored in acid-rich tissues and acidic organelles [15].

The solubility of components refers to the ability of components to dissolve in dispersed media to free state, and it is related to the properties of the solvent. If the solubility of components in the gastrointestinal tract is poor, it will directly affect the absorption of them and then the clinical efficacy. The solubility of components is often expressed as water solubility and lipid solubility. It is generally considered that the components with higher polarity are better water solubility, such as polysaccharide, flavonoid glycosides, and anthraquinone glycosides. The components with less polarity often have strong lipid solubility, such as volatile oil, etc.

The stability of the components is important to ensure effectiveness. The unstable changes of components will not only reduce the overall efficacy but also may produce toxicity, so their chemical stability should be controlled. Many factors affect the stability of components, such as temperature, humidity, pH, light, oxygen, and solvent. For example, the polarity of the solvent is produced by the uneven distribution of charge in the covalent bond, and the solvent with larger polarity increases the instability of the component and produces a certain hydrolysis reaction.

2.2.2.2 ADME Properties and Pharmacokinetic Characteristics of Components

The absorption, distribution, metabolism, and excretion of components in vivo reflect the law of interaction between components and the body. The components are interrelated whole when transporting in vivo and are different from that of monomer ingredients. It is not scientific to study the pharmacokinetic process of one of them, but it is also difficult to study the pharmacokinetic properties of components from the whole [16].

The absorption of drugs in the body mainly includes two processes, dissolution and penetration, and the components have good solubility and permeability to be absorbed by the body through the gastrointestinal epithelial cell mucosa into the blood circulation. The permeability of components is often characterized by the oil-water partition coefficient, and the value can indicate the lipophilicity and hydrophilicity of drugs to predict the difficulty of drug transmembrane transport. Generally, components with large logP values often have strong lipid solubility and good gastrointestinal permeability. Furthermore, the absorption of the components is also affected by the pH in the gastrointestinal tract, and the components with a certain weak acid or weak basic are in a dissociation state at a certain pH, thus affecting the absorption of them.

The main factors affecting the distribution of components are the physicochemical, physiological, and pathological characteristics of various parts of the body, among which the physicochemical properties are the key to predict the distribution such as acid and basic, lipid solubility, etc. The distribution of weak acidic and weak basic components is affected by the pH of extracellular fluid. The weak acidic components are easy to be dissociated in the extracellular fluid and hard to enter the tissue. The weak basic components are rarely dissociated and easy to enter the tissue under the pH of the blood. Moreover, the lipid solubility can also affect the distribution of components. The liposoluble small molecular components usually enter the brain through the blood-brain barrier (BBB) more easily. When transported to a cell membrane, the components with high lipid solubility easily access to intracellular and be accumulated in adipose tissue.

The chemical structure of some components will be changed under the action of various enzymes and body fluids to produce metabolites. Metabolites are more polar than the original drug, so it is easy to be expelled from the body. The integrity of metabolism will also be affected by the chiral of components. The stereoselectivity and chiral conversion of chiral components to substrates and products all affect the whole metabolic characteristics of the components. Besides, the difference in the metabolic clearance rate of enantiomers within the components can also be manifested by different metabolic pathways.

The excretion of components greatly affects the efficacy and the duration of it. There are several main excretion pathways such as renal excretion and bile excretion. When the excretion rate of a certain component increases, the amount of medicine retained in the blood and the efficacy decrease. In general, water-soluble and small molecular components are often eliminated by renal excretion. Lipophilic components are easily reabsorbed in glomerular filtration, while water-soluble components will be rapidly excreted in urine. Bile excretion is an important process for organic anions and cations that are too polar to reabsorb in the intestine. Besides, the acidity and basicity of the components also affect their excretion. For the weak acidic components, alkalinity can increase their degree of dissociation, resulting in reduced reabsorption and increased renal clearance. For the weak basic components, the degree of dissociation of them will be reduced in the environment with high pH value, resulting in the increase of reabsorption and the decrease of renal clearance.

Because of the extensive metabolism of components in organisms, the analysis of the changes of these components in vivo is most challenging. The traditional theory and technologies that follow the classical metabolism and excretion of chemical drugs are not suitable for TCM [17]. The emergence of new theories, such as "syndrome and treatment drug metabolic kinetics" and "syndrome differentiation drug metabolic kinetics," has promoted the development of drug metabolic dynamics of TCM. However, due to the complex composition of TCM, its pharmacokinetics still faces many problems and challenges [18]. By integrating the pharmacokinetic parameters between different levels, and combining the "dispersion" analysis method to compare the pharmacokinetics of each monomer, the overall ADME character of components structure can be clarified.

2.2.2.3 Pharmaceutical Properties of Components

The pharmaceutical properties of components include micrometric properties, surface properties, fluidity, hygroscopicity, etc. The components have different condensed forms, thus showing macroscopic pharmaceutical properties, which are an important theoretical basis for guiding the formation of component preparations. During the preparation process, the components often exist in the form of solid powder and liquid solution. The key forming techniques are granulation, pill making, tablet pressing, mixing liquid, or 3D printing [19]. Micromeritic properties have a great influence on the forming of dosage forms and drug release behavior, for example, the particle size of component powder may be positively correlated with the pellet size [20]. In addition, the preparation course will also affect the pharmaceutical properties of components, such as the drying method of extracts [21]. The powder of the tanshinone component prepared by the spray drying method has a smaller particle size and narrow distribution, which is beneficial to improve the bioavailability [22]. The modification of the unfavorable properties of the components such as high adhesion and strong hygroscopicity can be guided by the scientific characterization of the pharmaceutical properties. At present, the related researches are not comprehensive [23], and the quantitative parameters need to be used for describing the pharmaceutical properties of components.

2.3 Unit Preparation Techniques for Components

Solubility and permeability are the two main factors affecting the bioavailability of components in preparations. Only the components with high solubility and permeability can be absorbed into the blood circulation [24]. Therefore, the two physical properties of components are the keys to improve bioavailability. The components are divided into four categories according to the biopharmaceutics classification system of components: I (high solubility, high permeability), II (low solubility, high permeability), III (high solubility, low permeability), and IV (low solubility, low permeability). The classification system presents important references for the formulation design of component preparations [25].

2.3.1 Solubilization of Difficult Soluble Components

For difficult soluble components, the unit preparation techniques should be used to modify the defects of the components to improve the solubility and permeability. Adding solubilizer and cosolvent in the preparation process, the solubility and dissolution rate of the components can be improved by solid dispersion technology [26], O/W microemulsion, self-microemulsion technology, inclusion technology [27], powder modification technology [28], liquid-solid compression technology, and nanotechnology. Insoluble components, whether absorbed through the digestive tract or injected, require the addition of excipients to improve their solubilities, such as the use of surfactants exceeding the critical micelle concentration to form micelles or the use of cyclodextrin saturation techniques. However, the high concentration of surfactants in the prescription will not always increase the drug loading significantly and may produce unpredictable side effects. For example, the use of Tween-80 in Chinese medicinal injection may have serious hemolysis [29], and this problem may be solved by changing the excipients instead of Tween-80, such as polysaccharides without side effects and with high biocompatibility.

2.3.2 *Strategies to Improve or to Promote the Permeability of Components*

For less permeable components, biological barriers need to be overcome to perform better. According to the composition or mechanisms of the barriers, they can be divided into the mucosal barrier, cell membrane barrier, etc. or be divided into the mechanical barrier, biochemical barrier, immune barrier, etc.

2.3.2.1 Increasing Mucosal Permeability of Components

Reducing the viscosity or elasticity of the mucosal layer can promote the absorption of components, for example, the composition of bile acids within a certain amount of surfactant can promote absorption by reducing the viscosity of the mucous membrane. Components with different pH and solubility parameters may interact with penetrant, forming diverse micelles to promote the absorption of components. Besides, for the mucosal diseases, the unit drug delivery system is designed according to the adhesion of components, which can adhere to the colon mucosa and increase the releasing time and local concentration, thus exerting better efficacy [30]. The component preparations can also be designed according to the characteristics of the mucosa and the physical properties of components, such as the curcumin nanocrystals with different size which can be transported from the mucous membrane to improve the solubility and absorption rate [31].

2.3.2.2 Promoting Cellular Permeability of Components

Cell barrier is composed of cells and intercellular space, such as blood-brain barrier (BBB), placental barrier, blood vessel wall, lymphatic wall, and various organ cells in vivo. Cell barrier has a high selective permeability through the efflux proteins on cells and tight junction proteins between the cells [32] to hinder the transportation of components. Generally, the small hydrophilic molecules are more likely to enter the blood through the gap of intestinal epithelial cells, and the small liposoluble molecules are easier to pass through the cell barrier. The permeability of components could be improved by using auxiliary components in TCM. Therefore, the component preparations for the treatment of brain or gynecological diseases could be more effective. Actually, there are many components that can be used as brain penetration enhancers to be developed in resuscitation-inducing aromatic herbs [33].

2.3.2.3 Other Ways to Improve the Permeability of Components

The mucus, intestinal flora, and immune system are also the barriers in the body of component delivery. The mucus is continuously secreted on the surface of the intestinal mucosa. This mucus layer is a mechanical obstacle that affects the absorption of components. For example, airway mucus is the first obstacle affecting the absorption of components [34]. The viscosity of mucus can be reduced by dilution to promote the absorption. The intestinal flora may act with the components, and the enzyme metabolism system of intestinal epithelial cells will also become the biochemical barrier [35]. Generally, the components are biotransformed after being absorbed, however, they can be controlled by promoting or inhibiting the intestinal flora and intestinal enzyme activity, such as the glycosides and the main original components in Gegen Qinlian Decoction, can be decomposed into small molecule and liposoluble components to enhance their absorption [36].

2.3.3 New Ideas for the Design of Component Unit Preparation

For the components with poor solubility and permeability, it is necessary to improve them, and the usual ways are given by using surfactants, solubilizing agents, and absorbent promoters [37]. To date, membrane-piercing peptide composite micelles [38], self-microemulsion technology [39], phospholipid composite technology [40], biological adhesion technology [41], and nanotechnology can be used to increase the solubility, bioavailability, and absorption rate of the components. Besides, the synergy between components and the application of carriers can also play a key role.

2.3.3.1 Utilization of Physicochemical Synergy Between Components

The synergy between components can improve the solubility and permeability of components simultaneously. The synergy between components can be divided into three aspects [42]: physicochemical interaction, pharmacokinetic interaction, and pharmacodynamic interaction. Generally, components containing aromatic rings or hydroxyl groups can form a self-assembly structure, and without harsh reaction conditions, complex synthesis process or any modification, only rely on the physicochemical interaction between the components, such as through hydrogen bonding, electrostatic, π-π stacking, metal complexation and so on [43, 44]. The common ones are liposomes, self-microemulsions, nano-micelles, solid lipid nanoparticles, cochleate, etc. [45]. Interaction between components can enhance the ability of transmembrane transport, such as glycyrrhizic acid, which can improve the solubility and the permeability of berberine to Caco-2 cells [46]. The berberine and rhein could be self-assembled into antibacterial nanoparticles [47], resulting in transport synergy and pharmacodynamic synergy. It is reflecting the thought of "unification of drug and excipient."

2.3.3.2 Using Suitable Carrier to Transport Components

There are many kinds of drug carriers including micelles, liposomes, nanoparticles, and so on, which can be divided into microspheres (1–250 μm) and colloidal (10–1000 nm) drug loading systems according to their particle size. The carriers have different pathways and processes (Fig. 2.3). Ideally, the carrier should have the following characteristics: sufficient components carrier volume; safely deliver components to the target sites and maintain an effective concentration; control the release rate of components at the target site; keep components with sufficient biological activity after being carried; targeted localization; good biocompatibility, can be degraded and removed in vivo in time; non-antigenicity and non-pyrogen; low-risk to form thrombus; long effective period and easy to store.

I, flows through the gastrointestinal tract after oral administration; II, M cells or intestinal cyst areas attached to Peyer's patches; III, transport from mesenteric lymphatic channels; IV, flows in lymphatic vessels and is intercepted by lymph nodes (not shown); V, transport in lymph and blood. A, blood flow; B, extravasation

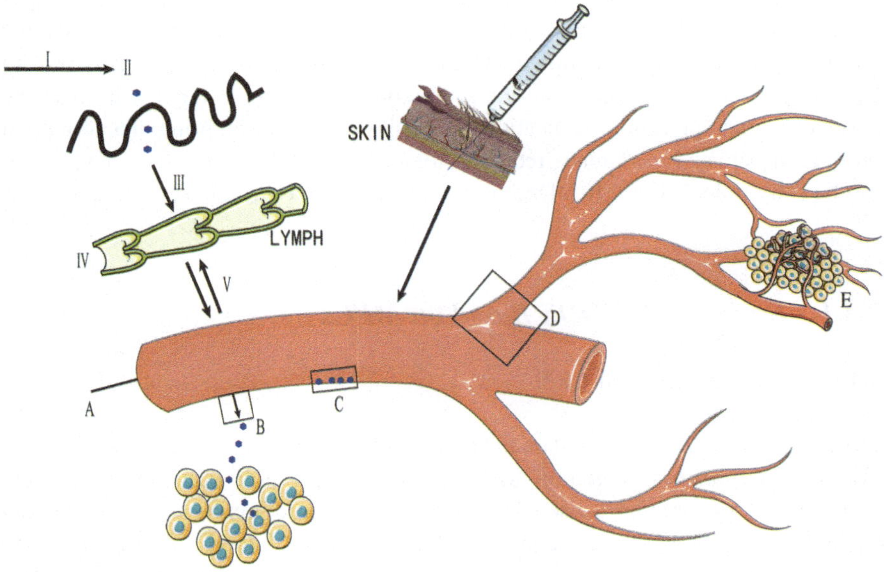

Fig. 2.3 Transport area of carrier particle flow

into tissue; C, attachment to a capillary wall; D, deposition at the vascular bifurcation; E, transport to a tumor. Complex routes of particulate flow (including subcutaneous pathways) include lymph, blood, and intestinal fluid (Torchilin. Nano particulates As Drug Carriers, 2006).

Polymers and other carriers can overcome the disadvantages of poor water solubility of components, such as nano-micelles formed by amphiphilic polymers with a hydrophobic core and solvation shell, which is a self-assembly structure to complete the solubilization and encapsulation of drugs. The degradable materials as the drug carriers, such as polyglycolic acid (PGA) and polylactic acid (PLA) [47], have good biocompatibility. Nano-micelles can not only enhance the ability of component to penetrate through physiological barriers but also easily penetrate leaky vascular tissues (tumor, embolism, etc.) and can also make components escape monocyte phagocytosis and have the effect of "invisibility" [48]. Besides, dendrimer is a new type of carrier with the advantages of highly branched structure, controllable size, and no immunogenicity. The cochleate [44] formed by the combination of phosphatidylserine and positive ions is also a safe and reliable drug carrier.

2.4 Design of MCDDS

Theoretical basis: The medicine properties and compatibility theory of TCM suggest that TCM plays an important role in both treating primary cause and alleviating symptoms by the synergistic action between drugs. Because the physical properties of diverse components are different, and the single dosage form has no advantages of synergistic action, the design of MCDDS must consider the distribution of components in vivo and the regularity of releasing time. Because of the clinical needs, the idea of "syndrome differentiation treatment" in TCM theory is highly consistent with that of "precision medicine," and the multi-component should be able to meet the needs of clinical precision medication. TCM should follow the principles of mutual promotion between medicines, reducing toxicity, and enhancing efficiency, which can be fully reflected by MCDDS based on traditional TCM theory (Fig. 2.4).

2.4.1 Design of MCDDS Based on MPCs

2.4.1.1 Design Based on CFN

The design of MCDDS is based on the accurate diagnosis of cold-heat syndrome of a disease. The modern research on the mechanism of febrile disease showed the heat syndrome of pneumonia caused by bacteria, virus, endotoxin, and other factors could be divided into four stages of "Wei, Qi, Ying, Blood" according to the symptoms and severity of the disease. There are latent periods, high fever, water-liquid metabolism disorder, and blood vessel injury bleeding as the main

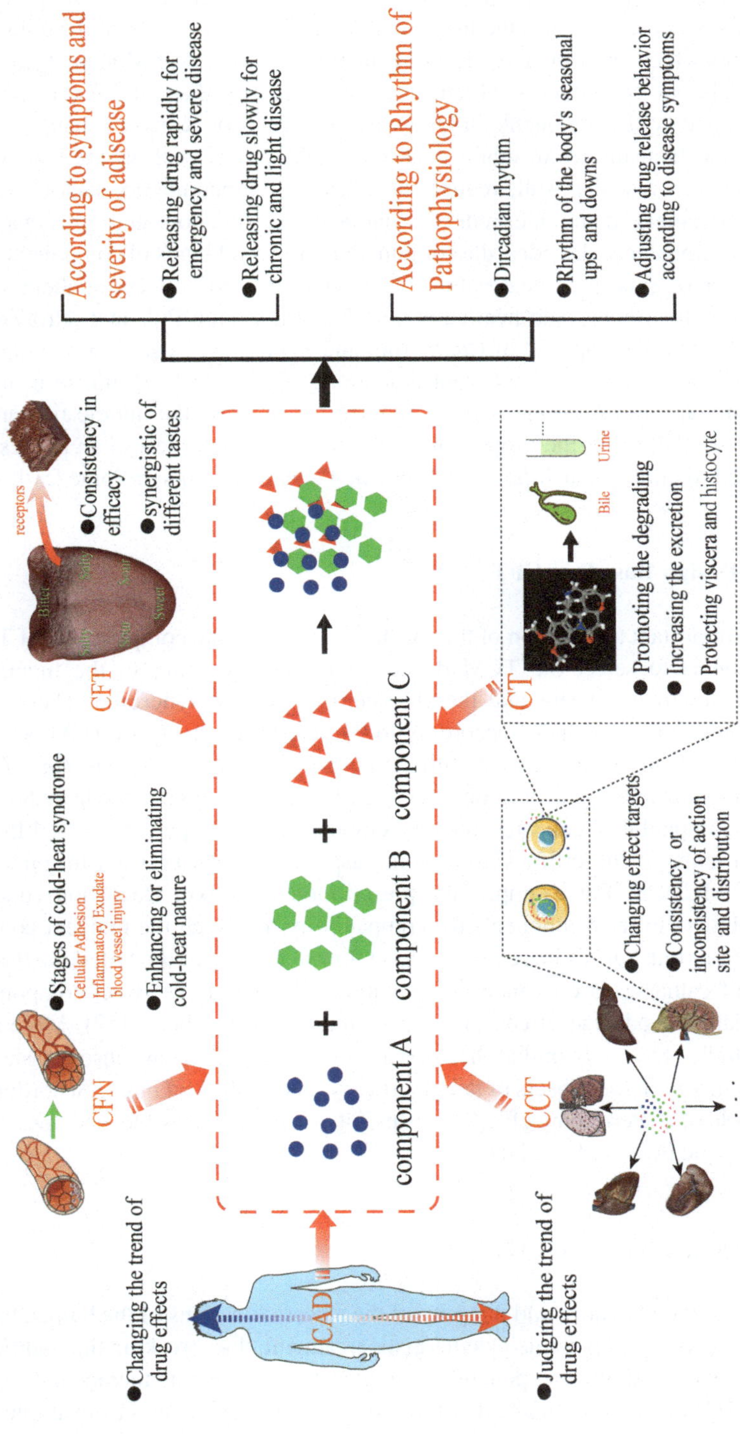

Fig. 2.4 Design of MCDDS based on the MPCs and characteristics of a disease

characteristics, respectively [49]. So we can correspondingly choose the pungent-cool components which enter the lung meridian in Sangju Decoction, the cold-cool components which enter the large intestine meridian in Dahuang Mudan Decoction, or the cold-cool components which enter the lung meridian in Maxing Shigan Decoction and cold components in Qingying Decoction or Xijiao Dihuang Decoction. The mechanisms are to inhibit leukocyte adhesion or peel off the leukocytes attached to the vascular wall, reduce the release of inflammatory factors, repair capillary basement membrane, reduce inflammatory exudation, and other ways to regulate the imbalance. Besides, the combination of several kinds of components can change their original cold-heat nature or alleviate the side effects of them when combined with stronger cold-heat nature, such as the Zuojin Pills and retro-Zuojin Pills; the former is composed of *Coptis* root and *Evodia rutaecarpa* at 6:1, and the latter shows the contrary. *Coptis* root is a strong bitter-cold to eliminate heat and purging fire, and *Evodia rutaecarpa* is pungent-hot to warm the middle Jiao and to remove cold. Adjusting the proportion of the two decoction pieces can be, respectively, used to cure stomach-heat syndrome and stomach-cold syndrome [50].

2.4.1.2 Design Based on CFT

The most important application of the five tastes theory in the compatibility of TCM prescription is to select the TCM decoction pieces according to the functional characteristics of five tastes and the characteristics of the syndrome. There were several compatibility methods according to the five tastes theory of TCM, such as *Xin Gan Hua Yang* (forming yang with the pungent and sweet), *Ku Xin Tong Jiang* (dispersing stagnation and purging heat with bitter and pungent medicinals), etc. [51]. The compatibility indicates that the combination of components with different tastes can enhance the efficacy from some aspects and can be used to guide the design of MCDDS. For example, the prescription of Xiexin Decoction contains pungent, bitter, sweet components for compatibility, in which the pungent component can carry out "Qi" to increase the blood flow velocity and the bitter one has the function of catharsis to eliminate inflammation. The adding of sweet components can alleviate the adverse effects of strong pungent on the body [52]. Moreover, modern studies have shown that there exists consistency between sensory taste and five tastes theory in the aspects of target, efficacy, and biological basis. According to the principle of "determining effect by tastes," it is scientific, feasible, and applicable for guiding the design of MCDDS.

2.4.1.3 Design Based on CCT

According to the relevance and integrity of the viscera functions of the human body, the components can play a role of synergistic treatment, thus breaking the traditional thinking mode of "single component and single target." Selecting therapeutic targets based on TCM theory can make the drug delivery more accurate. For example, the lesion sites of asthma are at the lungs, but the large intestine, spleen, or kidney will be selected as the targets according to the relationship between the lung, spleen, kidney, and large intestine [53] in the aspects of immunity and respiratory [54]. Besides, modern studies have shown that the components exert effects not only by binding to the target protein, but also by physicochemical reaction. For example, mirabilite, which has a cathartic effect, makes the intestinal tract produce high osmotic pressure and increases the intestinal volume.

2.4.1.4 Design Based on CAD

The theory of ascending and descending is one of the basic rules to guide the clinical practice of TCM. The designing of MCDDS could be guided by the ascending or descending characteristics of the disease. For example, for blood collapse, gastric prolapse, and other symptoms with downward tendency can be treated through hemostasis or increasing ligament tension, moreover, the components of astragalus, ginseng, which can "tonifying qi," could be used according to the theory of TCM. If the therapeutic target is in the lung, the *Platycodon grandiflorum* saponins with lifting properties could be used together [55]. Hypertension with upward tendency can be treated using the *Haematitum* with sinking properties. For complex diseases with dual tendency, the treat method of dual regulation may have a better effect. For example, at the beginning of diphtheria, the active component of mulberry leaves was used for heat dissipation, and it was supplemented by gypsum, *Ophiopogon japonicus*, and other cold components with sinking properties for cough [56]. Besides, it is necessary to pay special attention to the combination of ascending components and descending components. A small amount of sinking components in a large number of floating components often show the characteristics of ascending. This phenomenon indicates that the CAD will change in some cases and it should be mastered and used in the design of MCDDS.

2.4.1.5 Design Based on CT

Characterizing the CT is important for the safety of MCDDS. TCM prescriptions often reduce or eliminate the toxicity through compatibility. Modern toxicological studies have shown that the main mechanisms of reducing toxicity through compatibility are the decoction process to change the toxic components; reducing the content of toxic components greatly; changing the pharmacokinetic properties of toxic components, such as accelerating their metabolism and excretion rate; and improving the body immunity and protecting tissues to reduce the degree of damage. The components are extracted from TCM and refined, and a large number of invalid components have been removed in the process, resulting in a decrease in toxicity. For the toxic active components, the toxicity can be reduced by combining with certain component. The arrow patchouli C, metabolized from epimedin C, presents the toxic. The toxicity of arrow patchouli C could be reduced after combining with *Morinda officinalis* decoction. The mechanism was that the metabolic rate of toxic components was slowed down, thus reducing the duration time of side effects [57]. In conclusion, the safety of MCDDS was raised by applying the theory of CT.

2.4.2 Design Based on the Characteristics of a Disease

The TCM theory holds that the physiological activities of the human body have a strong time rhythm, such as circadian rhythm, *Zi Wu Liu Zhu* (*midnight-noon and ebb-flow doctrine*), "correspondence between five visceras and seasons," and so on. In line with the modern medical science [58], the transformation of a disease between the viscera has different characteristics in every stage. The rate and sustained time of drug release should be controlled according to the priorities of a specific disease and physiological rhythm. The principle adopted is that a disease should be cured from severe to mild.

2.4.2.1 According to the Priority of Syndromes of a Disease

As early as the pre-Qin period, the pills, plaster, etc. recorded in the *Huang Di Nei Jing* (*Huangdi's Internal Classic*) are the embryonic forms of sustained-release system and are very suitable for treating chronic diseases. The studies of the controlled-release preparation of TCM began in the 1990s, and it belongs to the third-generation TCM dosage form characterized by controlled releasing time. The releasing time of the components in pellets or capsules prepared with the water-insoluble skeleton is prolonged, such as the Tongmai Pills. Some components were designed to release rapidly and exert their efficacy, such as puerarin flavonoid, *Salvia miltiorrhiza* phenolic acid, and *Ligusticum chuanxiong* phenolic acid, while tanshinone were designed to release slowly for protecting cardiomyocytes. Therefore, the combination of quick-acting and long-acting drugs through procedural drug release can achieve the goal of alleviating both symptoms and causes [59]. A membrane-controlled sustained-release preparation of components was prepared by coating technology. The coating material and thickness were selected according to the CPP, such as pH, lipid solubility, and purpose to delay drug release [60]. According to the dissolution and absorption characteristics of the water-insoluble and water-soluble layer, the two-layer sustained-release tablets were prepared [61]. The osmotic release system is to control the releasing time by the water transmitting the semi-permeable membrane and forming osmotic pressure difference inside and outside the membrane [62]. For example, osmotic pump tablets of composite *Salvia miltiorrhiza* were prepared by using effervescent technology and osmotic pump technology with cellulose acetate as coating material containing the pore-forming agent to realize controlled release [63].

2.4.2.2 According to the Rhythm of Pathophysiology

In recent years, more and more attention has been paid to the time characteristics of component delivery systems. The MCDDS will be perfect if designed according to the rhythm of physiology and pathology. For example, tetramethylpyrazine phosphate for angina pectoris is designed to be taken before bedtime at night, after 5–6 h intervals, and released before the highest frequency of angina attacks in the early morning of the next day [64]. The release of an MCDDS is a procedural process, while simultaneous release [65] is only one of the special cases. The release rate, the amount of release, and absorption of each component should follow the TCM theory.

At present, under the impetus of artificial intelligence and 3D printing technology [66], MCDDS will be more intelligent, whose main characteristics is to increase the sensitivity to the vivo environment, and automatically adjusting drug release behavior according to pathological state and physiological rhythm. The release behaviors of drug could be triggered by proteases and pH produced by tumor microenvironment [67] or be triggered by near-infrared photothermal effect [68]. The MCDDS may also have the function of automatic monitoring and automatic interrupting drug release behavior [69].

2.4.3 Difficulties in the Design of MCDDS

The screening and targeted delivery of active sites are current research hotspots. Tumor targeting delivery system should be considered: the overall selection of targets according to the function of viscera; multiple resistance of tumor tissue; high specificity and affinity of tumor tissue to components; stability of components, which is conducive to prolonging drug half-life in vivo; tumor pathogenesis and its microenvironment; and utilizing appropriate carrier or carrier surface modification to enhance the precision of targeting. The tumor does not belong to the normal tissue of the human body, but the tumor cells themselves are the special cell barrier system. P-glycoprotein (P-gp) on the tumor cell membrane, one of the factors to produce multidrug resistance (MDR), can hinder the entry of components into the tumor cells. The MCDDS containing the components of P-gp activity inhibitory can overcome this problem [70].

The tissues and organs which are related to immunity could be simultaneously selected as the targets of the MCDDS aiming to kill tumor cells. The therapeutic effects of an MCDDS designed based on multi-viscera may be better [71]. Besides, the extraction process of TCM is a mostly chiral environment; as a result, enantiomers with the same physical properties in the non-chiral environment cannot be distinguished. The design of MCDDS inevitably needs to solve the problem of the "chirality" of components. However, whether the chiral components have strong physiological activity in a specific configuration and how to design the targeted delivery system of them need to be further studied.

2.5 Establishing a Scientific Evaluation System for MCDDS

The evaluations of MCDDS are an important step to ensure the overall curative effects of component preparations and are also the key link for designing the drug delivery system. Establishing a scientific and reasonable evaluation system of the MCDDS is important to guarantee the effectiveness and safety of clinical drug use.

2.5.1 *The Evaluations of MCDDS in Vitro*

The fundamental feature of TCM theory is the holistic view and "syndrome differentiation and treatment." The evaluation system of the MCDDS should always maintain the character. The evaluations in vitro of MCDDS were mainly aimed at the drug release units. Except for the general evaluation methods such as oar, basket, and cup recorded in the *Chinese Pharmacopoeia* (edition 2020), Kobayashi [72] established the continuous dynamic biomimetic system for drug dissolution/absorption (DDASS), characterized by simultaneous investigation of drug release and absorption in vitro, and the evaluation system considered the interaction between the components. The release/dissolution kinetics theory of the compound group was put forward by Jiwen Zhang et al. based on the overall spectral characteristics of the compound group of TCM, and the content of the compound group in dissolution medium was calculated by the Kalman filter method [73]. The evaluation method is simple and intuitive, and its application in evaluating MCDDS is comparatively scientific. In the future, the drug release behaviors of MCDDS will be more complicated; therefore, the combination of modern detection techniques, big data processing, and intelligent computing will be helpful for developing the evaluation system [5].

2.5.2 *The Evaluations for MCDDS in Vivo*

The evaluation methods of TCM preparations are often based on the content of single ingredient, which lacks scientific. The evaluation methods in vivo for the delivery system based on the principle of pharmacokinetics, using blood drug concentration method, biological effect method, and others, will be better. In recent years, the developed fingerprint characteristic peak [74], TCM compound group [73], quality weight method [75], statistical moment total kinetics [76], integrated pharmacokinetics [77], and other evaluation methods have gradually broken through the thinking mode of single-ingredient evaluation. It is an innovation to evaluate the bioavailability and safety of MCDDS by examining blood concentration, peak time, and bioavailability. However, there may still be some defects using pharmacokinetic methods in vivo, such as whether the content of active components in the preparation or the concentration in plasma is completely positive related to the efficacy. Guangji Wang has developed a theoretical method for the study of multi-component pharmacokinetics of TCM. It is the "target cell pharmacokinetics-pharmacology combination study" [17], which provides a new idea for the accurate evaluation of MCDDS in vivo.

2.5.3 The Evaluations for Toxicity and Side Effects of MCDDS

Safety evaluations of MCDDS should include the entire process from the raw materials of the component preparation to the pre-clinical study. In the production process, there are certain safety problems, such as the establishment of a pesticide and detection system of heavy metal. In recent years, to solve the contradiction that the resources of TCM are in short supply, the cultivation industry has been developed, followed by the problem of exceeding pesticides and heavy metals. At present, it is urgent to establish sensitive analysis methods about pesticide residue and heavy metal content standards for component preparation. The misunderstanding is that the safety is equal to non-toxic and toxic is equal to forbidden. The view seriously hindered the development of component preparations. There are many toxic components with strong activity. But there is also a situation where the components refined from TCM may lead to new toxicity due to the separation from their original overall environment, such as chiral isomers [78]. Therefore, it is necessary to strengthen the modern toxicological evaluation of toxic components and strictly control their dosage. It could also be toxic when several non-toxic components were used simultaneously in the normal dosage range. In this case, it is necessary to establish a drug-induced toxic injury evaluation system based on pre-clinical toxicity kinetics. Besides, the correlation between the exposure of components in cells and the safety is rarely be studied, but the evaluation systems of clinical safety need to be improved.

2.6 Conclusions and Prospects

The MCDDS is based on components, which integrates the traditional TCM theory with the preparations, and it embodies the characteristics of drug use based on the holistic view of TCM. One of the goals of developing MCDDS is to achieve accurate targets of active components. Its essence is to study the distribution of multi-component in vivo, and the key is to find the right targets. The component unit preparation technology can overcome various biological barriers by using new carriers to change the physical properties of components and their interactions. The second goal is to make the components release regularly, and the essence is to study the amount of drug release changing over time. The MCDDS designed according to the rhythm characteristics of physiology or pathology is more scientific.

It is urgent to establish a scientific evaluation system, and the final purpose of developing MCDDS is to serve the clinic. The most obvious characteristic of MCDDS is that it takes the component as the preparation unit and it is beneficial to develop MCDDS characterized by the thinking mode of TCM theory. In addition, modern Chinese medicine technologies such as Computer Aided Drug Design (CADD) and Multidimensional Quantitative Structure-Activity Relationship (MD QSAR) have all contributed to the design of MCDDS. In a word, MCDDS are still developing and improving, and it will be promoted by the integration of the interdisciplinary knowledge and the application of new technologies.

Acknowledgments The study was supported by the National Key R&D Program of China (Grant No. 2018YFC1706900); National Natural Science Foundation of China (81573620); and Project for Innovative Research Team of "Double First-Class" Construction of Chinese Pharmaceutical University (CPU2018GY11; CPU2018GF07).

References

1. Cuggino, J. C., Blanco, E. R. O., Gugliotta, L. M., Alvarez, L. C. I., & Calderón, M. (2019). Crossing biological barriers with nanogels to improve drug delivery performance. *Journal of Controlled Release, 307*, 221–246.
2. Zhang, J. M., Liao, W., He, Y. X., He, Y., Dong, Y., et al. (2013). Study on intestinal absorption and pharmacokinetic characterization of diester diterpenoid alkaloids in precipitation derived from Fuzi–Gancao herb-pair decoction for its potential interaction mechanism investigation. *Journal of Ethnopharmacology, 147*(1), 128–135.
3. Huang, Q., Wang, L., Yu, H., & Ur-Rahman, K. (2019). Advances in phenylboronic acid-based closed-loop smart drug delivery system fordiabetic therapy. *Journal of Controlled Release: Official Journal of the Controlled Release Society, 305*, 50–64.
4. Chen, T., Li, J., Chen, T., Sun, C. C., & Zheng, Y. (2017). Tablets of multi-unit pellet system for controlled drug delivery. *Journal of Controlled Release: Official Journal of the Controlled Release Society, 262*, 222–231.
5. Yu, D. H., Liu, D., Jia, X. B., Sun, H., Zhang, Z. H., et al. (2012). Construction of evaluation systems for traditional Chinese medicine multiple drug delivery system on basis of component level. *China Journal of Chinese Materia Medica, 37*(15), 2338–2343.
6. Hu, Y. N., Wang, M., Cao, J., Wang, Y., & Qiao, Y. J. (2016). Forecasting platform construction for properties of herbs components. *China Journal of Traditional Chinese Medicine and Pharmacy, 31*(3), 965–967.
7. Wang, J., Chen, Y., Yuan, Z. M., & Lv, J. (2016). Differences in effective mechanisms of Coptidis Rhizoma and bile processed Coptidis Rhizoma on heat. *China Journal of Chinese Materia Medica, 41*(14), 2638–2645.

8. Zou, G. F., Xiong, C. C., Chen, Y. F., Guo, L., Tao, S. H., et al. (2017). Heat-clearing herbs based on property theory of traditional chinese medicine. *Chinese Journal of Experimental Traditional Medical Formulae, 23*(6), 229–234.
9. Du, R. C., Wang, Y. J., Wu, F., Feng, Y., Xu, D. S., et al. (2013). Discrimination of traditional Chinese medicinal materials with different tastes based on electronic tongue. *China Journal Chinese Materia Medica, 38*(02), 154–160.
10. Wang, J., & Liang, M. X. (2012). Thoughts and methods of modern research on channel distribution of Chinese herbs. *Modernization of Traditional Chinese Medicine and Materia Medica-World Science and Technology., 14*(1), 1237–1241.
11. Liu, R. P., Li, X. J. Y., Huang, N. N., Fan, M. Y., & Song, R. (2020). Chapter Eleven – Toxicity of traditional Chinese medicine herbal and mineral products. *Advances in Pharmacology, 87*, 301–346.
12. Yu, Y., Zhao, L. J., Lin, X., Wang, Y. J., & Feng, Y. (2020). A model to simultaneously evaluate the compressibility and compactibility of a powder based on the compression ratio. *International Journal of Pharmaceutics, 577*, 119023.
13. Zheng, X., Wu, F., Hong, Y., Shen, L., & Feng, Y. (2019). Improvements in sticking, hygroscopicity, and compactibility of effervescent systems by fluid-bed coating. *RSC Advances, 9*(54), 31594–31608.
14. Charifson, P. S., & Walters, W. P. (2014). Acidic and basic drugs in medicinal chemistry: A perspective. *Journal of Medicinal Chemistry, 57*, 9701–9717.
15. Yun, Y. E., & Edginton, A. N. (2013). Correlation-based prediction of tissue-to-plasma partition coefficients using readily available input parameters. *Xenobiotica, 43*, 839–852.
16. Liu, C. X. (2005). Difficultyand hot points on pharmacokinetics studies of traditional Chinese medicine. *Acta Pharmacologica Sinica, 05*, 395–401.
17. Wang, G. J. (2019). Targeting endothelial senescence by natural products to improve vascular health. Chinese medicines. *Chinese Journal of Pharmacology Toxicology, 33*(09), 643.
18. Gu, J. F., Feng, L., Zhang, M. H., Qin, D., & Jia, X. B. (2014). New exploration on effect of characteristics of traditional Chinese medicine components structure on multi-ingredient / component pharmacokinetics. *China Journal of Chinese Materia Medica, 39*(14), 2782–2786.
19. Lee, J. W., & Cho, D. (2015). 3D Printing technology over a drug delivery for tissue engineering. *Current Pharmaceutical Design, 21*(12), 1606–1617.
20. Xiong, Z. W., Luo, Y., Liao, Z. G., Zhao, G. W., Li, Z., et al. (2014). Correlations between micromeritic properties of mixing powders of Danshen extract and formability of their pellets. *China Journal of Chinese Materia Medica, 39*(22), 4317–4323.
21. Liang, X. L., Zhang, P., Liao, Z. G., Zhao, G. W., Lai, J., et al. (2010). Effect of drying technology on pharmaceutical characterization of Radix Pueraria extracts. *Chinese Pharmaceutical Journal, 45*(10), 756–760.
22. Ding, D. M., Zhang, Z. H., Jiang, Y. R., Sun, E., & Wang, J. (2014). Micromeritic properties of tanshinone IIA spray drying powder. *Chinese Traditional and Herbal Drugs, 45*(10), 1398–1401.
23. Feng, Y., Ling, X., Shen, L., & Hong, Y. L. (2013). Pharmaceutical study on multi-component traditional Chinese medicines. *China Journal of Chinese Materia Medica, 38*(05), 629–632.
24. Liu, D., Jia, X. B., & Xiao, W. (2013). Study on solubility of ginkgolide components with mass fraction weight coefficient method. *China Journal of Chinese Materia Medica, 38*, 1865–1870.
25. Jia, X. B., Yang, B., Feng, L., Shi, X. H., Wang, H., et al. (2018). Research frontiers of Chinese medicine pharmaceutics: Foundations and key issues of components preparation technology. *Acta Pharmacologica Sinica, 53*(12), 1943–1953.
26. Cong, W. J., Shen, L., Xu, D. S., Zhao, L. J., Ruan, K. F., et al. (2014). Solid dispersion tablets of breviscapine with polyvinylpyrrolidone K30 for improved dissolution and bioavailability to commercial breviscapine tablets in beagle dogs. *European Journal of Drug Metabolism and Pharmacokinetics, 39*(3), 203–210.

27. Pan, Y., Qian, D., Liu, P., Zhang, W., Zhu, Z. H., et al. (2017). The influence of essential oils from Xiang-Fu-Si-Wu Decoction on its non-volatile components and its application for pharmacokinetics in normal rats. *Journal of Chromatography B, 1060*, 221–230.
28. Zhang, D. K., Lin, J. Z., Liu, J. Y., Qin, C. F., Guo, Z. P., et al. (2013). Powder modification technology used for the preparation of the hydrophilic decoction pieces of Indigo Naturalis and the modification principle. *Acta Pharmaceutica Sinica, 48*(7), 1148–1155.
29. Li, Y. K., & Zhang, J. Y. (2011). Improvement and enhancement of traditional Chinese medicine injections. *China Journal of Chinese Materia Medica, 36*(14), 1905–1909.
30. Zeeshan, M., Ali, H., Khan, S., Khan, S. A., & Weigmann, B. (2019). Advances in orally-delivered pH-sensitive nanocarrier systems; an optimistic approach for the treatment of inflammatory bowel disease. *International Journal of Pharmaceutics, 558*, 201–214.
31. He, Y., Liang, Y., Mak, J. C. W., Liao, Y., Li, T., et al. (2020). Size effect of curcumin nanocrystals on dissolution, airway mucosa penetration, lung tissue distribution and absorption by pulmonary delivery. *Colloids and Surfaces B: Biointerfaces, 186*, 110703.
32. Salama, N., Eddington, N., & Fasano, A. (2006). Tight junction modulation and its relationship to drug delivery. *Advanced Drug Delivery Reviews, 58*(1), 15–28.
33. Liang, J. M., Gao, C. F., Zhu, Y., Huang, Q., Zhu, Y. Z., et al. (2018). Natural brain penetration enhancer-modified albumin nanoparticles for glioma targeting delivery. *ACS Applied Materials & Interfaces, 10*(36), 30201–30213.
34. Alqahtani, S., Roberts, C. J., Stolnik, S., & Bosquillon, C. (2020). Development of an in vitro system to study the interactions of aerosolized drugs with pulmonary mucus. *Pharmaceutics, 12*(2), 145.
35. Ke, Z. C., Yang, N., Hou, X. F., Wang, A. D., Feng, L., et al. (2016). Metabolism of paeoniflorin by rat intestinal flora in vitro. *China Journal of Chinese Materia Medica, 41*(20), 3839–3845.
36. Ling, X., Xiang, Y., Chen, F., Tang, Q., Zhang, W., et al. (2018). Intestinal absorption differences of major bioactive compounds of Gegenqinlian Decoction between normal and bacterial diarrheal mini-pigs in vitro and in situ. *Journal of Chromatography B, 1083*, 93–101.
37. Zhu, Z. T., Pan, J. H., Wu, X. H., & Jang, Z. T. (2017). Screen absorption enhancer for intranasal administration preparations of paeoniflorin based on nasal perfusion method in rats. *China Journal of Chinese Materia Medica, 42*, 493–497.
38. Fan, B., Jin, M. J., Huang, W., Wang, Q. M., & Gao, Z. G. (2016). The development of cellpenetrating peptides in drug delivery system. *Acta Pharmaceutica Sinica, 51*, 264–271.
39. Wei, J., He, H. L., Zheng, C. L., & Zhu, J. B. (2011). Chitosan-coated ophthalmic submicro emulsion for pilocarpine nitrate. *Acta Pharmaceutica Sinica, 46*, 990–996.
40. Yu, F., Li, Y., Chen, Q., He, Y., Wang, H. Y., et al. (2016). Monodisperse microparticles loaded with the self-assembled berberine-phospholipid complexbased phytosomes for improving oral bioavailability and enhancing hypoglycemic efficiency. *European Journal of Pharmaceutics and Biopharmaceutics, 103*, 136–148.
41. Jiao, J. J., Sun, L. L., Guo, Z. Y., Hou, S., Holyst, R., et al. (2016). Antibacterial and anticancer PDMS surface for mammalian cell growth using the Chinese herb extract paeonol (4-methoxy-2- hydroxyacetophenone). *Scientific Reports, 6*, 38973.
42. Li, Y., Meng, Q., Yang, M., Liu, D., Hou, X., et al. (2019). Current trends in drug metabolism and pharmacokinetics. *Acta Pharmaceutica Sinica B, 9*(6), 1113–1144.
43. Li, Z. T., & Zhang, D. W. (2017). *Hydrogen bond molecular recognition and self-assemblyM* (Vol. 4). Chemical Industry Press.
44. Gao, C., Kewalramani, S., Valencia, D. M., Li, H. H., McCourt, J. M., et al. (2019). Electrostatic shape control of a charged molecular membrane from ribbon to scroll. *Proceedings of National Academy of Sciences of United States of America, 116*(44), 22030–22036.
45. Chen, Y. X. (2010). *Molecular pharmaceutics* (Vol. 1). Hunan Normal University Press.
46. Wang, N. Q., Zhang, L., Yang, X. Y., & Du, G. H. (2019). Toxicity and application evaluation of animal toxic Chinese medicines. *Chinese Journal of Pharmacology and Toxicology, 33*(09), 721.

47. Tian, X. H., Wang, P. L., Li, T., Huang, X. M., Guo, W. B., et al. (2019). Self-assembled natural phytochemicals for synergistically antibacterial application from the enlightenment of traditional Chinese medicine combination. *Acta Pharmaceutica Sinica B*. https://doi.org/10.1016/j.apsb.2019.12.014
48. Ma, W. Z., Wang, J. L., & Tu, M. F. (2015). Preparation characterization and antitumor activity in vitro of berberine hydrochloride polymeric micelles. *China Journal of Chinese Materia Medica, 40*(21), 4182–4188.
49. Hang, J. Y. (2020). The mechanisms underlying the beneficial effects of Ma-Xing-Shi-Gan-Tang on pulmonary interstitial edema and the beneficial effects of Yiqifumai on shock. *Modernization of Traditional Chinese Medicine and Materia Medica-World Science and Technology*, 1–9. http://kns.cnki.net/kcms/detail/11.5699.R.20200221.1125.002.html
50. Zhao, P., Xu, J., Zhang, T. J., Xu, H. Y., & Niu, C. J. (2011). Exploration on scientific connotation of compatibility of Zuojin Wan based on "disease-syndromes-formulas-medicines" binding mode. *China Journal of Chinese Materia Medica, 36*(23), 3380–3385.
51. Zhang, T. J., & Liu, C. X. (2015). Identification of Chinese materia medica and its chemical biology characterization path on five taste theory. *Chinese Traditional and Herbal Drugs, 46*(01), 1–6.
52. Liu, M., Wu, D. X., Li, J., Hou, N., Zhang, Y. L., et al. (2019). Nature-effect relationship research between pungent and bitter taste of traditional Chinese medicine for promoting blood circulation and removing blood stasis based on nature combination. *China Journal of Chinese Materia Medica, 44*(2), 218–223.
53. Zhen, H. T., Fan, Y. M., Yuan, H. X., & Yuan, B. (2018). Effects of intestinal flora on immune function base on the theory of "superficies-interior relationship between lung and large intestine" of traditional Chinese medicine. *Lishizhen Medicine and Materia Medica Research, 29*(05), 1170–1172.
54. Deng, X. F., Wu, Q. F., Tang, L., Zeng, Z. F., Xu, L., et al. (2018). Clinical efficacy of Jinshui Liujunjian combined with breathing exercises in treatment of Pneumoconiosis in stable phrase with syndrome of deficiency of lung, spleen and kidney. *Chinese Journal of Experimental Traditional Medical Formulae, 24*(02), 158–163.
55. Wang, K., Zhang, B. L., Cui, Y. W., Ma, Y., & Jiang, F. (2018). Literature study in Jiegeng Radix Platycodonis. "Taking Herbs Bottom-up". *Journal of Traditional Chinese Medicine, 59*(4), 271–275.
56. Gao, K. L., & Hao, H. (2018). BAI Changchuan's Experiences in the treatment of exogenous fever disease with sweating, dispersing, purging and preventing methods. *Journal of Traditional Chinese Medicine, 59*(20), 1730–1734.
57. Ling, J., Wang, M., Chen, Y., Song, J., & Sun, E. (2018). Analysis of Folium Epimedium toxicity in combination with Radix Morindae Officinalis based on zebrafish toxicity/metabolism synchronization. *Acta Pharmaceutica Sinica, 53*(01), 74–83.
58. Firsov, D., & Bonny, O. (2018). Circadian rhythms and the kidney. *Nature Reviews. Nephrology, 14*(10), 626–635.
59. Huang, Y. (2011). *The construction of multi-drug delivery system of Tongmai micro-pellets*. Jiangsu University.
60. Wu, B., Liu, Z. H., Lin, M. Z., Yang, H. D., & Song, H. T. (2015). Advance in studies on film-controlled synchronized release multi-component preparation of Chinese materia medica for oral. *Chinese Traditional and Herbal Drugs, 46*(12), 1853–1857.
61. Liao, Z. G., Liang, X. L., Ping, Q. N., Jiang, Q. Y., & Yang, M. (2009). Formula design and optimization of Guizhi fuling doublelayers sustained-release tablet. *Chinese Traditional and Herbal Drugs, 40*(4), 553–557.
62. Bai, Z. Y., Shao, S. Y., Xu, X. Y., & Zhang, J. F. (2016). Application of osmotic pump technology in Chinese materia medica preparation. *Chinese Traditional and Herbal Drugs, 47*(09), 1619–1624.
63. Li, Y., Hou, S., Bi, Y., Yu, Z., Cai, Z., et al. (2007). Novel two-step release system for the traditional Chinese medicine compound Danshen. *Yakugaku Zasshi, 127*(9), 1473–1484.

64. Zhen, Q., Wang, F., Yang, M., Hu, P. Y., Yue, P. F., et al. (2011). Study on the theory of time-oriented medication and the system of pulse release of traditional Chinese medicine. *Journal of Chinese Medicinal Materials, 34*(2), 309–312.
65. Yue, P. F., Wu, B., Zheng, Q., Hu, P. Y., & Yang, M. (2010). Innovation and discussion on evaluation pattern of synchronism/asynchronism release characterization of sustained and controlled release preparations for Chinese herbal formula. *Chinese Traditional and Herbal Drugs, 41*(9), 1413–1417.
66. Talebian, S., Foroughi, J., Wade, S. J., Vine, K. L., Pirouz, A. D., et al. (2018). Biopolymers for antitumor implantable drug delivery systems: Recent advances and future outlook. *Advanced Materials*, 30(31). https://doi.org/10.1002/adma.201706665
67. Chen, W., Luo, G., Qiu, W., Lei, Q., Liu, L., et al. (2016). Tumor-triggered drug release with tumor-targeted accumulation and elevated drug retention to overcome multidrug resistance. *Chemistry of Materials, 28*(18), 6742–6752.
68. Wang, F., Yuan, Z., McMullen, P., Li, R., Zheng, J., et al. (2019). Near-infrared-light-responsive lipid nanoparticles as an intelligent drug release system for cancer therapy. *Chemistry of Materials, 31*(11), 3948–3956.
69. Ohdo, S. (2010). Chronotherapeutic strategy: Rhythm monitoring, manipulation and disruption. *Advanced Drug Delivery Reviews, 62*(9-10), 859–875.
70. Liu, H. Y. (2015). Research progress on Chinese materia medica for reversing tumor multidrug resistance. *Chinese Traditional and Herbal Drugs, 46*(07), 1096–1102.
71. Yang, B., Yu, G. H., Li, M. Y., Gu, H. M., Chen, Y. P., et al. (2019). Mechanism of flavonoid components in Astragali Radix in inhibiting tumor growth and immunoregulation in C57BL /6 tumor bearing mice based on "invigorating Qi for consolidation of exterior". *China Journal of Chinese Materia Medica, 44*(23), 5184–5190.
72. Kobayashi, M., Sada, N., Sugawara, M., Ken, I., & Katsumi, M. (2001). Development of a new system for prediction of drug absorption that takes into account drug dissolution and pH change in the gastro-intestinal tract. *International Journal of Pharmaceutics, 221*(1–2), 87–94.
73. Zhang, J. W., Chen, L. B., Gu, J. K., Ge, W. H., & Yang, M. (2008). Novel theory and methods for chemomic multi-component release/dissolution kinetics of traditional Chinese medicine. *Chinese Journal of Natural Medicines, 6*(1), 48–52.
74. Zhang, W., Song, H. T., & Zhang, Q. (2010). Evaluation on in vitro release of gastric floating sustained-release preparation of Tripterygium wilfordii by HPLC fingerprints. *Chinese Traditional and Herbal Drugs, 41*(03), 376–380.
75. Amidon, G. L., Lennernas, H., Shah, V. P., & Crison, J. R. (1995). A theoretical basis for a biopharmaceutic drug classification: The correlation of in vitro drug product dissolution and in vivo bioavailability. *Pharmaceutical Research, 12*, 413–420.
76. He, F. Y., Deng, K. W., Liu, W. L., Shi, J. L., Wu, Y., et al. (2013). Experimental studies on pharmacokinetics of three components in Buyanghuanwu injection on base of total quantum statistical moment. *China Journal of Chinese Materia Medica, 38*(02), 253–262.
77. Zhang, F., Zhang, Y., Du, W., Zhu, M., Zhang, S., et al. (2019). Integrating pharmacokinetics study, network analysis, and experimental validation to uncover the mechanism of Qiliqiangxin capsule against chronic heart failure. *Frontiers in Pharmacology, 10*. https://doi.org/10.3389/fphar.2019.01046
78. Cao, S. Q., Wang, X., Shang, Y. M., Xu, F., & Liu, G. X. (2015). "Efficacy Theory" may help to explain characteristic advantages of traditional Chinese medicines. *China Journal of Chinese Materia Medica, 40*(17), 3435–3443.

Chapter 3
Sustained-Release Drug Delivery Systems of Chinese Medicines

Xiao Zheng, Teng Guo, Fei Wu, Lan Shen, and Xiao Lin

Abstract The bioactive micromolecules (e.g., alkaloids, glycosides, phenolic acids, and so on) and macromolecules (typically, polysaccharides) from Chinese medicines have exhibited potent efficacies (e.g., anti-tumor, anti-inflammation, antivirus, anti-ischemia, etc.). However, their unfavorable pharmacokinetic profiles (like rapid clearance, low bioavailability, and short half-time) together with their different undesirable physicochemical properties (e.g., low water solubility and poor stability for the micromolecules and low lipophilicity for the macromolecules) often significantly compromise their curative efficacies. Complexity of TCM compound recipes in chemical constitution and action mechanism is another issue. The development of Chinese medicine pharmaceutics needs to learn from the achievements of modern science and technology aiming to develop the theory and technology of sustained release of Chinese medicines. The combination with the clinical medication of Chinese medicines is the premise of preparing modern preparations of Chinese medicines to meet the needs of clinical prevention and treatment. Therefore, the developments in sustained-release drug delivery systems (DDSs) of Chinese medicines, especially synchronous or orderly sustained release of TCM compound recipes, are of significance in improving their drug-like properties and the treatment efficiencies in the clinic. On the other hand, the establishment of the objective quality evaluation system has been the key to ensuring the safety and effectiveness of such sustained-release preparations of Chinese medicines. In this chapter, the recent reports in this field were summarized to provide an informative reference for relevant readers.

Keywords Chinese medicine · TCM compound recipes · Pharmacokinetics · Sustained release · Drug delivery

X. Zheng · T. Guo · F. Wu · L. Shen · X. Lin (✉)
School of Pharmacy, Shanghai University of Traditional Chinese Medicine, Shanghai, China
e-mail: linxiao@shutcm.edu.cn

N. Feng, Z. Yang (eds.), *Novel Drug Delivery Systems for Chinese Medicines*,
https://doi.org/10.1007/978-981-16-3444-4_3

3.1 Introduction

In recent years, a variety of bioactive ingredients have been extracted from Chinese medicines, most of which are isolated from the root, stem, rhizome, fruit, and bark parts of the medicinal plants. According to the size of their molecular weight, they could be categorized into micromolecules (e.g., bioactive alkaloids, glycosides, phenolic acids, etc.) and macromolecules (e.g., bioactive polysaccharides, tannins, etc.). Recently, a wide spectrum of bioactivities has been found in such Chinese medicine-derived ingredients. Particularly, many of them possess anti-tumor efficacies by inhibiting the formation of microtubule of tumor cell's mitotic spindle, blocking DNA relegation through binding to topoisomerase, and inducing an arrest of the cell cycle at the G1 phase [1, 2]. What's more, they also possess a series of potent treatment efficiencies of anti-inflammation, antivirus, anti-ischemia, immunosuppression, and so on [3–5].

However, most of such ingredients show poor drug-like properties, thus leading to the decreased curative efficacies. On the one hand, the treatment efficiencies of Chinese medicine-derived bioactive micromolecules are mainly restricted by their undesirable physicochemical properties (like low water solubility and poor chemical stability) and baneful pharmacokinetic (PK) profiles (e.g., low bioavailability, rapid clearance, etc.). For example, the active moiety of 10-hydroxycamptothecine is easy to be degraded in physiological pH [2]. On the other hand, unlike the above micromolecules, the Chinese medicine-derived macromolecules (typically polysaccharides) often exhibit high hydrophilicity because they are rich in polar groups. But, the poor pharmacokinetic behaviors (e.g., poor oral absorption and rapid elimination via the kidneys) always severely limit their administration effectiveness and patient compliance [6, 7]. In general, it could be seen that the rapid elimination in vivo is the same problem for both Chinese medicine-derived micromolecules and macromolecules and, thus, needs to be solved urgently. Therefore, developments in sustained-release drug delivery systems (DDSs) of Chinese medicines are of significance in improving their drug-like properties (especially prolonging the in vivo retention time) and the corresponding curative efficacies in the clinic, which is summarized in Fig. 3.1.

On the other hand, as a multi-component whole, the effect of TCM compound recipes is not the result of single or several components, but the synergetic effect of each component. The development of Chinese medicine pharmaceutics needs to learn from the achievements of modern science and technology aiming to develop the theory and technology of sustained release of TCM compound recipes. The combination with the clinical medication of Chinese medicines is the premise of preparing modern preparations of TCM compound recipes to meet the needs of clinical prevention and treatment [8]. Synchronous sustained release of TCM compound recipes is a research idea of modern sustained-release preparation of Chinese medicine based on the studies of traditional Chinese herbal decoction. The "procedural release" from modern sustained-release preparations of TCM compound recipes not only conforms to the characteristics of Chinese medicine but also

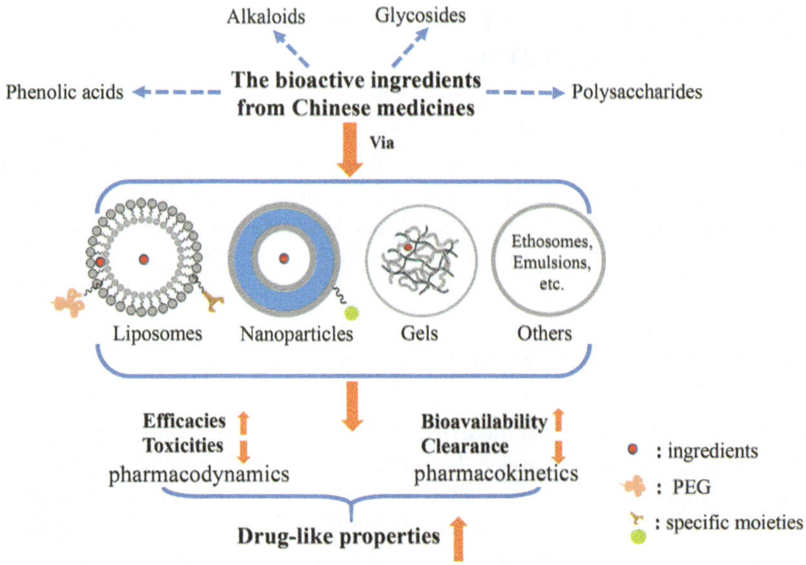

Fig. 3.1 Improvement of drug-like properties of Chinese medicine-derived ingredients via specific drug delivery systems

balances the release amount, release rate, and intake of each component in the drug release unit [9, 10].

In history, there have already been some records related to the embryonic form of sustained-release preparations, like "Pills act slowly, and thus treat the disease slowly and sustainedly over a long period (Li Dongyuan, 1180–1251)"; "Due to the difficulty in disintegration and dissolution, waxed pills exert their effect slowly or avoid toxic medicines from harming the spleen and stomach (Li Gao, 1180–1251)"; "Chinese medicines with high toxicity must use the dosage form of pills (*Su Shen Liang Fang* (*Fine Prescriptions of Su's and Shen's*), *Song* Dynasty)"; and so on. With continuous efforts, some modern sustained-release Chinese medicine preparations have also been successfully approved for marketing in China, such as sustained-release tablet of *Leigongteng* (*Tripterygium wilfordii*) and sustained-release tablet of *Zhengqing Fengtongning* (sinomenine hydrochloride extracted from *Qingfengteng* (*Sinomenii Caulis*)).

Besides, to ensure the safety and effectiveness of sustained-release DDSs of Chinese medicine, it is quite important to establish the objective quality evaluation system for them, which is beneficial to further promote the development of such DDSs, as well. Thus, in this chapter, the recent reports in the field of sustained-release DDSs of Chinese medicine and the quality evaluation systems for them were summarized with the aim of providing an informative reference for relevant readers.

3.2 Sustained Delivery of Various Bioactive Ingredients from Chinese Medicine

So far, a variety of novel DDSs (e.g., liposomes, nanoparticles, gels, emulsions, ethosomes, microspheres, etc.) have been utilized to deliver the problematic Chinese medicine-derived ingredients to prolong their release in vivo, thus improving their drug-like properties and the corresponding curative efficacy.

3.2.1 Sustained Delivery of Bioactive Alkaloids

The Chinese medicine-derived bioactive alkaloids are a type of nitrogen-containing small molecules with the molecular weight being generally less than 1 kDa [2]. Although a lot of bioactivities have been found in such alkaloids, their applications in the clinic are severely restricted due to their poor drug-like properties (e.g., short plasma half-lives, potential degradation). Therefore, long-acting DDSs (e.g., liposomes, nanoparticles, ethosomes, etc.) are desired to load such alkaloids due to their advantages of improving patient compliance, reducing administration frequency, and minimizing adverse effects [11].

Recently, a variety of liposomes, including normal liposomes, long-circulating liposomes, and active liposomes (containing components that provide a selective and controlled release of the liposome), have been developed to deliver the Chinese medicine-derived alkaloid to prolong their in vivo retention time and, thus, enhance their curative efficacy. For example, vincristine (VCR), a vinca alkaloid, has been indicated to possess the potent anticancer ability for a long time particularly in hematologic malignancies and solid tumors [12]. Unluckily, its neurotoxicity and baneful PK behaviors (such as a rapid and extensive distribution phase followed by a long elimination phase) have severely restricted its application in the clinic [13]. Using the delivery of normal liposomes, the in vivo release of VCR could be significantly prolonged [14]. However, this type of liposomes might be easily ingested by the mononuclear phagocyte system (MPS). Therefore, the loaded active substance would leak out and then be rapidly degraded [15]. To resolve this undesirable problem, long-circulating liposomes (also called "stealth liposomes") have recently been developed, which can exhibit their long-lasting capabilities by importing a hydrophilic polymer, notably polyethylene glycol (PEG), onto lipid surfaces. During the preparation process of such long-circulating liposomes, suitable long-circulating materials play a vital role. For example, the in vitro assays showed that the VCR-loading amount of such liposomes made up of chitosan was only about 1/2 of that achieved by the polyethylene glycol-1,2-distearoyl-sn-glycero-3-phosphatidylethanolamine (PEG-DSPE) or PEG-poly-lactide-*co*-glycolide (PEG-PLGA) formulation. Moreover, in terms of the in vivo PK behavior, the $AUC_{0-\infty}$ of VCR from the PEG-DSPE formulation was substantially larger (approximately 2.3-fold) than the PEG-PLGA or chitosan formulation. Overall, PEG-DSPE appeared to be the best long-circulating material among the three studied [16]. What's more, to further enhance the targeting capabilities, several specific moieties (e.g., Arg-Gly-Asp (RGD)) were labeled to these liposomes. For instance, to further improve the efficacy of oxymatrine on anti-hepatic fibrosis, Chai et al. (2012) designed an oxymatrine-loaded RGD-labeled liposome (OM-RGD-L) [17]. After intravenous administration to SD rats, the collagen area values and serum alkaline phosphatase (ALP) for OM-RGD-L groups decreased by 20.9% and 89.0%, respectively, compared to those achieved by the OM liposome. Moreover, in another study, the berberine-encapsulated liposomes modified with poly(*N*-isopropylacrylamide-*co*-methacrylic acid-*co*-octadecyl acrylate) could realize the pH- and thermo-triggered behavior [18]. In a word, the delivery of Chinese medicine-derived alkaloids by various liposomes has exhibited some great advantages of (1) improving their PK profiles, (2) enhancing their treatment efficacies, and (3) boosting their physicochemical properties. However, due to deficient knowledge about the action mechanism, structure-efficacy relationship, and/or in vivo course of such alkaloids, it is relatively difficult to find out a tailor-made liposome to specifically deliver them.

Besides, some novel nanocarriers as DDSs could be utilized to deliver some bioactive alkaloids to make them more prone to enter lesion tissues or organs and, thus, improve their efficacies of treating the corresponding diseases and decreasing their adverse reactions. Among such nanocarriers, solid nanoparticles (NPs) (e.g., polymeric NPs, solid lipid NPs) are one of the typical representatives to be used to deliver the alkaloids to achieve a long-acting behavior. The bioactive alkaloids could be loaded into the core or onto the shell of such particles to be delivered [19]. For example, the biodegradable poly(D,L-lactide-*co*-glycolide) (PLGA) was utilized to deliver ligustrazine to produce ligustrazine-loaded NPs [20]. After intravenous administration to New Zealand white rabbits, the relatively stable drug concentration could be maintained for about 21 days after C_{max} was reached. Moreover, the occurrence of proliferative vitreoretinopathy (PVR) in the NP group was markedly lower than that in the free drug group (12.5% at day 35 vs. 100% at day 14). In another investigation, solid lipid NPs (SLNs) were believed to be quite suitable to deliver several alkaloids with high toxicity, like aconitine [21]. The results showed that after topical administration to SD rats, the C_{max}, T_{max}, and AUC_{0-10h} values of aconitine-loaded SLNs were enhanced by 256, 400, and 126% in comparison to those achieved by the tincture, respectively. Namely, a more long-acting release behavior was achieved and, thus, remarkably decreased the toxicity of aconitine. On the whole, the above NPs showed their particular benefits of delivering the problematic alkaloids, not only improving their bioavailability and treating efficiencies but also reducing their toxicity. What's more, other novel carriers (e.g., gels and ethosomes) were also designed to load some alkaloids (e.g., tetrandrine and ligustrazine) to achieve an excellent sustained-release profile [22, 23]. For instance, Ma et al. designed a kind of calcium alginate gel beads to load tetrandrine, which was orally administrated to healthy dogs [22]. The in vivo assays showed that the T_{max} value was prolonged 2.27-fold compared to the tetrandrine tablet with the same dosage (30 mg/kg). Namely, a prolonged-release manner was achieved by such gel systems. Besides, the ethosomes could facilitate the delivery of some Chinese medicine-derived alkaloids (e.g., ligustrazine) into deep skin layers, which could not only significantly extend their release in vivo but also enhance their capability of skin penetration [23].

3.2.2 Sustained Delivery of Bioactive Glycosides

Another kind of representative of micromolecular ingredients derived from Chinese medicine is bioactive glycosides. They also exhibit potent curative efficacies of anti-inflammation, antivirus, anticancer, antibiosis, and so on [4, 24–26]. However, just like the problematic Chinese medicine-derived alkaloids, several undesirable properties (e.g., poor solubility, poor stability, and rapid elimination) of such glycosides also severely restrict their application in the clinic [27]. Therefore, the development of modern DDSs is of significance in improving their drug-like properties and, thus, treatment efficiencies in the clinic, too [28].

Nowadays, it has been found that a series of novel nanocarriers (e.g., nanoemulsions, NPs, microspheres, proliposomes, etc.) have been applied to delivering these Chinese medicine-derived glycosides through oral and/or intravenous administration to extend the in vivo release, thus reducing their administration times, increasing their treatment efficiency, and improving their patient adaptability [29]. In oral controlled-release, DDSs, microemulsions, and/or nanoemulsions acquired a great of achievements [30, 31]. For example, after *Panax notoginseng* saponins (PNS) were loaded into water-in-oil nanoemulsion, the oral bioavailability of PNS was significantly improved and exhibited a 2.58-fold increase in comparison to its water solution group [30]. In the meanwhile, the results of absorption kinetics in rat intestine showed that the absorption of three kinds of main components of PNS increased by about fivefold than the PNS solution. What's more, Wang et al. also found that the absorption of paeoniflorin microemulsion was better than its solution in the intestine [31]. Furthermore, pH-responsive nanocarriers offered another platform for increasing the bioavailability of these drugs. For example, a kind of pH-responsive nanoparticles, consisting of mesoporous silica nanoparticle cores and poly(acrylic acid) (PAA) shell layers, was utilized to encapsulate bioactive salidroside (extracted from *Rhodiola rosea*) [32]. The results showed that it could regulate the uptake and release of salidroside due to the PAA layers exhibiting either the opened or closed states at different pH values. Moreover, it was also found that the amphiphilic chitosan derivative-based liposome was also quite suitable to load salidroside, which exhibited higher encapsulation efficiency and slower sustained-release rate compared with other traditional liposomes (phosphatidylcholine/cholesterol liposome). On the other hand, several DDSs (e.g., microspheres and NPs) by injection could be also used to deliver some problematic glycosides derived from Chinese medicines (especially for the insoluble and unstable ones) to achieve the controlled release. For instance, Yang and Wang prepared a kind of collagen microspheres to enwrap steroidal saponins from Maidong (*Ophiopogon japonicus*) to achieve the purpose of sustained-release [33]. After administration, the assays showed that these microspheres could not only significantly sustain the release of the saponins but also be effective in improving the osteogenic potential. In another investigation, after being modified with mPEG-PLA, the ginsenoside Rh2 loaded in liposomes significantly prolonged its retention in the bloodstream and presented the more potent activity on suppressing tumor growth without any significant toxicity compared to the ones without modification [34].

Besides, some biological adhesive systems and in situ gel-forming systems could be also utilized to deliver these bioactive glycosides via the mucosal delivery route to sustain their release in vivo and, thus, improve their treatment efficiency [35, 36]. For example, Wu et al. used carbopol which acted as the gelling agent combined with hypromellose as a viscosity-enhancing agent to prepare baicalin-containing in situ pH-triggered gelling systems. After ophthalmic delivery, the in situ gelling systems could support sustained drug release over 8 h, and there was no irritation to eye tissues. Moreover, the AUC and C_{max} values of such a gelling system were 6.1-fold and 3.6-fold higher than the control solution, respectively [36]. In another study, to achieve better buccal adhesion of astragaloside, a kind of astragaloside-loaded mucoadhesive sustained-release tablets was prepared. By selecting the excipient prescription, this tablet could help astragaloside achieve satisfactory bioadhesive and sustained-release capability.

Generally, it shows that DDSs containing the bioactive glycosides can achieve various treatment purposes and reduce the corresponding side effects of these drugs. With the further development of novel and suitable DDSs and nanotechnology, we will eventually achieve the maximum treatment effect of these bioactive glycosides.

3.2.3 Sustained Delivery of Bioactive Phenolic Acids

Bioactive phenolic acids (e.g., ferulic acid, usnic acid, salvianolic acid B, etc.) extracted from Chinese medicines were also a kind of micromolecular components. Recently, a variety of bioactivities (e.g., anti-bacteria, anti-hyperalgesia, antioxidation, anti-inflammation, etc.) have been found from such phenolic acids [3, 37–39]. However, similarly, the poor bioavailability and chemical stability extremely limited their clinical use [3, 37–39]. Thus, the advance of DDSs may provide a kind of feasible strategy to help them improve their drug-like properties.

Recently, to overcome the barriers of such phenolic acids in an application, various novel DDSs (e.g., NPs, gels, liposomes, etc.) have been designed to deliver them. Generally, such delivery could be categorized into three main manners: oral, transdermal, and intravenous administration. In oral delivery, several NPs and nanostructured lipid carriers (NLCs) have been used to load ferulic acid and/or *trans*-cinnamic acid (TCD) to improve their undesirable properties [40–42]. For example, TCD, a kind of main ingredient extracted from cinnamon, has a variety of potent bioactivities (e.g., anticancer, antioxidant, antibacterial effects, etc.) [43]. Particularly, it could be used to cure tuberculosis by indirectly combining with DNA to adjust the expression of some genes and then prevent the tumor cells from growing and proliferating [44]. However, its low oral bioavailability and poor water solubility severely limit the clinical use of TCD. To solve such limitation, TCD was loaded into a kind of NPs (TCD-NPs) using liquid antisolvent precipitation [40]. The in vitro results exhibited that the dissolution rate of TCD-NPs was much faster than that of parent TCD (86.0 ± 3.8% vs. 51.5 ± 1.3% at 2 h) due to the reduced crystallization of TCD loaded into NPs. And, the TCD-NPs also showed a more potent diphenylpicrylhydrazyl radical scavenging activity. Moreover, the in vivo assays showed that the AUC_{0-24h} of TCD-NPs was about 2.16-fold higher that of parent TCD (2.85 ± 0.08 vs. 1.32 ± 0.04 mg/L·h). In general, the improvements in dissolution rate, bioavailability, and antioxidant activity may be owing to the higher specific surface area, amorphous state, and smaller particle size of TCD in NPs. What's more, ferulic acid (FA), a ubiquitous hydroxycinnamic acid, is another representative phenolic acid derived from Chinese medicine. It also displays a variety of therapeutic effects (especially anti-diabetic effect) [45]. However, its poor gastrointestinal stability and short plasma retention time severely restrict its application. To improve such undesirable properties, Panwar et al. used a kind of chitosan NPs to encapsulate FA (FA-NPs) [41]. After oral administration to healthy Wistar albino rats, the T_{max} of FA-NPs was fourfold larger than that of free FA (60 vs. 15 min) at an equal dose. On the other hand, the C_{max} of FA-NPs only accounted for about 30% of free FA (0.549 vs. 1.774 μg/ml). Namely, the plasma retention time in vivo of FA was significantly extended using the encapsulation of NPs. In another investigation, nanostructured lipid carriers were also used to deliver FA to prolong its release in vivo [42].

In transdermal delivery, various novel carriers (e.g., microemulsion- or nanoemulsion-based gel and nanofibrous scaffold) have been used to deliver pseudolaric acid B (PAB) and FA to extend their release. For instance, to improve the water solubility of PAB, Tao et al. prepared a kind of PAB-loaded microemulsion-based gel (PAB-ME-GE) [46]. The dermal pharmacokinetics studies showed that the real-time PAB concentrations of the skin of SD rats dealt with PAB-ME-GE were all much higher than those achieved from PAB-loaded gel in the period of 12 h, which indicated that the skin permeability of PAB-ME was significantly increased compared to the gel. Moreover, the bioavailability of PAB-ME-GE was remarkably improved in comparison to the gel, too (AUC_{0-12h}: 41.95 ± 8.89 vs. 13.90 ± 2.22 μg/ml). In general, such novel carriers not only significantly enhanced the skin permeability of PAB but also improved its dermal bioavailability by solubilizing it into microemulsion and developing ME-GE for its dermal delivery. In another investigation, a similar nanoemulsion-based gel (NE-GE) was utilized to deliver FA [47]. After administration, NE-GE also made FA achieve a sustained-release profile and improved skin permeability. What's more, another novel carrier (i.e., nanofibrous scaffold) was also used to encapsulate FA to sustain the release of FA up to 48% till 120 h [48].

Furthermore, in intravenous delivery, some novel DDSs (e.g., hydrogels and liposomes) have been developed to deliver the Chinese medicine-derived phenolic acids (e.g., salvianolic acid B and FA) to overcome their shortcomings. For example, after FA was loaded into a kind of injectable hydrogel, the preparation not only sustained FA release in vivo but also effectively decreased the oxidative stress-induced damage of Cisd2-deficient murine under oxidative stress [49]. A similar sustained-release profile of salvianolic acid B could also be obtained by the liposome encapsulation [3].

In general, it can be concluded that such novel DDSs provide promising approaches for the effective delivery of these bioactive phenolic acids from Chinese medicine.

3.2.4 Sustained Delivery of Bioactive Polysaccharides

Polysaccharides (PSs) are not only one of the four basic substances that constitute lives but also one of the important representatives of bioactive macromolecule ingredients derived from Chinese medicine (e.g., *Ophiopogonis Radix* PS, *Astragali Radix* PS, *Dioscoreae Rhizoma* PS, *Antrodia camphorata* PS, etc.). They have been found to have a wide spectrum of bioactivities, like immunomodulation, anti-tumor, anti-virus, anti-ischemia, antioxidation, anti-inflammation, and so on [5, 6]. Though playing an important role in various biological processes, PS-based drugs cover only a limited area in clinical treatment. This is due to a series of reasons (e.g., costly and time-consuming preparation, lack of their structure-function relationship knowledge, need of long-term administration for exerting their efficacy, etc.) [50]. Among these reasons, poor drug-like properties of PSs (e.g., poorly oral absorption and rapid elimination by kidneys) severely limit their administration effectiveness and compliance. Therefore, it is urgent and needed to develop effective delivery systems to improve their pharmacological action and/or to reduce the administration frequency for ultimately improving patient benefits.

So far, a variety of novel DDSs (e.g., NPs, liposomes, in situ forming systems (ISFSs), etc.) have been applied to delivering Chinese medicine-derived bioactive PSs to improve their drug-like properties and curative efficiencies. For example, to overcome the negative attributes hampering the clinical use of Chinese yam PS, PLGA-based NPs were utilized to encapsulate this PS [51]. The in vitro tests revealed the achievement of slowed release and improved immunomodulatory activities of CYPS by this nanoencapsulation. In another study, after being delivered by chitosan-silica NPs, *Antrodia camphorata* PS showed certain preferable effects on damaging the membrane of hepatocarcinoma cells and inducing cell death compared to the equivalent solution of the PS [52]. Such results provide a basis for further investigating the in vivo behavior and efficacy of these NPs. Besides the NPs, liposomes were also a suitable strategy to be used to deliver PS. For example, Wang et al. used long-circulating liposomes (LC) to enwrap the bioactive Radix Ophiopogonis PS (ROPS) via the reverse-phase evaporation method [53]. The results showed the ROPS loaded into LC exhibited a 45-times increase in plasma half-life compared to the raw ROPS. Moreover, the targeting efficacy and exposure in infarcted rat myocardia achieved by the LC-loaded ROPS were both significantly improved.

Besides, some novel ISFSs have been used singly or in combination with the chemical conjugation techniques to deliver PSs for prolonging their in vivo release. For example, after astragalus PS was encapsulated by poloxamer (P)-based thermoresponsive ISFSs, an in vitro sustained-release profile of approximately 5.5 days was obtained, together with about 16.3% initial burst release [54]. In another investigation, two kinds of ISFSs (i.e., hydrophilic P-based ISFSs and hydrophobic PLGA- or sucrose acetate isobutyrate (SAIB)-based ISFSs) were utilized to deliver ROPS [55]. The results showed that the two hydrophobic ISFSs "40% $PLGA_{30k}$ in *N*-methyl-2-pyrrolidone (NMP)" and "30% $PLGA_{50k}$ in NMP" exhibited low but lasting blood levels of ROPS for about 4 days after subcutaneous administration at a dose of 200 mg/kg compared to the day-long sustained release of hydrophilic P-based ISFSs (like 24% P407/10% P188) administrated at the same dose. Therefore, such hydrophobic ISFSs might be more hopeful for the long-term treatment and/or precaution of myocardial ischemia [55]. To conquer the initial burst release and achieve further long-lasting delivery of ROPS, the hydrophobic solvent mixture of 90% benzyl benzoate and 10% co-solvent (NMP, triacetin, or benzyl alcohol) was used to replace NMP in the ISFS, which reduced 3.7–8.0-times initial burst release and remarkably prolonged the plasma exposure of ROPS from ~4 days to ~10–15 days [56]. On the other hand, longer-lasting delivery could be achieved by the combination of ISFMs and chemical conjugation techniques [6]. For example, by loading 20 kDa PEG mono-modified ROPS in the ISFS "40% PLGA30k in NMP," an almost monthly smooth rat blood exposure was obtained [57]. In another study, it was found that weeks- to months-long (16–60-day) smooth drug delivery of ROPS could be achieved by varying the level (10–30%) and MW (10–50 kDa) of PLGA or by employing a moderate MW conjugate (~20 or ~30 kDa) [11]. As a whole, for PSs that are highly hydrophilic and need to be used at a high dose per administration, more than one long-lasting delivery technologies might be needed for the achievement of the month(s)-long delivery per dosing.

3.2.5 Others

Other kinds of bioactive ingredients derived from Chinese medicine (e.g., coumarins, terpenes, and flavonoids) could also be loaded into some novel carriers to achieve the purpose of sustained delivery. On the whole, such delivery could be categorized into three approaches (i.e., transdermal, intravenous, and oral delivery). In transdermal delivery, several carriers (like nanostructured lipid carriers, liquid crystals, ethosomes, and nano-vesicles) have been mainly utilized to encapsulate the Chinese medicine-derived coumarins (e.g., psoralen, osthole, etc.) and terpenes (e.g., triptolide, andrographolide, etc.) [58–63]. For example, after topical administration of psoralen-loaded ethosomes to SD rats, the skin sites' peak concentration and AUC of psoralen were approximately 3.37- and 2.34-fold higher than those of psoralen from the tincture, respectively [58]. Similarly, the AUC and C_{max} of the osthole-loaded ethosome also remarkably increased compared to the osthole-loaded transfersomes. Moreover, the in vitro studies exhibited that the osthole encapsulated into ethosomes significantly enhanced the transdermal flux and decreased the lag time across porcine ear skin [59]. In another study, a kind of cubic and hexagonal liquid crystals was used to deliver one of the lactones (i.e., triptolide) to improve the in vivo bioavailability and enhance its anti-arthritic efficacies via transdermal administration [60]. What's more, the novel carriers delivering the Chinese medicine-derived terpenes (e.g., oleanolic acid) and flavonoids (e.g., scutellarin) were mainly using intravenous approach. For example, Zhang et al. prepared a kind of codelivery of oleanolic acid- and gentiopicrin-loaded nanostructured lipid carriers (NLCs) using the film-ultrasonic method. The results showed that compared with the oleanolic acid- or gentiopicrin-loaded NLCs alone, both the drug concentrations of oleanolic acid- and gentiopicrin-loaded NLCs persisted for a significantly longer time in plasma with a linear decrement following second-order kinetics [61]. Furthermore, some liposomes could be utilized to deliver the Chinese medicine-derived flavonoids (e.g., breviscapine) to achieve their sustained-release profile using oral approach [63]. The corresponding consequences were summarized in Table 3.1.

3.3 Sustained-Release Preparations of TCM Compound Recipes

Different from the single components extracted and separated from Chinese medicine, the material basis of TCM compound recipes is multi-component, for which it exerts multi-processed, multi-targeted, and comprehensive regulation. With the in-depth development of material science and pharmaceutical science, it has become a difficult but hot spot in the research on the application of the sustained-release technology to the TCM compound recipe. At present, oral sustained-release preparations of Chinese medicine can be divided into matrix type, membrane-controlled type, osmotic pump type, and gastric retention type according to mechanisms of the drug release [64]. The principle of sustained release was shown in Table 3.2. The preparation technologies mainly include multi-layer sustained- and controlled-release coating technology, multi-layer controlled-release technology, multiparticulate site-controlled release technology, functional reserving technology, etc., which is showed in Fig. 3.2.

3.3.1 Membrane-Controlled Type

Due to the differences in the properties of various effective components of the TCM compound recipes, and in the pH values of the human gastrointestinal tract, hydroxypropyl methylcellulose (HPMC), acrylic resin, and other excipients as coating materials dissolving under different pH values are used for the preparation

Table 3.1 Sustained-release DDSs for representative bioactive ingredients from Chinese medicine to improve their drug-like properties and curative efficacy

Delivery approach	Name	Bioactivities	Existing problems	DDSs and achieved improvements	References
Oral	Tetrandrine	Having the efficacies of anti-cancer and anti-inflammation; treating hypertension and pneumosilicosis	Poor water solubility and low oral bioavailability	Gels: T_{max} ↑ 1.27-fold, $T_{1/2}$ ↑ 0.58-fold, C_{max} ↓ 24.4%, 12 h of sustained release in vitro	[2, 22]
				The nanocapsules: $AUC_{(0–24h)}$ ↑ 1.08-fold, $MRT_{(0–24h)}$ ↑ 0.1-fold, T_{max} ↑ 1.56-fold	
	Panax notoginseng saponins	Having the efficacies of inhibiting the apoptosis of myocardial cells, resistance to myocarditis, anticancer	Low oral bioavailability	Nanoemulsion: Oral bioavailability ↑ 2.58-fold; the absorption of three kinds of main components ↑ five-fold	[29, 30]
	Trans-cinnamic acid	Having potent bioactivities of anti-cancer, antioxidant, and antibacterial effects; curing tuberculosis	Low oral bioavailability and poor water solubility	Nanoparticles: $AUC_{0–24h}$ ↑ 2.16-fold; dissolution rate ↑ 1.67-fold; DPPH radical scavenging activity ↑	[40]
Intravenous	Vincristine	Curing non-Hodgkin's lymphoma, acute lymphoblastic leukemia, hematologic malignancies, and other solid tumors	Extensive distribution and long elimination; severe neurotoxicity	Liposome: Therapeutic index ↑, target tumor ↑, individual dose ↑ over two-fold, CL ↓ 40.4%, C_{max} ↑ 52.3%, AUC ↑ 73.1%, MRT ↑ 56.6%, $T_{1/2}$ ↑ 55.6%	[2, 14, 16]
				PEG-coated liposome: $T_{1/2}$ of PEG-DSPE formulation ↑ 0.4-fold compared to the market, 12 h of retardation in the clearance from blood	
	Steroidal saponins of *Ophiopogon japonicus*	Treating bone and joint diseases, nerve damage, and hematischesis	Short terminal half-life	Microspheres: Initial burst release ↓, linear release over the first 8 days; ALP ↑, bone regeneration and bone formation ↑	[29, 33]
	Ferulic acid	Improving cardiovascular functions and possessing an anti-diabetic effect		Hydrogel: Oxidative stress-induced damage ↓, endogenous ROS ↓, cell	[49]

			Poor gastrointestinal stability and short plasma retention time	viability ↑; sustained release of ferulic acid	
	Radix Ophiopogonis PS	Having the efficacies of hypoglycemic and anti-obesity effects and treating and preventing the ischemia-reperfusion injury	Short $T_{1/2}$, ~0.5 h, and MRT, 0.65 h; low oral bioavailability, 1.7%	Liposome: Immunoregulatory activities and adjuvanticity ↑	[6, 11, 56]
				PEG-coated liposome: $T_{1/2}$ ↑ 45-fold; targeting delivery ↑	
				Mono-PEGylation: $T_{1/2}$ ↑ 32- to 100-fold; targeting delivery, therapeutic effect, and administration compliance ↑	
				ISFS: day(s)- to week(s)-long sustained delivery; administration compliance ↑	
				ISFS + mono-PEGylation: Week(s)- to month(s)-long sustained delivery; administration compliance ↑	
Transdermal	Aconitine	Having the efficacies of anti-inflammation and analgesia; treating neuronal disorders	High toxicity; limited oral administration, short elimination half-time	The SLNs: C_{max} ↑ 2.56-fold, $AUC_{(0-10h)}$ ↑ 1.26-fold, T_{max} ↑ three-fold than the ethanol tinctures, the $AUC_{(0-10h)}$ and C_{max} of the SLNs in scapular region > abdomen > chest; the toxicity ↓; transdermal permeability ↑	[2, 21]
	Taxifolin glycoside	Treating atopic dermatitis and inhibiting microbial antigen-stimulated, dendritic cell-mediated allergic responses	Low water solubility	Elastic liposomes: the amount of taxifolin glycoside skin permeated ↑ 9.4-fold compared to the solution; recovery of AD-induced NC/Nga mice ↑; AD-associated immune responses serum interleukine-4,	[29, 64]

(continued)

Table 3.1 (continued)

Delivery approach	Name	Bioactivities	Existing problems	DDSs and achieved improvements	References
				immunoglobulin E, and interferon gamma were regulated	
	Pseudolaric acid B	Having the efficacies of fungicidal activity against *Candida albicans* and antifungal activity against azole-resistant *Candida* species	Poor water solubility	Microemulsion-based gel: AUC_{0-12h} ↑ 3.0-fold, real-time pseudolaric acid B concentrations ↑ compared to pseudolaric acid B-loaded gel in the period of 12 h; in vitro skin permeability ↑	[46]

Note: $T_{1/2}$ half-life, C_{max} maximum plasma concentration, T_{max} the time taken to reach C_{max}, *AUC* area under the concentration-time curve, *MRT* mean residence time, *DPPH* diphenylpicrylhydrazyl, *CL* clearance, *PEG* polyethylene glycol, *DSPE* distearoylphosphatidylethanolamine, *ALP* alkaline phosphatase, *ROS* reactive oxygen species, *ISFS* in situ forming system, *SLNs* solid lipid nanoparticles, *AD* atopic dermatitis

Table 3.2 Technologies of modern sustained-release preparations of TCM compound recipes

Preparation process	Principle	Application	References
Multi-layer tablet compressing technology	Retardation of different excipients	*Guizhi Fuling* double-layer sustained-release tablet	[65]
Matrix-type sustained-release technique	Sustained release of matrix materials	*Pueraria lobata* and *Uncaria rhynchophylla* compound sustained-release tablets; extencap of decoction of *Gastrodia* and *Uncaria*	[66, 67]
Osmotic pump technology	Driving force from osmotic pressure	Osmotic pump tablets for *Fuzi Lizhong*; osmotic pump tablet of compound *Danshen*	[68, 69]
Multiparticulate site-controlled release technology	Dissolution at different pH from different coating materials	Gradient-release pellets for *Guanxin Suhe* and *Shexiang Baoxin*	[70, 71]
Multiparticulate time-controlled release technology	Successive swelling of swelling layer and controlled-release layer	Compound recipe *Shuxiong* sustained-release capsules; compound *Danshen* sustained-release capsule	[72, 73]

of coated pellets for site-controlled release. Specifically, the coating membranes could be dissolved under the conditions of pH $= 1.2$, pH ≥ 5.5, or pH ≥ 6.8, corresponding to rapid disintegration at the stomach, duodenum, or small intestine, respectively. Once these coated pellets are mixed in a certain proportion and filled into capsules, then they have sustained release with pH-dependent properties, which ensures that the various components of the compound recipes can be released simultaneously, showing sustained-release characteristics overall. Tang et al. [70] coated Guanxin Suhe pellets with HPMC, HPMCP HP-55, and Eudragit L100/S100, respectively. Three kinds of coated pellets were mixed in the ratio of 1:1:1 to prepare Guanxin Suhe sustained-release capsules, realizing pH-dependent gradient release at the stomach, duodenum, jejunum, and ileum. The T_{max} of Guanxin Suhe pills and Guanxin Suhe sustained-release capsules were 0.42 and 1.08 h, respectively, which indicated that pH-dependent gradient release microspheres could achieve better sustained-release effect in vivo. Song et al. [71] used HPMC 60RT-5, Eudragit L30D-55, and L100-Eudragit S100 as coating materials to prepare heart-protecting musk pellets by fluid-bed coating technology and then filled different coated pellets into capsules in a certain proportion. The γ-scintigraphic tracer evaluation demonstrated that various coated pellets disintegrated at the stomach, duodenum, jejunum, and ileum, respectively; and the release similarity factor f_2 value of total ginsenosides and borneol (water-soluble and fat-soluble, respectively) in the capsule reached 79.6, realizing the similar release rates of components with different physical and chemical properties.

The drug-loaded pellets or tablets are coated with a swelling layer and controlled-release layer in turn, and then the pellets or tablets with different thicknesses of

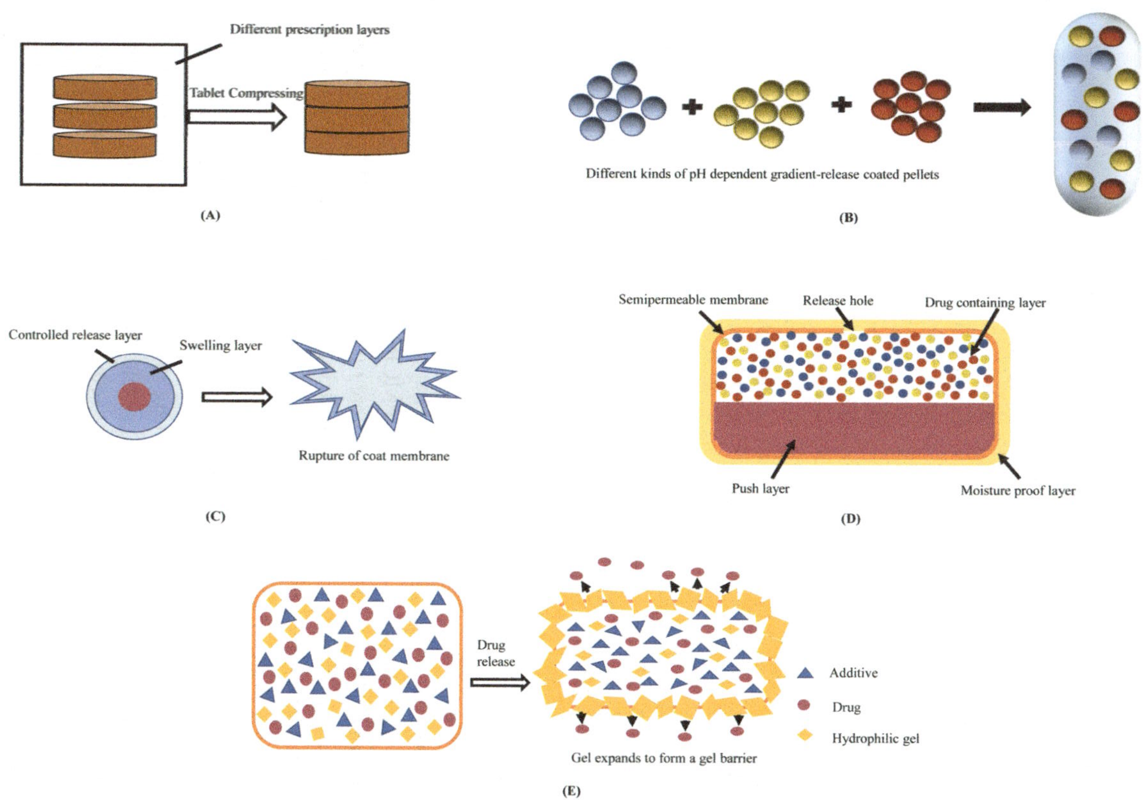

Fig. 3.2 The technologies of sustained- and controlled-release preparation of TCM compound recipes. (**a**) Multi-layered sustained-release tablets; (**b**) multiparticulate site-controlled release capsules; (**c**) multiparticulate time-controlled release pellets; (**d**) osmotic pump tablets; (**e**) gastric retention tablets

controlled-release layer are mixed into the capsules. The swelling layer gradually expands with the infiltration of water. Drugs rapidly release when the swelling pressure is large enough to break controlled-release coating. Pellets or tablets with different thickness of controlled-release layer have different lag time. Pellets or tablets with different lag time can release drug in turn at different time, showing the characteristics of synchronous release on the whole. A certain proportion of HPMC 60RT-5 and sodium dodecyl sulfate (SDS) was combined with low-substituted hydroxypropyl cellulose (L-HPC), respectively, to form the coating solution of *Shuxiong* sustained-release capsules. The coating of pellet-containing heart was used as the swelling layer, and the ethyl cellulose aqueous dispersion coating was used as the controlled-release layer. Equal weight of pellets coated with different controlled-release layer was filled into the hard capsules. In artificial gastric and intestinal fluid, the f_2 values of hydroxysafflor yellow A and *Panax notoginseng* saponins, hydroxysafflor yellow A and ferulic acid, and *Panax notoginseng* saponins and ferulic acid were 90.1, 77.3, and 87.0, respectively. The release profiles of these three compositions from Shuxiong sustained-release capsules showed no significant difference with a characteristic of synchronously sustained release [72].

3.3.2 Matrix Type

The matrix-type sustained- and controlled-release preparations mainly include hydrophilic gel frame, insoluble frame, and erosive frame. Wu et al. [66] used HPMC as a hydrophilic gel frame and prepared *Pueraria lobata* and *Uncaria rhynchophylla* compound sustained-release tablets by wet granulation. When 22% HPMC K4M was used as a matrix material and 18% lactose was used as diluent, the preparation showed good in vitro release characteristics for 12 h. Liu et al. [67] prepared the extencap of *Gastrodia* and *Uncaria* Decoction with ethyl cellulose (EC) as an insoluble matrix material, achieving constant drug release for 12 h in vitro, and the drug release mechanism was consistent with zero-order release. Liao et al. [65] divided the extracts of six herbs in *Guizhi Fuling* Decoction into two groups: water-soluble (the extract of *Paeoniae Radix Alba*, *Moutan Cortex*, *Cinnamomi Ramulus*, and *Persicae Semen*) and water-insoluble layer drugs (ethanol extracts and water-extraction alcohol-precipitation of *Poria cocos*, paeonol, essential oil-cyclodextrin complexes of *Cinnamomi Ramulus*). HPMC K4M and EC 20 were used, respectively, as matrix materials to prepare *Guizhi* (*Cinnamomi Ramulus*) and *Fuling* (*Poria*) compound double-layer sustained-release tablets. The cumulative release rates of paeonol, amygdalin, and paeoniflorin were 82%, 91%, and 90%, respectively, within 12 h. Compared with paeonol in water-insoluble layer, the f_2 values of amygdalin and paeoniflorin in water-soluble layer were 68 and 64, respectively. The drug release of hydrophilic gel frame preparation and insoluble frame preparation is mainly due to passive diffusion. The drug release rate is not only controlled by the frame but also related to the physical and chemical properties of the drug. The drug release rate of the soluble skeleton mainly depends on the dissolution rate of the excipients and is not affected by the physicochemical factors such as drug solubility, which provides a new idea for the synchronous and sustained release of all components of Chinese medicine. However, the drug release from erosive frame preparations mainly depends on the erosion rate of excipients and is not affected by physicochemical properties such as drug solubility, providing a new idea for the synchronous release of various component in TCM compound recipes.

3.3.3 Osmotic Type

Osmotic-type preparations often release drug in zero order for a long time with the utilization of osmotic pressure. Therefore, the drug concentration in blood is stable, and the effect is persistent in vivo. The core is covered with a semi-permeable membrane, and the drug dissolves into a saturated solution with the infiltration of water, thus forming an osmotic pressure difference between the inside and outside of the membrane. Consequently, the drug release from the pores is driven by osmotic pressure [74].

According to the acidic nature of *Fuzi Lizhong* prescription, sodium chloride and sodium bicarbonate were added as osmotic active substances and solubilizers in the core to prepare *Fuzi Lizhong* effervescent osmotic pump tablets by Li et al. [68]. The release test in vitro showed that sodium bicarbonate reacted with acidic components and then produced carbon dioxide gas when water penetrated into the core, which guaranteed the continuous and complete drug release in the effervescent osmotic pump tablets, and the cumulative release rate reached 96.9% after 14 h. In addition, osmotic pump tablets were coated with HPMC as a blocking agent to solve the problem of too high drug release rate, which changed the drug release curve from non-constant release to constant rate release. Compound *Danshen*, containing phenolic hydroxyl and carboxyl phenolic acids and triterpenoid saponins, is weakly acidic. Xue et al. [69] directly added sodium bicarbonate as an effervescent agent, sodium chloride and mannitol as penetration enhancers, and HPMC as a blocking agent to form the core of the tablets. Then the core was coated with CA membrane containing porogen to prepare effervescent osmotic pump tablet (EOPT) of compound Danshen. The changes in structure and osmotic pressure in core showed that the drug release was driven by osmotic pressure in EOPT. Driving force was composed of three osmotic pressures, including the osmotic pressure of saturated solution formed by osmotic active substances such as sodium chloride and mannitol, the air pressure formed by the reaction of drugs with sodium bicarbonate, and the expansion pressure formed by the blocking agent. In addition, the similarity factor analysis showed that all the active components were released synchronously in zero order. Fang et al. [75] prepared gastric retention two-compartment osmotic pump tablet (TCOPT) containing total alkaloids extracted from *Huanglian* (*Coptidis Rhizoma*) and *Wuzhuyu* (*Euodiae Fructus*), which was composed of a pushing layer and a drug layer. The pushing layer contained light porous microspheres, making the apparent density of the tablet less than water. Due to the buoyancy, the tablets floated in the gastric fluid, and the water permeated into the drug layer to form an ointment-like drug suspension, which pushed the layer to absorb water and expand and simultaneously pushed the drug layer out of the hole. Based on the single-factor experiments, the formulation was optimized by orthogonal design. In the formulation, the mixture of PEO:HPMC (4:1) was used as the booster layer swelling agent, NaCl was used as the booster layer permeating agent, PEO was used as the suspension agent, and PEG 400 was used as the porogen of CA membrane. The preparation with osmotic pressure as release mechanism has the characteristics of synchronous and zero-order release. The sustained release driven by osmotic pump can realize the synchronous release of each component in TCM compound recipes, which conforms to the characteristics of traditional decoction to a certain extent. However, it is a fact that the drug release only driven by osmotic pressure cannot completely follow the release rule of TCM compound recipes, and thus it is still necessary to explore the preparation technology of controlled-release preparation [76].

3.3.4 Intragastric Floating Type

Intragastric floating can prolong the retention time of drugs in the stomach by floating and biological adherence, thereby extending the absorption of drugs. Intragastric floating type is widely used in sustained-release preparations of Chinese medicine. It utilizes hydrophilic gel materials to rapidly expand and form gel in the stomach or uses light materials with low density or gas generation to reduce the specific gravity of preparations and thus floats in gastric fluid for a long time. In addition, hydrophilic colloid expands in the gastric fluid and forms a colloidal barrier on the outer layer of the drug. The drug can be slowly diffused into the gastric juice through the colloidal barrier and absorbed by the body, thus maintaining a stable blood drug concentration [77]. Based on "drug-supplement combination" theory, Du et al. [78] prepared *Shaoyao Gancao* compound intragastric floating sustained-release tablets with chitosan as the main molding excipient and konjac glucomannan, HPMC, carbomer, sodium alginate, microcrystalline cellulose, and sodium bicarbonate as auxiliary excipients. The continuous release time of *Shaoyao Gancao* compound intragastric floating tablets was more than 8 h, the duration of floating was more than 12 h, and the initial floating time was less than 1 min. Shen et al. [79] utilized the dried extract of *Beishashen* (*Glehniae Radix*), *Maidong* (*Ophiopogonis Radix*), *Shihu* (*Dendrobii Caulis*), *Maiya* (*Hordei Fructus Germinatus*), *Baishao* (*Paeoniae Radix Alba*), and *Gancao* (*Glycyrrhizae Radix et Rhizoma*) together with excipients of hydroxypropyl methylcellulose, sodium bicarbonate, octadecanol, microcrystalline cellulose, etc., to prepare gastric floating sustained-release tablets by direct compression technique. The release of the tablets in vitro was stable at 80% within 10 h, indicating that the preparation had good floatability and stable drug release. Zhou et al. [80] developed *Zuojin* intragastric floating sustained-release tablet based on the hydrodynamic balanced controlled-release system (HBS). With

HPMC, sodium carboxymethylcellulose (CMC Na), octadecanol, and polyethylene glycol 6000 (PEG 6000) as excipients, a uniform design method was used to optimize the preparation. It was shown that the in vitro drug release conformed to Higuchi equation and there was a good correlation between the release amount and the release time. In addition, it was found that the drug release mechanism of sustained-release tablets was the result of diffusion of hydrophilic gel layer and the erosion of matrix materials; therefore, it was concluded that *Zuojin* intragastric floating sustained-release tablet had the characteristics of sustained release and long floating time.

3.4 The Quality Evaluation of Sustained-Release DDSs of Chinese Medicines

The sustained-release DDSs of Chinese medicines have the advantages of (1) reducing the frequency and dosage of administration, (2) keeping steady-state plasma concentration, and (3) exhibiting the smaller difference between $C_{\max}$ and $C_{\min}$ than ordinary preparations. Therefore, they have been one of the research focuses in the Chinese medicine field in recent years [81]. However, it is quite difficult to establish the objective quality evaluation system for such sustained-release DDSs due to the complicated chemical components and unclear medicinal material basis of Chinese medicine. This has become one of the important obstacles to their development. Therefore, it is quite meaningful to discuss how to establish an effective quality evaluation system for sustained-release DDSs of Chinese medicine.

On the whole, the integrated quality evaluation system for sustained-release DDSs of Chinese medicine should be comprised of six parts, i.e., evaluations of active/index component(s), fingerprint, in vitro release characteristics, pharmacokinetics, PK-PD (pharmacokinetics-pharmacodynamics) and IVIVC (in vivo-in vitro correlation), and safety.

Firstly, in the process of choosing an active/index component(s) as a quality control index, it is important to select suitable chemical ingredients. And, the desirable components should possess two kinds of characteristics as below. One is pharmacodynamic relevance, which means that the selected components can represent the curative efficacy of Chinese medicine to a certain degree. The other is testability, which means that the chosen components can be used to establish stable and feasible detection methodology [82]. Secondly, the fingerprint technique, one of comprehensive and quantifiable quality control modes for Chinese medicine, can take nearly all representative chemical ingredients contained in Chinese medicine as an evaluation index and, thus, effectively overcome drawbacks of the current quality control mode of Chinese medicine preparations. Thirdly, in the process of evaluating the in vitro release characteristics of Chinese medicine, the release profiles of either one or several index components or effective parts of Chinese medicine are used to evaluate the in vitro release profile of the whole Chinese medicine. For example, Zhu et al. regarded tanshinone IIA, salvianolic acid B, and ginsenoside Rg1 as index components to evaluate the in vitro release profile of compound Danshen sustained-release tablets [83]. Fourthly, in the process of evaluating the pharmacokinetics of Chinese medicine, some researchers suggest that serum pharmacochemistry of Chinese medicine should be determined due to the medicinal material basis of Chinese medicine being the chemical constituents existing in blood [82]. In some studies, about ten kinds of blood transitional components had been determined by the UPLC/MS technique after oral administration of Dachuanxiong prescription to SD rats. And, regarding such components as index components to research the PK profile of Dachuanxiong prescription multi-unit DDSs (including rapid- and sustained-release units) is believed to be able to better reflect the whole PK characteristics of the multi-component the compound recipes [84]. This is of significance for establishing a reliable quality evaluation system for Chinese medicine. Fifthly, as for the PK-PD evaluation of Chinese medicine, the current way is mainly to establish the correlation between "the PK data of one or several bioactive ingredients in the preparations" and "the PD data of one or several pharmacodynamics indexes" in one or more experimental animal models. Lastly, due to the increased drug dosage in sustained-release DDSs of Chinese medicine (especially those containing toxic substances), the corresponding safety must be taken into consideration.

3.5 Conclusion

The novel sustained-release preparations of Chinese medicine have shown their immense advantages in the delivery of the bioactive micromolecules (mainly including alkaloids, glycosides, and phenolic acids) and macromolecules (especially, polysaccharides) derived from Chinese medicine, resulting in not only the improved PK behaviors of these ingredients but also the reduced adverse effects and enhanced curative efficacies. Especially, the T_{max} and AUC values of these ingredients loaded into sustained-release DDSs (e.g., liposomes, nanoparticles, gels, in situ forming systems, etc.) were both much larger than those of the free drugs with the equal administration dosage, while their C_{max} values were significantly decreased using three major kinds of delivery approaches (i.e., oral, intravenous, and transdermal delivery). Namely, such bioactive micromolecules and macromolecules achieve both the capability of long-lasting release and improved bioavailability, which plays a vital role in reducing administration frequency, increasing treatment efficiency, and ultimately improving their patient compliance. These novel DDSs for sustained-release make both the Chinese medicine-derived micromolecules and macromolecules achieve a long-lasting blood profile. Besides, a part of these DDSs is more prone to improve the low water solubility and weak chemical stability of the micromolecules, whereas some prefer to improve the low oral absorption of the macromolecules due to their different physical and chemical natures.

For TCM compound recipes, it is unapt to use one or several components as representative research objects, because it is a multi-component whole and its efficacy is often the synergism of the pharmacological effects from various substances. In addition, the physicochemical properties of each component are also relatively complex. Consequently, the research on the formulation design and selection of sustained-release preparations of TCM compound recipes needs to be strengthened. In the design, the close connection with the guidelines of Chinese medicine is necessary, aiming to realize the "procedural release" of multiple components in TCM compound recipes. Namely, the release of multiple components of Chinese medicines should be orderly. Meanwhile, their absorption should be guaranteed, so that each drug release unit can play the optimal integration effect in the target site. In various types of sustained-release preparations of TCM compound recipes, membrane-controlled preparations can more easily realize the synchronous release by different coating materials with different thickness. According to differences in physicochemical properties of drugs such as drug solubility, the appropriate matrix materials can synchronize the release of each unit. Osmotic-type preparations are not affected by environmental pH, gastrointestinal peristalsis, and other factors, can achieve zero-order release, and often have good in vitro and in vivo correlation. However, because the solubility and dissolution rate of active substances in TCM compound recipes are greatly different, the drug release may be inconsistent and incomplete. By prolonging the retention time of drugs in the stomach, intragastric floating technology can not only prolong the duration but also improve the absorption of drugs, especially for drugs with specific absorption in the stomach and duodenum.

As a whole, due to the deficient knowledge about the action mechanism, structure-efficacy relationship, and/or in vivo course of bioactive components, it's still a relatively new field to develop DDSs for them. With the achievements of their structural attributes and the in vitro and in vivo properties, some tailor-made DDSs might be designed and developed for them, which could further improve their drug-like properties and curative efficacies and ultimately accelerate the pace of their clinical application. For TCM compound recipes, the research in sustained-release preparations is still in the early stage, lacking a large number of clinical or biological studies to support. Meanwhile, it will be a great challenge to apply the technology for single components to TCM compound recipes with large dosage and complex components.

Besides, it is quite important to establish a reliable quality evaluation system for ensuring the safety and effectiveness of sustained-release preparations of Chinese medicine. So far, owing to the complicated chemical components and action mechanisms of Chinese medicine, it is still very challenging to establish a comprehensive and objective quality evaluation system for such preparations. Luckily, as the rapid advance of science and technology and the mutual penetration between different disciplines, a series of new theories and new methods would continue to emerge and promote the continuous improvement of the quality evaluation system for such sustained-release preparations.

References

1. Douer, D. (2016). Efficacy and safety of vincristine sulfate liposome injection in the treatment of adult acute lymphocytic leukemia. *The Oncologist, 21*(7), 840–847.
2. Zheng, X., Wu, F., Lin, X., Shen, L., & Feng, Y. (2018). Developments in drug delivery of bioactive alkaloids derived from traditional Chinese medicine. *Drug Delivery, 25*(1), 398–416.
3. Singh, M., Devi, S., Ran, V. S., Mishra, B. B., Kumar, J., & Ahluwalia, V. (2019). Delivery of phytochemicals by liposome cargos: Recent progress, challenges and opportunities. *Journal of Microencapsulation, 36*(3), 215–235.
4. Dai, D., Zhang, C. F., Williams, S., Yuan, C. S., & Wang, C. Z. (2017). Ginseng on cancer: Potential role in modulating inflammation-mediated angiogenesis. *The American Journal of Chinese Medicine, 45*(1), 13–22.
5. Dong, Q. Q., Lin, X., Shen, L., & Feng, Y. (2016). The protective effect of herbal polysaccharides on ischemia-reperfusion injury. *International Journal of Biological Macromolecules, 92*, 431–440.
6. Li, Z., Wang, L. N., Lin, X., Shen, L., & Feng, Y. (2017). Drug delivery for bioactive polysaccharides to improve their drug-like properties and curative efficacy. *Drug Delivery, 24*(2), 70–80.
7. Venturoli, D., & Rippe, B. (2005). Ficoll and dextran vs. globular proteins as probes for testing glomerular permselectivity: Effects of molecular size, shape, charge, and deformability. *American Journal of Physiology - Renal Physiology, 288*(4), F605–F613.
8. Yue, P. F., Wu, B., Zheng, Q., Hu, P. Y., & Yang, M. (2010). Innovation and discussion on evaluation pattern of synchronism/ asynchronism release characterization of sustained and controlled release preparations for Chinese herbal formula. *Chinese Traditional and Herbal Drugs, 41*(9), 1413–1417.
9. Xia, H. J., Zhang, Z. H., Liu, D., Yu, D. H., & Jia, X. B. (2013). Establishment of modern multicomponent sustained-release preparations of oral traditional Chinese medicines. *China Journal of Chinese Materia Medica, 38*(19), 3400–3404.
10. Yang, Y. T., Tao, Y. Q., Tang, W. H., Li, S., Shi, J. L., Zhou, Y. Q., Liu, W. L., & He, F. Y. (2016). Investigation on supramolecular mechanism of multi-component overall control in Chinese medicine controlled sustainedrelease preparation. *China Journal of Chinese Materia Medica, 41*(24), 4675–4679.
11. Wang, L. N., Zheng, X., Wu, F., Shen, L., Lin, X., & Feng, Y. (2018). Delivery of radix ophiopogonis polysaccharide via sucrose acetate isobutyrate-based in situ forming systems alone or combined with its mono-PEGylation. *Drug Delivery, 25*(1), 267–277.
12. Silverman, J. A., & Deitcher, S. R. (2013). Marqibo (R) (vincristine sulfate liposome injection) improves the pharmacokinetics and pharmacodynamics of vincristine. *Cancer Chemotherapy and Pharmacology, 71*(3), 555–564.
13. Silverman, J. A., Reynolds, L., & Deitcher, S. R. (2013). Pharmacokinetics and pharmacodynamics of vincristine sulfate liposome injection (VSLI) in adults with acute lymphoblastic leukemia. *Journal of Clinical Pharmacology, 53*(11), 1139–1145.
14. Nakamura, K., Yoshino, K., Yamashita, K., & Kasukawa, H. (2012). Designing a novel in vitro drug-release-testing method for liposomes prepared by pH-gradient method. *International Journal of Pharmaceutics, 430*(1-2), 381–387.
15. Chen, J., Yan, G. J., Hu, R. R., Gu, Q. W., Chen, M. L., Gu, W., Chen, Z. P., & Cai, B. C. (2012). Improved pharmacokinetics and reduced toxicity of brucine after encapsulation into stealth liposomes: Role of phosphatidylcholine. *International Journal of Nanomedicine, 7*, 3567–3577.
16. Zhang, J., Chen, Y. C., Li, X., Liang, X. L., & Luo, X. J. (2016). The influence of different long-circulating materials on the pharmacokinetics of liposomal vincristine sulfate. *International Journal of Nanomedicine, 11*, 4187–4197.

17. Chai, N. L., Fu, Q., Shi, H., Cai, C. H., Wan, J., Xu, S. P., & Wu, B. Y. (2012). Oxymatrine liposome attenuates hepatic fibrosis via targeting hepatic stellate cells. *World Journal of Gastroenterology, 18*(31), 4199–4206.
18. Zhou, W. T., An, X. Q., Wang, J. Z., Shen, W. G., Chen, Z. Y., & Wang, X. Y. (2012). Characteristics, phase behavior and control release for copolymer-liposome with both pH and temperature sensitivities. *Colloids and Surfaces A: Physicochemical and Engineering Aspects, 395*, 225–232.
19. Liu, Y., & Feng, N. P. (2015). Nanocarriers for the delivery of active ingredients and fractions extracted from natural products used in traditional Chinese medicine (TCM). *Advances in Colloid and Interface Science, 221*, 60–76.
20. Zhang, X. M., Wei, J. H., Ma, P. K., Mu, H. J., Wang, A. P., Zhang, L. M., Wu, Z. M., & Sun, K. X. (2015). Preparation and evaluation of a novel biodegradable long-acting intravitreal implant containing ligustrazine for the treatment of proliferative vitreoretinopathy. *The Journal of Pharmacy and Pharmacology, 67*(2), 160–169.
21. Zhang, Y. T., Han, M. Q., Shen, L. N., Zhao, J. H., & Feng, N. P. (2015). Solid lipid nanoparticles formulated for transdermal aconitine administration and evaluated in vitro and in vivo. *Journal of Biomedical Nanotechnology, 11*(2), 351–361.
22. Ma, Y., Li, W. Z., Guan, S. X., Lai, X. P., & Chen, D. W. (2009). Evaluation of tetrandrine sustained release calcium alginate gel beads in vitro and in vivo. *Yakugaku Zasshi Journal of Pharmaceutical Society of Japan, 129*(7), 851–854.
23. Liu, X. Y., Liu, H., Zeng, Z. W., Zhou, W. H., Liu, J. Q., & He, Z. W. (2011). Pharmacokinetics of ligustrazine ethosome patch in rats and anti-myocardial ischemia and anti-ischemic reperfusion injury effect. *International Journal of Nanomedicine, 6*, 1391–1398.
24. Yu, C. H., Zhang, Z. Y., Zhang, H. J., Zhen, Z., Galway, T., Wang, Y. W., Yuan, C. S., & Wang, C. Z. (2013). Pretreatment of baicalin and wogonoside with glycoside hydrolase: A promising approach to enhance anticancer potential. *Oncology Reports, 30*(5), 2411–2418.
25. Song, J., Yeo, S. G., Hong, E. H., Lee, B. R., Kim, J. W., Kim, J., Jeong, H., Kwon, Y., Kim, H., Lee, S., Park, J. H., & Ko, H. J. (2014). Antiviral Activity of Hederasaponin B from Hedera helix against Enterovirus 71 Subgenotypes C3 and C4a. *Biomolecules & Therapeutics, 22*(1), 41–46.
26. Yang, S. H., Ahn, E. K., Lee, J. A., Shin, T. S., Tsukamoto, C., Suh, J. W., Mei, I., & Chung, G. (2015). Soyasaponins Aa and Ab exert an anti-obesity effect in 3T3-L1 adipocytes through downregulation of PPAR gamma. *Phytotherapy Research, 29*(2), 281–287.
27. Puglia, C., Lauro, M. R., Tirendi, G. G., Fassari, G. E., Carbone, C., Bonina, F., & Puglisi, G. (2017). Modern drug delivery strategies applied to natural active compounds. *Expert Opinion on Drug Delivery, 14*(6), 755–768.
28. Ajazuddin, S. S. (2010). Applications of novel drug delivery system for herbal formulations. *Fitoterapia, 81*(7), 680–689.
29. Li, L., Feng, Y., Hong, Y. L., Lin, X., & Shen, L. (2018). Recent advances in drug delivery system for bioactive glycosides from traditional chinese medicine. *The American Journal of Chinese Medicine, 46*(8), 1791–1824.
30. Liu, Z. D., Zhang, Q., Ding, L. L., Li, C. H., Yin, Z. P., Yan, G. Q., Pi, J. X., Li, J. W., Li, N., & Qi, D. L. (2016). Preparation procedure and pharmacokinetic study of water-in-oil nanoemulsion of Panax notoginseng saponins for improving the oral bioavailability. *Current Drug Delivery, 13*(4), 600–610.
31. Wang, C., Yuan, J., Yang, Z. Y., Nie, X. X., Song, L. H., & Wei, W. (2012). Pharmacokinetics of paeoniflorin microemulsion after repeated dosing in rats with adjuvant arthritis. *Die Pharmazie, 67*(12), 997–1001.
32. Peng, H. L., Dong, R. C., Wang, S. Q., Zhang, Z., Luo, M., Bai, C. Q., Zhao, Q., Li, J. H., Chen, L. X., & Xiong, H. (2013). A pH-responsive nano-carrier with mesoporous silica nanoparticles cores and poly(acrylic acid) shell-layers: Fabrication, characterization and properties for controlled release of salidroside. *International Journal of Pharmaceutics, 446*(1-2), 153–159.

33. Yang, C. R., & Wang, J. H. (2014). Preparation and characterization of collagen microspheres for sustained release of steroidal saponins. *Materials Research-Ibero-American Journal of Materials, 17*(6), 1644–1650.
34. Xu, L. Q., Yu, H., Yin, S. P., Zhang, R. X., Zhou, Y. D., & Li, J. (2015). Liposome-based delivery systems for ginsenoside Rh2: In vitro and in vivo comparisons. *Journal of Nanoparticle Research, 17*(10), 13.
35. Cai, J., & Wang, S. (2012). Optimization of excipient prescription of astragaloside buccal mucoadhesive sustained-release tablets and determination of its in-vitro dissolution rate. *Journal of Guangzhou University of Traditional Chinese Medicine, 29*(3), 310–314.
36. Wu, H. Y., Liu, Z. D., Peng, J. J., Li, L., Li, N., Li, J. W., & Pan, H. (2011). Design and evaluation of baicalin-containing in situ pH-triggered gelling system for sustained ophthalmic drug delivery. *International Journal of Pharmaceutics, 410*(1-2), 31–40.
37. Francolini, I., Giansanti, L., Piozzi, A., Altieri, B., Mauceri, A., & Mancini, G. (2019). Glucosylated liposomes as drug delivery systems of usnic acid to address bacterial infections. *Colloids and Surfaces. B, Biointerfaces, 181*, 632–638.
38. Heep, G., Almeida, A., Marcano, R., Vieira, D., Mainardes, R. M., Khalil, N. M., & Sarmento, B. (2019). Zein-casein-lysine multicomposite nanoparticles are effective in modulate the intestinal permeability of ferulic acid. *International Journal of Biological Macromolecules, 138*, 244–251.
39. Jia, H. J., Jia, F. Y., Zhu, B. J., & Zhang, W. P. (2017). Preparation and characterization of glycyrrhetinic-acid loaded PEG-modified liposome based on PEG-7 glyceryl cocoate. *European Journal of Lipid Science and Technology, 119*(7), 9.
40. Li, W. G., Zhao, X. H., Sun, X. L., Zu, Y. G., Liu, Y., & Ge, Y. L. (2016). Evaluation of antioxidant ability in vitro and bioavailability of trans-cinnamic acid nanoparticle by liquid antisolvent precipitate. *Journal of Nanomaterials, 2016*, 11.
41. Panwar, R., Raghuwanshi, N., Srivastava, A. K., Sharma, A. K., & Pruthi, V. (2018). In-vivo sustained release of nanoencapsulated ferulic acid and its impact in induced diabetes. *Materials Science & Engineering, C: Materials for Biological Applications, 92*, 381–392.
42. Zhang, Y. T., Li, Z., Zhang, K., Yang, G., Wang, Z., Zhao, J. H., Hu, R. F., & Feng, N. P. (2016). Ethyl oleate-containing nanostructured lipid carriers improve oral bioavailability of trans-ferulic acid ascompared with conventional solid lipid nanoparticles. *International Journal of Pharmaceutics, 511*(1), 57–64.
43. Kopp, C., Singh, S. P., Regenhard, P., Müller, U., Sauerwein, H., & Mielenz, M. (2014). Trans-cinnamic acid increases adiponectin and the phosphorylation of AMP-activated protein kinase through G-protein-coupled receptor signaling in 3T3-L1 adipocytes. *International Journal of Molecular Sciences, 15*(2), 2906–2915.
44. Tsai, C. M., Sun, F. M., Chen, Y. L., Hsu, C. L., Yen, G. C., & Weng, C. J. (2013). Molecular mechanism depressing PMA-induced invasive behaviors in human lung adenocarcinoma cells by cis- and trans-cinnamic acid. *European Journal of Pharmaceutical Sciences, 48*(3), 494–501.
45. Nomura, E., Kashiwada, A., Hosoda, A., Nakamura, K., Morishita, H., Tsuno, T., & Taniguchi, H. (2003). Synthesis of amide compounds of ferulic acid, and their stimulatory effects on insulin secretion in vitro. *Bioorganic & Medicinal Chemistry, 11*(17), 3807–3813.
46. Wan, T., Xu, T., Pan, J. T., Qin, M. Y., Pan, W. H., Zhang, G. G., Wu, Z. H., Wu, C. B., & Xu, Y. H. (2015). Microemulsion based gel for topical dermal delivery of pseudolaric acid B: In vitro and in vivo evaluation. *International Journal of Pharmaceutics, 493*(1-2), 111–120.
47. Harwansh, R. K., Mukherjee, P. K., Bahadur, S., & Biswas, R. (2015). Enhanced permeability of ferulic acid loaded nanoemulsion based gel through skin against UVA mediated oxidative stress. *Life Sciences, 141*, 202–211.
48. Poornima, B., & Korrapati, P. S. (2017). Fabrication of chitosan-polycaprolactone composite nanofibrous scaffold for simultaneous delivery of ferulic acid and resveratrol. *Carbohydrate Polymers, 157*, 1741–1749.

49. Cheng, Y. H., Lin, F. H., Wang, C. Y., Hsiao, C. Y., Chen, H. C., Kuo, H. Y., Tsai, T. F., & Chiou, S. H. (2016). Recovery of oxidative stress-induced damage in Cisd2-deficient cardiomyocytes by sustained release of ferulic acid from injectable hydrogel. *Biomaterials, 103*, 207–218.
50. Ernst, B., & Magnani, J. L. (2009). From carbohydrate leads to glycomimetic drugs. *Nature Reviews. Drug Discovery, 8*(8), 661–677.
51. Luo, L., Zheng, S. S., Huang, Y. F., Qin, T., Xing, J., Niu, Y., Bo, R. N., Liu, Z. G., Huang, Y., Hu, Y. L., Liu, J. G., Wu, Y., & Wang, D. Y. (2016). Preparation and characterization of Chinese yam polysaccharide PLGA nanoparticles and their immunological activity. *International Journal of Pharmaceutics, 511*(1), 140–150.
52. Kong, Z. L., Chang, J. S., & Chang, K. L. B. (2013). Antiproliferative effect of Antrodia camphorata polysaccharides encapsulated in chitosan-silica nanoparticles strongly depends on the metabolic activity type of the cell line. *Journal of Nanoparticle Research, 15*(9), 13.
53. Wang, L. N., Yao, C. X., Wu, F., Lin, X., Shen, L., & Feng, Y. (2015). Targeting delivery of Radix Ophiopogonis polysaccharide to ischemic/reperfused rat myocardium by long-circulating macromolecular and liposomal carriers. *International Journal of Nanomedicine, 10*, 9.
54. Yu, Z. G., Guo, F. X., Guo, Y. Y., Zhang, Z. R., Wu, F., & Luo, X. Q. (2017). Optimization and evaluation of astragalus polysaccharide injectable thermoresponsive in-situ gels. *PLoS One, 12*(3), 13.
55. Shi, X. L., Lin, X., Yao, C. X., Shen, L., & Feng, Y. (2015). Injectable long-acting in situ forming systems for Radix Ophiopogonis polysaccharide. *International Journal of Biological Macromolecules, 72*, 553–559.
56. Wang, L. N., Lin, X., Hong, Y. L., Shen, L., & Feng, Y. (2017). Hydrophobic mixed solvent induced PLGA-based in situ forming systems for smooth long-lasting delivery of Radix Ophiopogonis polysaccharide in rats. *RSC Advances, 7*(9), 5349–5361.
57. Shi, X. L., Lin, X., Zheng, X. W., Feng, Y., & Shen, L. (2014). Injectable long-acting systems for Radix Ophiopogonis polysaccharide based on mono-PEGylation and in situ formation of a PLGA depot. *International Journal of Nanomedicine, 9*, 5555–5563.
58. Zhang, Y. T., Shen, L. I. N., Zhao, J. H., & Feng, N. P. (2014). Evaluation of psoralen ethosomes for topical delivery in rats by using in vivo microdialysis. *International Journal of Nanomedicine, 9*, 669–678.
59. Meng, S., Zhang, C., Shi, W., Zhang, X. W., Liu, D. H., Wang, P., Li, J. X., & Jin, Y. (2016). Preparation of osthole-loaded nano-vesicles for skin delivery: Characterization, in vitro skin permeation and preliminary in vivo pharmacokinetic studies. *European Journal of Pharmaceutical Sciences, 92*, 49–54.
60. Shan, Q. Q., Jiang, X. J., Wang, F. Y., Shu, Z. X., & Gui, S. Y. (2019). Cubic and hexagonal liquid crystals as drug carriers for the transdermal delivery of triptolide. *Drug Delivery, 26*(1), 490–498.
61. Zhang, K. C., Lv, S. W., Li, X. Y., Feng, Y. F., Li, X., Liu, L., Li, S., & Li, Y. J. (2013). Preparation, characterization, and in vivo pharmacokinetics of nanostructured lipid carriers loaded with oleanolic acid and gentiopicrin. *International Journal of Nanomedicine, 8*, 3227–3239.
62. Wei, Y. F., Li, L. C., Xi, Y. F., Qian, S. A., Gao, Y. A., & Zhang, J. J. (2014). Sustained release and enhanced bioavailability of injectable scutellarin-loaded bovine serum albumin nanoparticles. *International Journal of Pharmaceutics, 476*(1-2), 142–148.
63. Zhou, Y., Ning, Q., Yu, D. N., Li, W. G., & Deng, J. (2014). Improved oral bioavailability of breviscapine via a Pluronic P85-modified liposomal delivery system. *The Journal of Pharmacy and Pharmacology, 66*(7), 903–911.
64. Tang, Q., Zhang, J. F., Hou, S. X., & Xu, X. Y. (2013). Progress in the study of oral sustained-release preparation of Traditional Chinese medicine. *Chinese Pharmaceutical Journal, 48*(12), 953–957.

65. Liao, Z. G., Liang, X. L., Ping, Q. N., Jiang, Q. Y., & Yang, M. (2009). Formula design and optimization of Guizhi Fuling double layers sustained-release tablet. *Chinese Traditional and Herbal Drugs, 40*(4), 553–557.
66. Wu, W., Tang, D., Song, B. L., & Tan, X. D. (2017). Preparation and in vitro release rate of pueraria lobata and uncaria rhynchophylla compound sustained-release tablets. *Chinese Archives of Traditional Chinese Medicine, 35*(1), 26–28.
67. Liu, W., Song, X. L., & Lin, C. (2008). Preparation of gastrodia and uncarra drink extencap and experiment of in vitro release. *Chinese Archives of Traditional Chinese Medicine, 26*(16), 2343–2345.
68. Li, X. D., Pan, W. S., Nie, S. F., & Wu, L. J. (2004). Studies on controlled release effervescent osmotic pump tablets from traditional Chinese medicine compound recipe. *Journal of Controlled Release, 96*(3), 359–367.
69. Xue, L. A., Li, Y. B., Guo, D. D., Yin, J. H., Liu, Y. C., & Hou, S. X. (2009). Study on preparation and release mechanism of effervescent osmotic pump tablet of compound Danshen. *China Journal of Chinese Materia Medica, 34*(7), 848–851.
70. Tang, X., Tian, X. L., & Ci, L. (2004). Preparation and evaluation of pH-dependent gradient-release pellets for TCM. *Drug Development and Industrial Pharmacy, 30*(10), 1079–1087.
71. Song, H. T., Guo, T., Zhang, R. H., Zheng, C. L., Ma, Y., Li, X., Bi, K. S., & Tang, X. (2002). Preparation of the traditional Chinese medicine compound recipe heart-protecting musk pH-dependent gradient-release pellets. *Drug Development and Industrial Pharmacy, 28*(10), 1261–1273.
72. Song, H. T., Zhang, Q., Wang, H. J., Guo, X. J., Chen, D. W., & He, Z. G. (2007). Preparation of the traditional Chinese medicine compound recipe Shuxiong sustained-release capsules by multiparticulate time-controlled explosion technology. *Die Pharmazie, 6*(5), 372–377.
73. Li, D., Song, H. T., Chu, Y., Chen, D. W., & He, Z. G. (2009). Preparation of compound Danshen sustained-release capsula by multiparticulate time-controlled release technology. *Chinese Traditional and Herbal Drugs, 40*(4), 544–548.
74. Bai, Z. Y., Shao, S. Y., Xu, X. Y., & Zhang, J. F. (2016). Application of osmotic pump technology in Chinese materia medica preparation. *Chinese Traditional and Herbal Drugs, 47*(9), 1619–1624.
75. Fang, Y., & Shi, Q. W. (2011). Studies on preparation and dissolution test in vitro of intragastric floating two-chamber osmotic pump tablets of total alkaloids of coptis chinensis and evodia rutaecarpa. *Chinese Medica Materia, 34*(5), 779–782.
76. Tian, Z., Zhang, J., Zhou, X., & Song, H. T. (2011). Advance in studies on synchronized and sustained-release preparations of multi-component of Chinese materia medica for oral. *Chinese Traditional and Herbal Drugs, 42*(10), 2130–2134.
77. Wu, Z. F., Wei, S. F., Zheng, Q., Yue, P. F., Hu, P. Y., & Yang, M. (2011). Evaluation of innovation on in vivo - in vitro correlation of gastric retenting drug delivery system for Chinese materia medica. *Chinese Traditional and Herbal Drugs, 42*(6), 1041–1045.
78. Du, P., Liu, W., Qing, Y. J., Yao, X. Y., Jin, Y., Chen, H. C., & He, L. (2018). Study on the traditional Chinese medicine compound sustained-release preparation based on the unification of medicines and excipients -- a case study of Shaoyao Gancao intragastric floating tablets. *Chinese Medica Materia, 41*(10), 2403–2407.
79. Shen, H., Zhu, L. Y., Li, B. Y., & Peng, H. L. (2012). Preparation and quality research of gastric floating sustained-release tablets of Fei's Qiwei Weiyin. *Chinese Traditional Patent Medicine, 34*(7), 1263–1266.
80. Zhou, Y. S., Song, H., Jia, Y. Y., Zhai, D. Y., & Duan, Q. H. (2005). Study on the floating sustained release tablets of Zuojin. *Chinese Traditional Patent Medicine, 27*(12), 1379–1381.

81. Chen, J., Lu, W. L., Gu, W., Lu, S. S., Chen, Z. P., & Cai, B. C. (2013). Skin permeation behavior of elastic liposomes: Role of formulation ingredients. *Expert Opinion on Drug Delivery, 10*(6), 845–856.
82. Wei, Y.-F., Lin, X., Zhang, N., & Feng, Y. (2010). Quality evaluation system for the oral sustained- and controlled-release drug delivery systems of traditional Chinese medicine. *Acta Pharmaceutica Sinica, 45*(4), 430–435.
83. Zhu, S. S., Yuan, X. J., & Li, Y. X. (2006). Study on the water-soluble composition release of compound Danshen sustained-release tablet. *China Journal of Chinese Materia Medica, 31*(1), 37–40.
84. Wei, Y., Lin, X., Zhang, N., & Feng, Y. (2011). UPLC-MS analysis of constituents of dachuanxiong fang active parts absorbed into blood. *China Journal of Chinese Materia Medica, 36*(9), 1245–1248.

Chapter 4
Transdermal Delivery of Chinese Medicine

Shaoping Yin, Mei Dong, Jie Dong, Wei Gu, Shanshan Lu, Junhong Yao, and Jun Chen

Abstract Transdermal delivery of Chinese medicine (TDCM) is an attractive and innovative drug delivery strategy with limited adverse effects, which has been widely accepted by patients and physicians for its flexibility, first-pass hepatic metabolism avoidance, faithful clinical efficacy, and unique prevention method. However, due to the poor physicochemical characteristics, the bioavailability of active components, and the unique structure of skin with a layer of the stratum corneum (SC), delivery of Chinese medicine via transdermal route is challenging. To overcome these barriers, lots of strategies have been attempted to enhance the percutaneous absorption and therapeutic efficacy of Chinese medicine, including application of penetration enhancers (PEs) such as essential oils (EOs), physical penetration enhancement techniques, and various nanocarriers. In this chapter, the mechanism of enhanced skin penetration, role of "four natures," and percutaneous absorption of EOs are elaborated from the perspectives of both modern medicine and traditional Chinese medicine (TCM). Other technologies to accelerate physical penetration including microneedles (MNs), iontophoresis, sonophoresis, and cupping therapy in TDCM are also discussed. Furthermore, we summarize the latest insights of liposomes, nanoparticles, and nanoemulsions for controlled and reliable TDCM. The transdermal evaluation techniques such as phospholipid vesicle-based permeation assay (PVPA) and transdermal microdialysis are also introduced. Overall, integration of the penetration enhancement techniques in TDCM is essential to improve the absorption and efficacy of Chinese medicine for its optimal applications of transdermal delivery.

S. Yin · M. Dong · J. Dong · W. Gu · S. Lu · J. Yao
Jiangsu Provincial Engineering Research Center of TCM External Medication Development and Application, Nanjing University of Chinese Medicine, Nanjing, China

J. Chen (✉)
Jiangsu Provincial Engineering Research Center of TCM External Medication Development and Application, Nanjing University of Chinese Medicine, Nanjing, China

School of Pharmacy, Nanjing University of Chinese Medicine, Nanjing, China
e-mail: chenjun75@njucm.edu.cn

N. Feng, Z. Yang (eds.), *Novel Drug Delivery Systems for Chinese Medicines*,
https://doi.org/10.1007/978-981-16-3444-4_4

Keywords Chinese medicine · Penetration enhancement · Nanocarriers · Transdermal delivery

4.1 Introduction

Transdermal delivery of Chinese medicine (TDCM) is classified as external therapy of traditional Chinese medicine (TCM), which was firstly described in the form of oracle bone inscriptions in about 1300 BC. Thanks to its flexible treatment, faithful clinical efficacy, and unique prevention method, TDCM has saved millions of Chinese people from various diseases and displayed its unique advantages. The application of acupuncture and theories of *Zangfu* (*viscera and bowels*) and meridians in *Huang Di Nei Jing* (*Huangdi's Internal Classic*) laid a theoretical foundation of TDCM. The practice of TDCM continued to evolve, obtaining its highest popularity in the late *Qing* dynasty with mature theoretical theory, as elaborated in the book *Li Yue Pian Wen* (*Rhymed Discourse for Topical Remedies*). This book is written based on *Wu Shiji*'s experience, and he summarized external therapy and clinical practice about decades. It was emphasized in this book that the same therapeutical principles could be applied for both transdermal and oral administration by the guidance of TCM theory [1]. Moreover, according to this book, TDCM should be applied specifically at the relevant acupuncture points to treat diseases, exerting therapeutic efficacy by not only percutaneous absorption of active ingredients from TDCM system but also the stimulation via acupoints. For example, the acupoint Chinese medicine patch has been proved to significantly improve the quality of life for the treatment of allergic rhinitis [2].

Chinese medicine preparations usually contain various active components (e.g., bioactive alkaloids, glycosides, phenolic acids, etc.). During the percutaneous absorption process, synergistic effect among different components is usually existed. Brucine with an analgesic and anti-inflammatory activity is an active alkaloid extracted from *Maqianzi* (*Strychni Semen*). It was found that the percutaneous absorption of brucine was significantly enhanced by other ingredients from the total alkaloid fraction (TAF) from *Maqianzi* [3]. Similar synergistic effects were also reported in other components extracted from Chinese medicine [4, 5].

Traditionally, topical application includes fumigation, ironing, hot compressed, and iontophoresis with Chinese herbs or their extracts, etc. [6]. Plaster, especially black plaster, is the most commonly used formulation to apply transdermal Chinese medicine preparations. According to *Wu Shiji*, almost all diseases can be treated with Chinese medicine transdermal plaster if they can be treated with oral administration of Chinese medicine decoction. The plaster is a sticky mass made from deep-fried, dried herbs that is added with red lead oxide (Pb_3O_4). The plaster is known to have a superior efficacy and a particular advantage to treat various diseases such as osteoarthritis (OA), the most common form of arthritis that causes pain, stiffness, and swelling. The ***Tongluo Qutong* Plaster** is the convenient preparation in Chinese medicine to improve symptoms which severely affect the quality of patients with

OA. The results of clinical trials have provided reliable evidence of its efficacy and safety [7]. Recently, with the development of functional polymers, the usage of plaster has gradually decreased as the new percutaneous formulation via using cataplasm normally reduce skin irritation reactions.

Cataplasm, also called Babu plaster or hydrogel patch, is a patch using water-soluble hydrogel polymers as matrix reinforcing materials. In addition to better water retention, biocompatibility, and biodegradability, such biomaterials used in cataplasm can also enhance drug loading capacity with rapid adhesion and sustained drug delivery through the skin, resulting in extensive applications in transdermal drug delivery of Chinese medicine. Some commercialized Chinese medicine and research reports about cataplasm preparations are listed in Table 4.1. *Xiaozhang* Plaster, a traditional Chinese herbal cataplasm containing *Dahuang* (*Rhei Radix et Rhizoma*), *Laifuzi* (*Raphani Semen*), concocted *Gansui* (*Kansui Radix*), *Chenxiang* (*Aquilariae Lignum Resinatum*), *Dingxiang* (*Caryophylli Flos*), *Bingpian* (*Borneolum syntheticum*), and *Shexiang* (*artificial Moschus*), has been investigated as an adjuvant in treating cirrhotic ascites. A clinical trial performed with 92 patients showed that *Xiaozhang* Plaster is safe and effective on relieving abdominal distention [10]. It should be noted that some active polysaccharide exacted from Chinese medicine can be used as hydrogel materials for the development of cataplasm [21].

Along with research on development of pharmaceutical vesicle and investigation on new excipients in TDCM preparations, novel TDCM systems and penetration enhancement techniques have been developed. The bioactive components such as alkaloids from Chinese medicine have exerted potent efficacies. However, a series of undesirable physicochemical characteristics (e.g., low solubility) and limited bioavailability have been found to confine their clinical uses via transdermal route. Until now, a lot of strategies have been used to enhance the percutaneous absorption and curative efficacies, such as the application of penetration enhancement techniques and nano-vesicles [22].

4.2 Chinese Medicine Essential Oils as Penetration Enhancers

For TDCM, the main penetration barrier is located in the outermost layer of the skin, stratum corneum (SC), with a unique hierarchical structure composed of multiple lipid bilayers and the embedded corneocytes [23]. To overcome this lipid-based barrier, penetration enhancers (PEs) are applied as one of the most commonly used strategies to improve the percutaneous absorption for the development of transdermal drug delivery system (TDDS). Various classes of PEs have been identified, including azone, surfactants, alcohols, fatty acids, pyrrolidones, sulfoxides, as well as essential oils (EOs) and their components (terpenes) [24]. Among these PEs, natural EOs extracted from Chinese medicine are now receiving increased attention

Table 4.1 The applications of Chinese medicine cataplasm

Name	Components	Application	References
Fufang Nanxing Zhitong cataplasm	*Dingxiang*, *Rougui* (*Cinnamomi cortex*), *Baizhi* (*Angelicae Dahuricae Radix*), *chuanxiong* (*chuanxiong Rhizoma*), etc.	Cold-dispelling, dehumidifying, blood-activating, and pain-relieving	[8]
Compound antimalarial ethosomal cataplasm	Artesunate-loaded ethosomes and febrifugine-loaded ethosomes	Malaria	[9]
Chinese herbal cataplasm *Xiaozhang* plaster	*Dahuang*, *Laifuzi*, *Gansui*, *Chenxiang*, *Dingxiang*, *Bingpian*, and *Shexiang*	Cirrhotic ascites	[10]
Majie cataplasm	*Mahuang* (*Ephedrae Herba*), *Kuxingren* (*Armeniacae semen Amarum*), *Baijiezi* (*white mustard seed*), *Yanhusuo* (*Corydalis Rhizoma*), and *Shengjiang* (*Zingiberis Rhizoma Recens*)	Allergic asthma and asthmatic punch from the neuroimmune system	[11, 12]
Rhizoma Drynariae cataplasm	*Gusuibu*(*Drynariae Rhizoma*)	Osteoporosis	[13]
Yiguanjian cataplasm	*Dihuang* (*Rehmanniae Radix*), *Beishashen* (*Glehniae Radix*), *Danggui* (*Angelicae Sinensis Radix*), *Maidong* (*Ophiopogonis Radix*), *Gouqi*(*Lycii Fructus*), *Dangshen* (*Codonopsis Radix*), and *Baizhu* (*Atractylodis Macrocephalae Rhizoma*)	Naloxone-induced opioid withdrawal syndrome	[14]
Lishui Xiaogu cataplasm	*Qianniuzi* (*Pharbitidis semen*), *Cheqianzi* (*Plantaginis semen*), *Dahuang*, *Yiyiren* (*Coicis semen*), *Gansui*, and *Muxiang* (*Aucklandiae Radix*)	Cirrhotic ascites	[15]
Cayenne pepper Cataplasm	Cayenne pepper (*Capsicum annuum* L.)and kaolin powder	Musculoskeletal diseases	[16]
Dinggui gel paste	*Qianghuo* (*Notopterygii Rhizoma et Radix*), *Yanhusuo*, *Duhuo* (*Angelicae Pubescentis Radix*), *Danggui*, *Moyao* (*Myrrha*), etc.	Athletic injury and painful joints	[17]
Sanqi hydrogel patch	*Sanqi* (*Notoginseng Radix et Rhizoma*), *Honghua* (*Carthami Flos*), *Xuduan* (*Dipsaci Radix*), *Cibotium barometz* (L.) J. Sm., *Wujiapi* (*Acanthopanacis cortex*), etc.	Activating blood circulation, removing blood stasis, relieving swelling and pain	[18]

(continued)

Table 4.1 (continued)

Name	Components	Application	References
Zhitong cataplasm	*Chuanxiong*, *Baizhi* (*Angelicae Dahuricae Radix*), *Xixin* (*Asari Radix et Rhizoma*), *Huajiao* (*Zanthoxyli Pericarpium*), etc.	Pain-relieving	[19]
Shangshi Zhitong cataplasm	*Shangshi Zhitong* liquid extract, *Dianqie Liujingao* (*belladonna* liquid extract), *Bohe* (*Menthae Haplocalycis Herba*), *Zhangnao* (*camphor*), etc.	Rheumatoid arthritis	[20]

as promising skin PEs for the transdermal or dermal delivery of hydrophilic and hydrophobic drugs [25, 26].

4.2.1 Mechanism of Penetration Enhancement

Similar to other PEs, EOs and their terpene constituents can improve permeation of different drugs from TDCM into the deeper skin layers using different mechanisms: (1) disintegration of intercellular lipid structure among SC corneocytes, (2) conformational modification of intracellular protein, and (3) enhancement of drug partitioning into SC [25].

In previous studies, the effects of penetration enhancement of six EOs (turpentine, *Angelica*, *Chuanxiong*, *Cyperus*, cinnamon, clove oils) extracted from Chinese medicine were investigated. It has been demonstrated that the investigated six EOs showed significantly higher penetration enhancement effect and lower topical toxicity compared with azone. These EOs promote drug permeation mainly by disturbing SC lipids [27].

For some kinds of EOs, increased skin blood flow can also be utilized in accelerating penetration. Frankincense and myrrh essential oil had been proved to promote skin permeation of *Chuanxiong* [28]. The mechanism was found to be related to increased blood flow which promote the diffusion of drugs from the epidermis to dermal capillaries, resulting in significantly enhanced transdermal permeation amounts of drugs.

The classical permeation experimental apparatus using Franz diffusion cells provides a reliable in vitro model for screening of PEs for TDCM formulations. However, it is labor-intensive and time-consuming. Recently, measurement of the changes in skin electrical resistance (SER) has been used as an efficient technique to screen effective PEs such as EOs [29, 30]. It has been proved that measurement of SER is a convenient method for evaluating the PEs, particularly via acting on SC lipids [31].

4.2.2 Role of "Four Natures"

The four natures of Chinese herbs, namely, cold, hot, warm, and cool, were believed to be strongly associated with skin penetration enhancement ability of EOs extracted from Chinese herbs [32, 33]. Four natures in terms of cold, hot, warm, and cool refer to the four properties of Chinese medicines. It reflects human body's effect of inclination of the ups and downs of *Yin* and *Yang* and the semi-interior phase change after the Chinese medicines acting on the body. By data mining, the relationship between penetration enhancement effect of EOs and drug properties especially four natures and five flavors was fully analyzed via a general linear model. Based on the findings in this literature, EOs used as PEs for TDDS were all sourced from acrid Chinese medicine, due to their positive drug nature which contribute to the enhanced skin penetration effect of essential oil. It should also be noted that four natures have the most significant effect on the penetration effect of EOs [32]. More research studies revealed that the order of penetration ability of EOs was hot>warm>cold and cool. The sesquiterpenoids from EOs may be the most correlated chemical components with the "four nature" drug properties and the abilities of penetration enhancement [33].

4.2.3 Percutaneous Absorption of EO Components

EOs are complex aromatic-smelling volatile mixtures of various components, especially monoterpenes and sesquiterpenes. The main components are monoterpene hydrocarbons, sesquiterpene hydrocarbons, their corresponding oxidized compounds, and phenylpropanoids. For EOs, the effects in analgesic, anti-inflammatory, antibacterial, anti-rheumatic, and blood circulation have been described. Consequently, besides the penetration enhancement, the percutaneous absorption of EO components is also known to be associated with its pharmacological effect, which means the application of EOs in transdermal drug delivery (TDD) formulations is in accord with the "unification of medicines and excipients" principle in TCM theory [34].

The cross-talking effects of each essential oil component may also affect percutaneous essential oil absorption [35]. The essential oil from *Huajiao* (*Zanthoxyli Pericarpium*) (*Z. bungeanum* oil) can remarkably increase the percutaneous absorption of drug molecules as a natural skin penetration enhancer. Its main terpene components include terpinen-4-ol, 1,8-cineole, and limonene. The penetration enhancement effect and the cell toxicity of *Z. bungeanum* oil on skin cells were examined and compared together with the analysis of its main terpene components. It showed that the three terpene compounds used individually had higher cell toxicity on HaCaT cells or CCC-ESF-1 cells compared to *Z. bungeanum* oil. The capacity of better permeation by all tested agents was determined as the following order: terpinen-4-ol≈1,8-cineole<limonene<*Z. bungeanum* oil [36]. Consequently, the pharmacokinetic characteristics of EO components should be further evaluated as well as its penetration enhancement effect. Galangal Essential Oil (GEO) from *Gaoliangjiang* (*Alpiniae Officinarum Rhizoma*) was used as PE for TDD of flurbiprofen (FP). The most abundant constituent of GEO was found to be 1,8-cineole (52.06%). Compared to azone, both significantly higher penetration ability and significantly reduced skin cell toxicity of GEO were found. Furthermore, the relative bioavailability of FP and 1,8-cineole remained at 96.58% and 85.49%, respectively, via transdermal administration when compared to oral administration of FP-GEO-microemulsion. It has also been reported that GEO constitutes possess good efficiency in percutaneous absorption [37].

4.3 Techniques in Increasing Physical Penetration

Aiming to increase skin penetration of active components and to promote the efficiency of TDCM, various strategies are applied to enhance the skin permeability. In addition to the PEs such as EOs, the physical disturbance of the SC layer is widely used in altering skin penetration. These physical techniques such as microneedles (MNs), iontophoresis, and sonophoresis are also applicable to TDCM. Moreover, some traditional techniques such as cupping therapy are proved to physically help the transdermal delivery of Chinese medicine.

4.3.1 Microneedles

The MNs are also known as minute needle arrays (usually 50–900μm), which are used to induce pores in the skin, therefore increasing TDCM into systemic circulation. At present, microneedles are commonly divided into solid MNs, hollow MNs, coated MNs, and dissolving MNs. The advantage of using MNs is that they are painless but also capable to deliver drug in the dermis through the penetration of SC via well-controlled length of MNs (Fig. 4.1). In addition, MNs are also able to increase drug absorption, simplify self-vaccination, avoid infection, and ease disposal [38].

In TCM, acupuncture is an originally Chinese practice of inserting fine needles through the skin at specific points (acupoint) to produce and transmit physiological and biochemical signals that can alter the local pathophysiological state of patients. But the pain caused by acupuncture needles limits its acceptance by patients. Therefore, the self-administered MNs can be alternative options as a painless replacement for acupuncture and deliver drugs across SC barrier. In a recent study, immunosuppressive rats were treated with acupuncture at *Zusanli* (ST36) acupoint using microneedles containing thymopentin. It was found that either MNs containing thymopentin or conventional acupuncture both showed faster immune

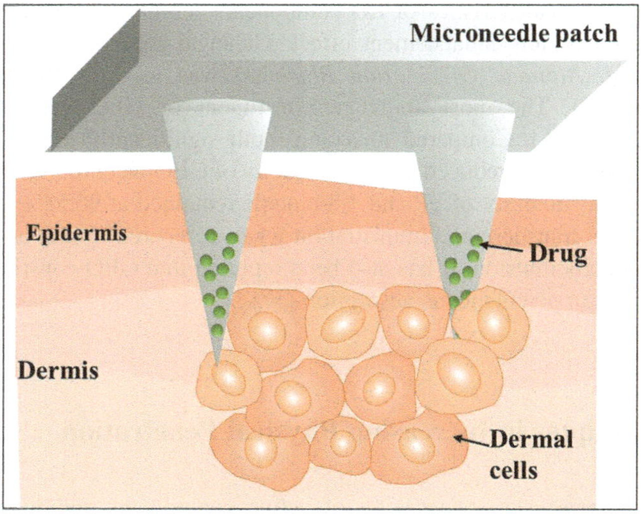

Fig. 4.1 The transdermal delivery mechanism of microneedle array patch

cell proliferation, effectively mitigating the anxiety caused by immune-suppression [39].

As a device for improving percutaneous absorption of TDCM, MNs offer a painless and minimally invasive route to cross the SC. MNs can promote the permeability of various Chinese medicine components. For example, sinomenine is an anti-inflammatory alkaloid extracted from *Qingteng* (*Sinomenium acutum*). By a casting method, the sinomenine hydrochloride (SH)-loaded MNs were prepared using polyvinylpyrrolidone and chondroitin sulfate. Transdermal pharmacokinetic study revealed that the area under the curve (AUC) values of SH following the administration of SH-MN were determined to be 1.43- and 1.63-fold higher compared to SH gel, respectively. Moreover, the needle tip was almost completely dissolved after 4 h, and the drug could reach a depth of 200μm under the skin. Therefore, SH-MN was proved to be a simple, effective, and safe strategy for the development of TDDS [40].

4.3.2 Iontophoresis

Iontophoresis is a technology that uses weak electrical current to stimulate drug-carrying ions to pass through intact skin on the patch of ionic drug absorption (Fig. 4.2). The iontophoresis equipment is usually composed of an electrode, a battery, a drug reservoir, and a control circuit. Under the effect of iontophoresis equipment, the skin appendages route is recognized as the main percutaneous absorption pathway of the drug. To further enhance percutaneous drug absorption

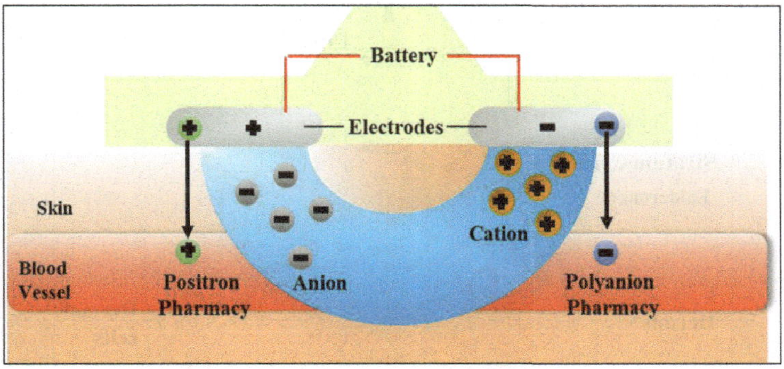

Fig. 4.2 The transdermal delivery mechanism of iontophoresis

and decrease possible side effects, iontophoresis is usually combined with PEs, electroporation, and sonophoresis for the development of TDDS [41].

In treating degenerative osteoarthropathy, the Chinese medicine iontophoresis was applied, and the clinical curative effect was evaluated on 296 cases. All patients were randomly divided into two groups, Chinese medicine iontophoresis group vs. control group. For the Chinese medicine iontophoresis group, the joint was treated by Chinese medicine iontophoresis and medium-frequency electrotherapy. For the control group, only medium-frequency electrotherapy was applied for the treatment of the joint. The total effective rates of the Chinese medicine iontophoresis group and the control group were determined to be 93.2% and 74.3%, respectively. Chinese medicine iontophoresis has great potential for the treatment of degenerative osteoarthropathy [42].

Iontophoresis with traditional Chinese herbal medicine was also reported to promote blood circulation and accelerate the growth of bony callus, providing a new therapeutic approach for promoting bone regeneration post fractures [43]. Moreover, combining acupuncture and Chinese medicine iontophoresis has been proved to be a potential treatment for chronic progressive cervical intervertebral disk disease [44] or rheumatoid arthritis [45].

4.3.3 Sonophoresis

Sonophoresis is the permeation of drug molecules through the skin using specific ultrasound frequency (Fig. 4.3). The ability of ultrasonic penetration can be affected by physical and chemical properties of the drug, coupling medium, energy density, and ultrasonic frequency. The mechanism of using low-frequency sonophoresis includes cavitation, thermal effects, radiation effects, acoustic microfluidic effects, lipid extraction, etc.. The percutaneous absorption of Chinese medicine can be significantly promoted by low-frequency sonophoresis. Therefore, Chinese researchers have investigated the penetration enhancement effect of Chinese

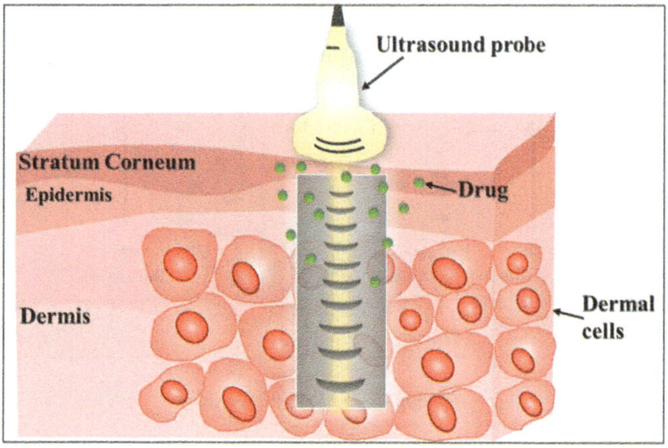

Fig. 4.3 The transdermal delivery mechanism of sonophoresis

medicine formula via using a low-frequency sonophoresis. Many studies showed that the therapeutic efficacy can be enhanced. The results of clinical trial including 110 eligible participants revealed that transdermal delivery of a Chinese medicine formula could be facilitated by low-frequency ultrasound to improve the efficacy of intrapleural administration of interleukin-2 [46].

Dachengqi Decoction (DCQD) is classical Chinese medicine formula composed of seven Chinese herbs. It has been widely used for the treatment of digestive diseases such as bowel obstruction. By transdermal administration, the low permeation of DCQD through the skin is regarded as a major concern. To enhance the skin penetration, sonophoresis was conducted using a working frequency of 40 kHz with 300 mW/cm^2 peak power, 100 mW/cm^2 pulse effective power, and over 12 cm^2 skin surface area. The modified *Dachengqi* Decoction (MDCQD) was applied locally at the site of Tianshu (S 25) or abdominal pain for 30 min, twice daily for 5 consecutive days. As demonstrated by the clinical studies, topical delivery of MDCQD at 100 g/day using sonophoresis was found to be effective in patients with refractory metastatic malignant bowel obstruction [47].

4.3.4 *Cupping Therapy*

Cupping therapy is one of the five TCM therapies (herbal medicine, acupuncture, moxibustion, massage, and cupping). Cupping therapy is believed to produce a negative pressure in the tank through the exhaust, resulting in the enlargement of the SC passages for TDD and overcoming the SC barrier for drug permeation. Based on cupping therapy, Fu's cupping therapy (FCT) has been developed as a comprehensive modernized innovation [48].

To evaluate the penetration effect of FCT, transdermal permeation of eight drugs with different molecular weights (MW) was compared with or without the application of FCT. It was found that FCT exerted a significantly improved effect on enhancing the percutaneous penetration of the selected log(P)-model drugs in addition to other two large MW drugs (ginsenoside Rg1 and notoginsenoside R1). Therefore, FCT can be considered as a novel method to improve the physical penetration, thus effectively enhancing the percutaneous absorption of drug molecules [49].

4.4 Nanocarriers for Transdermal Delivery of Chinese Medicine

Over the past decades, extraordinary advances have been made successfully on the development of novel TDDS by the encapsulation of active ingredients of Chinese medicine into a series of structurally deformable and stable nanocarriers. This provides an alternative strategy to efficiently deliver drug across the skin barrier [50]. Nanocarriers can promote the intercellular diffusion and transcellular transmission of medicine and also change the transdermal delivery mode of medicine, such as follicle targeting [50] (Fig. 4.4).

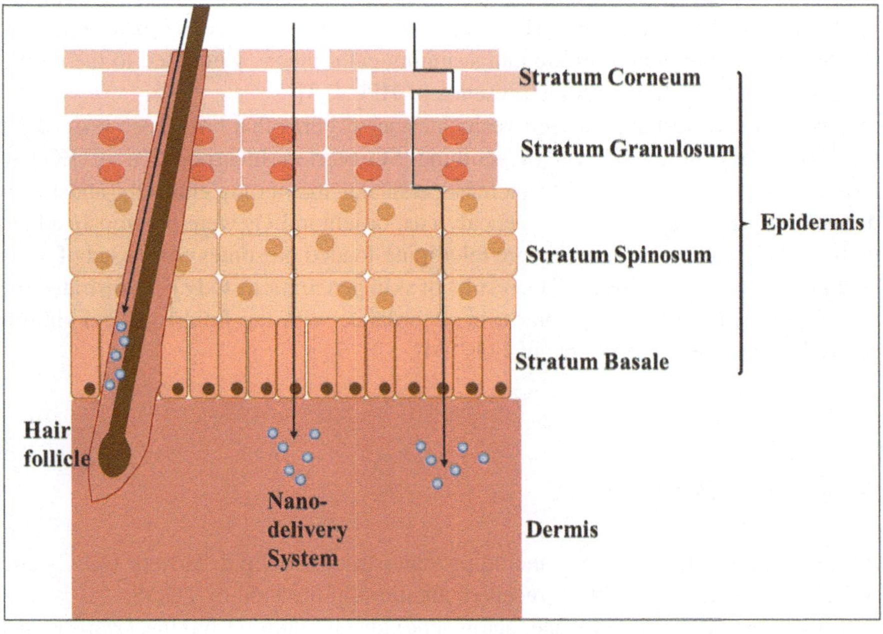

Fig. 4.4 Schematic diagram of transdermal penetration promoted by nanocarriers

4.4.1 Liposomes

Incorporation of CM ingredients within elastic liposomal vesicles has been proved to be one of the well-studied and popular routes for delivering active ingredients to systemic circulation. Various flexible liposomal nanocarriers have been developed including transfersomes, ethosomes, niosomes, etc. [51].

Cinnamic acid, an antioxidant and anti-inflammatory ingredient extracted from *Rougui* (*Cinnamomi Cortex*), was encapsulated into conventional liposomes and transfersomes. Different from conventional liposomes, an edge activator such as sodium deoxycholate is used as the component of lipid bilayer and increases the deformability of the vesicle. The transdermal flux of cinnamic acid from the optimized transfersomes was approximately threefold higher than that of conventional liposomes. In addition, the results of an in vivo microdialysis study demonstrated that the dermal drug concentrations in various skin regions following administration of transfersomes were much lower compared to those after administration of conventional liposomes [52].

Ethosomes are the vesicular carriers composed of phospholipids and relatively high concentration (20–40%) of alcohol. Ethosomes with elastic membrane can easily penetrate into the deep layers of the skin, allowing it for the application of TDDS. Curcumin was encapsulated into composite ethosomes composed of both saturated hydrogenated phosphatidylcholine (HPC) and unsaturated phosphatidylcholine (PC). The study showed that the vesicle stability and skin permeability of the composite ethosomes were significantly enhanced compared to the conventional ethosomes which were composed of PC or HPC only. Moreover, a significant interaction between saturated HPC and unsaturated PC molecules was found by molecular simulation and differential scanning calorimetry, which led to the reduction of PC peroxidation with the presence of HPC [53].

Niosomes are surfactant-based vesicular nanosystems that have been proved for their efficiency in TDDS via overcoming SC barrier. Incorporation of EOs in niosomes has been approved to increase vesicular membrane elasticity and transdermal delivery efficiency. Clove, eucalyptus, or lemon EOs were previously added in the vesicle composition to prepare felodipine-loaded niosomes composed of Span 60 and cholesterol (2:1, w/w). The results of skin penetration study demonstrated the superiority of EO-loaded niosomes, in accordance with the fluidizing and significantly better penetration effects of EOs [54].

4.4.2 Nanoparticles

Recently, nanoparticles (NPs) including nanostructured lipid carriers (NLC) and solid lipid nanoparticles (SLN) received attention in the field of TDDS.

Triptolide (TPL) is a diterpene lactone epoxide compound from the *Tripterygium wilfordii* Hook. F.. It can be widely used to treat inflammation, malignancy, depression, and autoimmune diseases. TPL was encapsulated into NLC and SLN, respectively. Both TPL-NLC and TPL-SLN were demonstrated to penetrate into the skin in a time-dependent manner. Moreover, the penetration of these nanoparticles was realized by changing the structure, thermodynamic properties, and components of the SC. Revealed by the parameters of the cumulative permeated amount and the skin penetration rate, the skin permeation of TPL-NLC was higher than TPL-SLN [55].

4.4.3 Nanoemulsions

Nanoemulsions are isotropic, transparent/translucent, heterogeneous systems of two immiscible liquids, normally consisting of an oily system dispersed in an aqueous system or an aqueous system dispersed in an oily system, forming droplets or oily phases of nanometric sizes. Now, the development of nanoemulsion-based semisolid dosage forms is an active area of TDDS [56].

Asiaticoside (ASI) is one of the triterpenoid components found in *Centella asiatica* that has promising neuroprotective properties. To enhance skin permeation, asiaticoside nanoemulsions (ASI-NEs) and asiaticoside nanoemulsions-based gels (ASI-NBGs) were prepared and examined with commercial cream of asiaticoside (ASI-C) in terms of transdermal drug delivery characteristics. The cumulative amounts of ASI permeated from ASI-NEs and ASI-NBGs at 12 h following application were determined to be (3504.30 ± 180.93) and (1187.40 ± 128.88)μg/cm^2, respectively, which are 6.57 and 2.23 times higher than the control group of ASI-C. In addition, the drug depositions of ASI in the skin following application of ASI-NEs and ASI-NBGs were determined to be (159.48 ± 7.47) and (120.53 ± 5.71)μg/cm^2, respectively, which are 5.93 and 4.48 times higher than that of ASI-C. Furthermore, the skin permeation mechanism of ASI-NEs and ASI-NBGs is related to affecting the SC ultrastructure and penetrating through the skin appendage route [57].

4.5 Transdermal Evaluation Technique

The phospholipid vesicle-based permeation assay (PVPA) model, an in vitro model, can mimic SC barriers for the evaluation the skin permeability of drugs. By mimicking both structure and composition of the SC barrier, the PVPA model was developed and proved to be a more efficient model for the prediction of drug permeation ability compared with the commercial EpiSkin® model [58].

After the optimization of the artificial PVPA, the penetration enhancement effect of menthol on five active compounds (ferulic acid, paeoniflorin, albiflorin, tetrahydrocolumbamine, and tetrahydropalmatine) from *Xiangfu Siwu* Decoction was investigated. The enhancement ratio ranking of the five active compounds determined by the optimized PVPA model was in accordance with observation on

Franz diffusion cell device using porcine ear skin. The comparable mechanisms of menthol which perturbs the SC lipid arrangement and extracts the SC lipids were demonstrated by attenuating total reflection-Fourier transform infrared spectroscopy (ATR-FTIR) analysis of PVPA model and porcine ear skin. The optimized PVPA model had been proved to possess great potential for the development of a more standardized, cheaper, and ethical approach for drug screening and Chinese medicine formulation development [59].

Being minimally invasive, transdermal microdialysis is used as a sampling and monitoring technique to measure drug concentrations in the extracellular fluid of the skin. It is usually used in preclinical and clinical dermal pharmacokinetic or pharmacodynamic assays [60]. By using transdermal microdialysis, the in vivo penetration-enhancing effect of EO from *Hujiao* (*Piperis Fructus*) was evaluated. The skin pharmacodynamics studies showed that the EO could enhance the percutaneous absorption of tetramethylpyrazine in a concentration-dependent manner and the enhancement ratio for 5% EO was 98.64 [61].

4.6 Conclusion

Applications of TDCM in China can trace back to 1300 BC, which present many advantages such as patient convenience, flexible treatment, local targeting, first-pass hepatic metabolism avoidance, faithful clinical efficacy, and unique prevention method. The effectiveness and safety of the conventional TDDS (e.g., plaster, powder, ointment, etc.) in the treatments of arthrophlogosis, dermatoses, and gynecological diseases have been widely accepted by physicians. Due to the physiologic barriers of the highly organized structure of skin, particularly SC, the penetration rate of the active components is still a challenging problem. The present chapter has reviewed and discussed the mechanism, four natures, and percutaneous absorption of EOs as the penetration enhancer in details. It is also been summarized that the rapid developments and advantages of physical penetration enhancement techniques (e.g., MNs, iontophoresis, sonophoresis, CT, etc.) and diverse novel nano-drug delivery systems (e.g., liposomes, NPs, nanoemulsion), which can be utilized to solve the penetration problems, thus increasing the bioavailability, targeting, efficacy, and circulation time of the active components. Based on this, we expect to present a potential guideline and foundation for the rational design of novel TDCM.

A reliable evaluation system is essential to estimate the effectiveness and safety of TDCM. Currently, artificial skin models such as PVPA model have received more attentions to replace the animal or human skin models to quantificationally evaluate the penetration ability of TDDS, which provide a reproducible strategy for TDCM optimization. Moreover, the advancements in external pharmaceutical formulation technology of Chinese medicine open new horizons for the experimental and clinical applications of transdermal microdialysis assay.

Since the efficacy of Chinese medicine is always in a combination of many active components, it is improper to simply apply the guidelines for chemical drugs to

Chinese medicine with complex components and desired dosage. Though myriad literatures have reported the potentials of physical penetration enhancement techniques and nanocarriers in penetration enhancement, their applications in TDCM are still challenges. It is necessary to confirm the physicochemical properties, interactions, action mechanisms, percutaneous absorptions, and in vivo fates of the active Chinese medicine components to design TDCM with programmed release and favorable penetration ability to ensure effective therapy. Overall, the progress of TDCM and modernization of TCM will be promoted by making full use of the modern technologies.

References

1. Wu, S. (2007). *Li Yue Pian Wen* (2nd ed.). China Press of Traditional Chinese Medicine.
2. Hsu, W. H., Ho, T. J., Huang, C. Y., Ho, H. C., Liu, Y. L., Liu, H. J., Lai, N. S., & Lin, J. G. (2010). Chinese medicine acupoint herbal patching for allergic rhinitis: A randomized controlled clinical trial. *The American Journal of Chinese Medicine, 38*(4), 661–673.
3. Chen, J., Wang, X., Qu, Y. G., Chen, Z. P., Cai, H., Liu, X., Xu, F., Lu, T. L., & Cai, B. C. (2012). Analgesic and anti-inflammatory activity and pharmacokinetics of alkaloids from seeds of Strychnos nux-vomica after transdermal administration: Effect of changes in alkaloid composition. *Journal of Ethnopharmacology, 139*(1), 181–188.
4. Kong, H., Qu, H. H., Qu, B. P., Zeng, W. H., Zhao, Y., Wang, X. Q., & Wang, Q. G. (2016). Correlation between the transdermal characteristics of pseudoephedrine and amygdalin in majiepingchuan in vitro. *Journal of Traditional Chinese Medicine, 36*(2), 238–242.
5. Ding, X., Sun, Y. M., Wang, Q., Pu, T. T., Li, X. H., Pan, Y. Q., & Yang, Y. (2016). Pharmacokinetics and pharmacodynamics of glycyrrhetinic acid with Paeoniflorin after transdermal administration in dysmenorrhea model mice. *Phytomedicine, 23*(8), 864–871.
6. Chen, W. H., Liu, X. X., Tong, P. J., & Zhan, H. S. (2016). Diagnosis and management of knee osteoarthritis: Chinese medicine expert consensus (2015). *Chinese Journal of Integrative Medicine, 22*(2), 150–153.
7. Xu, B. P., Yao, M., Tian, Z. R., Zhou, L. Y., Yang, L., Li, Z. J., Zhu, S., Wang, X. T., Lan, J. H., Wang, Y. J., & Cui, X. J. (2019). Study on efficacy and safety of Tong-luo Qu-tong plaster treatment for knee osteoarthritis: Study protocol for a randomized, double-blind, parallel positive controlled, multi-center clinical trial. *Trials, 20*(1), 377. https://doi.org/10.1186/s13063-019-3481-6
8. Li, Y., Du, S. Y., Lu, Y., Bai, J., Wang, Y. Z., Wang, Y., Xing, Y. S., & Xiao, W. (2013). Study on transdermal characteristics of compound Nanxing pain-relieving cataplasm and effects of gaultherolin in prescriptions. *Zhongguo Zhong Yao Za Zhi, 38*(16), 2601–2604.
9. Shen, S., Liu, S. Z., Zhang, Y. S., Du, M. B., Liang, A. H., Song, L. H., & Ye, Z. G. (2015). Compound antimalarial ethosomal cataplasm: Preparation, evaluation, and mechanism of penetration enhancement. *International Journal of Nanomedicine, 10*, 4239–4253.
10. Xing, F., Tan, Y., Yan, G. J., Zhang, J. J., Shi, Z. H., Tan, S. Z., Feng, N. P., & Liu, C. H. (2012). Effects of Chinese herbal cataplasm Xiaozhang Tie on cirrhotic ascites. *Journal of Ethnopharmacology, 139*(2), 343–349.
11. Ji, W., Zhang, Q., Shi, H., Dong, R., Ge, D., Du, X., Ren, B., Wang, X., & Wang, Q. (2020). The mediatory role of Majie cataplasm on inflammation of allergic asthma through transcription factors related to Th1 and Th2. *Chinese Medicine, 15*, 53.
12. Ji, W., Yu, X., Gao, Y., Ren, B., Zhang, S., Wang, Q., & Wang, X. (2020). Majie cataplasm provides a shield against asthmatic punch from the neuroimmune system. *Heliyon, 6*(5), e03896.

13. Guo, W., Shi, K., Xiang, G., Lu, D., Dou, H., Xie, C., & Chen, L. (2019). Effects of Rhizoma Drynariae cataplasm on fracture healing in a rat model of osteoporosis. *Medical Science Monitor, 25*, 3133–3139.
14. Gao, S., Gao, H., Fan, Y., Zhang, G., Sun, F., Zhao, J., Li, F., Yang, Y., & Wang, K. (2016). Yiguanjian cataplasm attenuates opioid dependence in a mouse model of naloxone-induced opioid withdrawal syndrome. *Journal of Traditional Chinese Medicine, 36*(4), 464–470.
15. Yang, X., Ru, S., Luo, L., Lv, X., Bai, W., Zhang, F., & Jiang, F. (2019). Efficacy and safety of umbilical therapy with the traditional Chinese medicine formulation Lishui Xiaogu cataplasm for cirrhotic ascites: Protocol for a randomized controlled trial. *Trials, 20*(1), 127.
16. Sarabon, N., Löfler, S., Cvecka, J., Hübl, W., & Zampieri, S. (2018). Acute effect of different concentrations of cayenne pepper cataplasm on sensory-motor functions and serum levels of inflammation-related biomarkers in healthy subjects. *European Journal of Translational Myology, 28*(1), 7333.
17. Zhu, L., Ma, J., & Tu, H. (2015). Comparison on release and transdermal behavior in vitro between Dinggui Gel Paste and Dinggui Huoluo Rubber Patch. *Chinese Traditional and Herbal Drugs, 46*(15), 2223–2227.
18. Zhang, C., Jia, C., Li, W., Zhao, F., Yu, Q., Yu, J., Wang, Y., & Yang, R. (2015). Preparation of Sanqi Hydrogel Patch used for setting a bone and study on its transdermal permeability in vitro. *Chinese Traditional and Herbal Drugs, 46*(5), 654–664.
19. Liu, C. M., Bai, J., Du, S. Y., Lu, Y., & Li, P. Y. (2013). Study on transdermal behavior of Zhitong cataplasm. *China Journal of Chinese Materia Medica, 38*(16), 2609–2613.
20. Wu, X. R., He, C., Wang, N. J., Zhang, Y. Y., Xi, C. X., & Xie, S. H. (2012). Experimental study on in vitro transdermal absorption of Shangshi Zhitong cataplasm. *China Journal of Chinese Materia Medica, 37*(7), 913–915.
21. Yan, J., Wang, Y., Zhang, X., Zhao, X. L., Ma, J. Z., Pu, X. Y., Wang, Y. G., Ran, F., Wang, Y. L., Leng, F. F., & Zhang, W. J. (2019). Snakegourd root/Astragalus polysaccharide hydrogel preparation and application in 3D printing. *International Journal of Biological Macromolecules, 121*, 309–316.
22. Zheng, X., Wu, F., Lin, X., Shen, L., & Feng, Y. (2018). Developments in drug delivery of bioactive alkaloids derived from traditional Chinese medicine. *Drug Delivery, 25*(1), 398–416.
23. Trommer, H., & Neuber, R. H. H. (2006). Overcoming the stratum corneum: The modulation of skin penetration. *Skin Pharmacology and Physiology, 19*(2), 106–121.
24. Parhi, R., Suresh, P., Mondal, S., & Kumar, P. M. (2012). Novel penetration enhancers for skin applications: A review. *Current Drug Delivery, 9*(2), 219–230.
25. Herman, A., & Herman, A. P. (2015). Essential oils and their constituents as skin penetration enhancer for transdermal drug delivery: A review. *The Journal of Pharmacy and Pharmacology, 67*(4), 473–485.
26. Chen, J., Jiang, Q. D., Wu, Y. M., Liu, P., Yao, J. H., Lu, Q., Zhang, H., & Duan, J. A. (2015). Potential of essential oils as penetration enhancers for transdermal administration of ibuprofen to treat dysmenorrhoea. *Molecules, 20*, 18219–18236.
27. Jiang, Q., Wu, Y., Zhang, H., Liu, P., Yao, J., Yao, P., Chen, J., & Duan, J. (2017). Development of essential oils as skin permeation enhancers: Penetration enhancement effect and mechanism of action. *Pharmaceutical Biology, 55*(1), 1592–1600.
28. Zhu, X. F., Luo, J., Guan, Y. M., Yu, Y. T., Jin, C., Zhu, W. F., & Liu, H. N. (2017). Effects of Frankincense and Myrrh essential oil on transdermal absorption in vitro of Chuanxiong and penetration mechanism of skin blood flow. *Zhongguo Zhong Yao Za Zhi, 42*(4), 680–685.
29. Karande, P., Jain, A., & Mitragotri, S. (2004). Discovery of transdermal penetration enhancers by high-throughput screening. *Nature Biotechnology, 22*, 192–197.
30. Ren, L., Chen, J. Y., Yao, J. H., Zhu, X. M., Dong, J., Gu, W., & Chen, J. (2018). Comparative study on the transdermal penetration enhancement effect of essential oils of interior-warming drugs based on electrical resistance of skin. *Journal of Nanjing University of Chinese Medicine, 34*(5), 474–479.

31. Zhu, X. M., Li, Y., Xu, F., Gu, W., Yan, G. J., Dong, J., & Chen, J. (2019). Skin electrical resistance measurement of oxygen-containing terpenes as penetration enhancers: Role of stratum corneum lipids. *Molecules, 24*(3), 523. https://doi.org/10.3390/molecules24030523
32. Yang, W. G., Chen, J., Liu, P., Jiang, Q. D., Wang, Y., Zhou, C., & Duan, J. A. (2015). Association between penetration enhancement effect of essential oils and drug properties of traditional Chinese medicines by data mining method. *Zhongguo Zhong Yao Za Zhi, 40*(23), 4609–4615.
33. Yang, W. G., Zhu, X. M., Wu, F. Y., Dong, Y. F., Xi, J. A., Chen, S. Y., & Chen, J. (2019). Research on correlation among "four natures" drug properties, penetration enhancement abilities and chemical components of essential oils from pungent Chinese herbs based on stepwise discrimination analysis method. *Chinese Traditional and Herbal Drugs, 50*(17), 4219–4224.
34. Zhang, D. K., Fu, C. M., Lin, J. Z., Ke, X. M., Zou, W. Q., Xu, R. C., Li, H., & Yang, M. (2017). Study on theory and application value of "unification of medicines and excipients" in Chinese materia medica preparations. *Zhongguo Zhong Yao Za Zhi, 48*(10), 1921–1929.
35. Schmitt, A. S., Schaefer, U. F., Doebler, L., & Reichling, J. (2009). Cooperative interaction of monoterpenes and phenylpropanoids on the in vitro human skin permeation of complex composed essential oils. *Planta Medica, 75*, 1381–1385.
36. Lan, Y., Li, H., Chen, Y. Y., Zhang, Y. W., Liu, N., Zhang, Q., & Wu, Q. (2014). Essential oil from Zanthoxylum bungeanum Maxim. and its main components used as transdermal penetration enhancers: A comparative study. *Journal of Zhejiang University Science B (Biomedicine & Biotechnology), 15*(11), 940–952.
37. Dong, J., Zhu, X. M., Wu, F. Y., Yang, B. Q., Feng, H., Dong, Y. F., Gu, W., & Chen, J. (2020). Development of galangal essential oil-based microemulsion gel for transdermal delivery of flurbiprofen: Simultaneous permeability evaluation of flurbiprofen and 1,8-cineole. *Drug Development and Industrial Pharmacy, 46*(1), 91–100.
38. Ye, Y., Yu, J., Wen, D., Kahkoska, A. R., & GZ. (2018). Polymeric microneedles for transdermal protein delivery. *Advanced Drug Delivery Reviews, 127*, 106–118.
39. Zhang, Q., Xu, C. C., Lin, S. Q., Zhou, H. B., Yao, G. T., Liu, H., Wang, L. L., Pan, X., Quan, G. L., & Wu, C. B. (2018). Synergistic immunoreaction of acupuncture-like dissolving microneedles containing thymopentin at acupoints in immune-suppressed rats. *Acta Pharmaceutica Sinica B, 8*(3), 449–457.
40. Shu, Z. X., Cao, Y. J., Tao, Y. T., Liang, X., Wang, F. Y., Li, Z., Li, Z. B., & Gui, S. Y. (2020). Polyvinylpyrrolidone microneedles for localized delivery of sinomenine hydrochloride: Preparation, release behavior of in vitro & in vivo, and penetration mechanism. *Drug Delivery, 27*(1), 642–651.
41. Bakshi, P., Vora, D., Hemmady, K., & Banga, A. K. (2020). Iontophoretic skin delivery systems: Success and failures. *International Journal of Pharmaceutics, 586*, 119584.
42. Geng, X. L., Sun, X. H., Zhang, J., Yang, J. B., & Liang, Q. D. (2015). Clinical curative effect observation of therapy of Chinese drug iontophoresis in treatment of degenerative osteoarthropathy. *Journal of Biological Regulators and Homeostatic Agents, 29*(1), 135–141.
43. Zhou, F. H., Zhao, M. J., & Zhao, H. Y. (2004). Iontophoresis with traditional Chinese herbal medicine accelerates the healing of bone fracture. *Di Yi Jun Yi Da Xue Xue Bao, 24*(6), 708–710.
44. Song, W. R., Pang, H. D., Cui, J. W., Lin, D. G., & Lin, J. H. (2020). Acupuncture combined with Chinese Medicine iontophoresis treatment for chronic progressive cervical intervertebral disk disease in a dog. *Complementart Medical Research, 9*, 1–7.
45. Fan, D. H., & Xia, B. (2007). Observation on therapeutic effect of heat needle combined with herb iontophoresis and western medicine on rheumatoid arthritis. *Zhongguo Zhen Jiu, 27*(10), 731–734.
46. Tian, A. P., Yin, Y. K., Yu, L., Yang, B. Y., Li, N., Li, J. Y., Bian, Z. M., Hu, S. Y., Weng, C. X., & Feng, L. (2020). Low-frequency sonophoresis of Chinese Medicine formula improves efficacy of malignant pleural effusion treatment. *Chinese Journal of Integrative Medicine, 26*(4), 263–269.

47. Tian, A. P., Yin, Y. K., Yu, L., Yang, B. Y., Li, N., Li, J. Y., Bian, Z. M., Hu, S. Y., Weng, C. X., & Feng, L. (2020). Topical delivery of modified Da-Cheng-Qi Decoction using low-frequency ultrasound sonophoresis for refractory metastatic malignant bowel obstruction: An open-label single-arm clinical trial. *Chinese Journal of Integrative Medicine, 26*(5), 382–387.
48. Xie, W. J., Zhang, Y. P., Xu, J., Sun, X. B., & Yang, F. F. (2017). Mechanism of transdermal penetration enhancement of Fu's cupping therapy: New physical penetration technology for transdermal administration with traditional Chinese Medicine (TCM) characteristics. *Molecules, 22*(4), 525. https://doi.org/10.3390/molecules22040525
49. Miao, Y. Y., Xu, J., Liu, Y., Yang, F. F., Zheng, X. X., Xie, W. J., & Zhang, Y. P. (2020). Evaluation of the Transdermal permeation effectiveness of Fu's cupping therapy on eight different types of model drugs. *Current Drug Delivery*. https://doi.org/10.2174/1567201817999201116192238
50. Kurmi, B. D., Tekchandani, P., Paliwal, R., & Paliwal, S. R. (2017). Transdermal drug delivery: Opportunities and challenges for controlled delivery of therapeutic agents using nanocarriers. *Current Drug Metabolism, 18*(5), 481–495.
51. Ashtiakr, M., Nagarsekar, K., & Fahr, A. (2016). Transdermal delivery from liposomal formulations - Evolution of the technology over the last three decades. *Journal of Controlled Release, 242*, 126–140.
52. Zhang, Y. T., Xu, Y. M., Zhang, S. J., Zhao, J. H., Wang, Z., Xu, D. Q., & Feng, N. P. (2014). In vivo microdialysis for the evaluation of transfersomes as a novel transdermal delivery vehicle for cinnamic acid. *Drug Development and Industrial Pharmacy, 40*(3), 301–307.
53. Li, Y., Xu, F., Li, X., Chen, S. Y., Huang, L. Y., Bian, Y. Y., Wang, J., Shu, Y. T., Yan, G. J., Dong, J., Yin, S. P., Gu, W., & Chen, J. (2021). Development of curcumin-loaded composite phospholipid ethosomes for enhanced skin permeability and vesicle stability. *International Journal of Pharmaceutics, 592*, 119936.
54. Eid, R. K., Easa, E. A., & El Maghraby, G. M. (2019). Essential oils in niosomes for enhanced transdermal delivery of felodipine. *Pharmaceutical Development and Technology, 24*(2), 157–165.
55. Gu, Y. W., Yang, M., Tang, X. M., Wang, T., Yang, D. S., Zhai, G. X., & Liu, J. Y. (2018). Lipid nanoparticles loading triptolide for transdermal delivery: Mechanisms of penetration enhancement and transport properties. *Journal of Nanobiotechnology, 16*(1), 68. https://doi.org/10.1186/s12951-018-0389-3
56. Rai, V. K., Mishra, N., Yadav, K. S., & Yadav, N. P. (2018). Nanoemulsion as pharmaceutical carrier for dermal and transdermal drug delivery: Formulation development, stability issues, basic considerations and applications. *Journal of Controlled Release, 270*, 203–225.
57. Peng, Q., Xie, W. L., Chen, J. Y., Jiang, T., Zhang, G. Q., Xu, Z. W., Zhang, J. N., & Zhang, L. (2018). Transdermal characteristics and mechanism of asiaticoside nanoemulsions and asiaticoside nanoemulsions-based gels. *Zhongguo Zhong Yao Za Zhi, 43*(9), 1857–1863.
58. Engesland, A., & ÀŠkalko-Basnet N, Flaten GE. (2015). Phospholipid vesicle-based permeation assay and EpiSkin® in assessment of drug therapies destined for skin administration. *Journal of Pharmaceutical Sciences, 104*, 1119–1127.
59. Ma, M., Di, H. J., Zhang, H., Yao, J. H., Dong, J., Yan, G. J., Qiao, H. Z., & Chen, J. (2017). Development of phospholipid vesicle-based permeation assay models capable of evaluating percutaneous penetration enhancing effect. *Drug Development and Industrial Pharmacy, 43*(12), 2055–2063.
60. Erdő, F., Hashimoto, N., Karvaly, G., Nakamichi, N., & Kato, Y. (2016). Critical evaluation and methodological positioning of the transdermal microdialysis technique. A review. *Journal of Controlled Release, 233*, 147–161.
61. Lan, Y., Yang, L., Shi, D. Y., Wang, Y. X., Wu, X. P., Xie, X., & Wu, Q. (2017). In vivo transdermal penetration enhancing activity of essential oil from Zanthoxyli Pericarpium by using microdialysis technique. *Zhongguo Zhong Yao Za Zhi, 42*(14), 2676–2682.

Chapter 5
The Contribution of Traditional Chinese Medicine Compound in Nasal Drug Delivery System

Xuechun Liu, Haiyan Hu, Ziqi Chen, Zekang Zhang, Changhai Wang, Yueying Zhao, and Yang Lu

Abstract The nasal drug delivery system (NDDS) has been used for a long time in China and has formed a complete theoretical framework and technique. There are many records in classic medical books about nasal administration, such as *Huang Di Nei Jing* (*Huangdi's Internal Classic*) and *Nan Jing* (*Classic of Difficult Issues*), which influenced and appealed to many researchers to study. With the assistance of natural sciences, such as anatomy and medical imaging, experts and scholars have accumulated a wealth of knowledge about the structure of the nasal cavity and revealed the underlying pathway for drug delivery to the site of disease. Nasal administration also has played a unique role in western medicine. To date, large bodies of dosage forms have been emerged in nasal administration, such as nasal drops, aerosols and sprays, microemulsions, gels and in situ gels, liposomes, and nanoparticles. This chapter introduces some efficient, controllable, and safe NDDS of some traditional Chinese medicine compounds prepared by modern pharmaceutical techniques. The theoretical basis and the historical evolution of NDDS in China and western countries were discussed. Eventually, we focus on the opportunities and challenges currently facing the NDDS in traditional Chinese medicine compounds.

Keywords Traditional Chinese medicine · Nasal administration · New dosage form · Modern pharmaceutical preparations technique

---

X. Liu · H. Hu · Z. Chen · Z. Zhang · C. Wang · Y. Zhao · Y. Lu (✉)
School of Chinese Materia Medica, Beijing University of Chinese Medicine, Beijing, China
e-mail: luyang@bucm.edu.cn

N. Feng, Z. Yang (eds.), *Novel Drug Delivery Systems for Chinese Medicines*,
https://doi.org/10.1007/978-981-16-3444-4_5

5.1 Nasal Therapy Under Traditional Chinese Medicine Theory

Recently, nasal administration has been considered as one of the drug administration modes that can be absorbed quickly and efficiently and introduced as a mode of administration for a long time in China.

Traditional Chinese medicine (TCM) has already given the mechanism of nasal drug administration on diseases from the perspectives of Guan Qiao-Zang Fu theory and Guan Qiao-Meridian theory in detail. TCM believes that the human body is an interconnected whole, which is indivisible in tissue structure, is coordinated in physiological functions, and affects each other in pathology and pathogenesis. Therefore, nasal administration can not only directly treat nasal lesions but also treat systemic diseases through the regulation of meridian and related organ transmission. As early as in the *Huang Di Nei Jing* (*Huangdi's Internal Classic*), there is a saying that "lung opening at the nose"; *Su Wen · Jin Gui Zhen Yan Lun* (the chapter "Discourse on the True Words in the Golden Chest" of the *Plain Questions*) also said that "open the orifice to the nose, hide the essence in the lungs." In *Ling Shu · Mai Du Pian* (*Miraculous Pivot chapter 17 The Measurements of the Vessels*), it states: "Lung Qi flows through the nose, lungs function well and nose can know the smell." *Nan Jing* (*Classic of Difficult Issues*) also documented that "Lung Qi passes through the nose, nose functions well will know the smell." Also, according to *Yi Lin Gai Cuo* (*Correction of Errors in Medical Classics*), it said "The nose passes through the brain, and the smell is attributed to the brain," and in *Chuang Yang Jing Yan Quan Shu* (*Complete Manual of Experience in the Treatment of Sores*), it said, "Because the nose is in the middle of the face, substance through the nose can quickly transfer into blood; nostril is the orifice of the lung, qi pass it can go up to the brain and go down to the lung." Hence, the mechanism of nasal drug delivery for treating diseases has a profound theoretical basis in traditional Chinese medicine.

Traditional Chinese medicine nasal therapy has a complete theoretical system; is easy for patients to use; has a rapid onset of action, low drug consumption, and low cost and price; and shows significant curative effect. It is especially suitable for the elderly and children. Therefore, it has been widely used by folks in China.

In the earliest existing ancient medical book *Wu Shi Er Bing Fang* (*Prescriptions for Fifty-two Diseases*), it is recorded that fresh fish and salt are applied externally to the nose to treat leprosy. Numerous expositions on the nose in the classic traditional Chinese medicine book *Huang Di Nei Jing* (*Huangdi's Internal Classic*) had initially laid the theoretical foundation for nasal therapy. *Ling Shu* (*Miraculous Pivot*) for the first time discussed the application of nasal medicine for the treatment of systemic diseases. Its record that using the grass to insert the nostril and induce the sneezing can stop hiccupping created a precedent therapy by sneezing. In the Eastern Han Dynasty, Zhang Zhongjing's *Shang Han Za Bing Lun* (*Treatise on Cold Damage and Miscellaneous Diseases*) had a record of treating sudden death by irrigating the nose with mashed scallion juice in first aid. *Zhou Hou Bei Ji Fang* (*Handbook of Prescriptions for Emergencies*) written by Ge Hong of east Jin dynasty, which was recorded the therapies, such as stabbing, plugging, or irrigating the nose with saponin, spring onion, scallion juice, leek juice, realgar, and other medicines. During the Sui and Tang Dynasties, Sun Simiao compiled *Qian Jin Yao Fang* (*Essential Prescriptions Worth a Thousand Gold for Emergencies*) and *Qian Jin Yi Fang* (*Supplement to the Essential Prescriptions Worth a Thousand Gold*), that were recorded many fragrant prescriptions; including Taiyi Liujin Powder, Xiaojinya Powder, and Dajinya Powder. Nasal therapies were widely used in the Song, Jin and Yuan dynasties, the book of *Tai Ping Sheng Hui Fang* (*Peaceful Holy Benevolent Prescriptions*) was recorded the powder of grinding alum, veratrum, coptis, and others into the nasal cavity for the treatment of infantile malnutrition. In the Ming Dynasty, the application of nasal therapy was more common. Many of the prescriptions for nasal therapy were included in the largest prescription in China, *Pu Ji Fang* (*Formulary of Universal Relief*). Besides, there are also hundreds of nasal prescriptions in *Ben Cao Gang Mu* (*Compendium of Materia Medica*). Such as the formula for treating migraine, "Zhi Ling Powder: realgar and asarum are divided into two equal powder parts, each of them blew into the nose with a dose of one-character size on the coins." In the Qing Dynasty, nasal therapy not only received an unprecedented universal application but also paid attention to the theoretical discussion of nasal therapy. *Li Yue Pian Wen* (*Rhymed Discourse for External Remedies*) summarized the experience of nasal administration in the past. The book contains the theory, method, prescription, and medicine, forming a relatively complete theoretical system of nasal medicine therapy, which was called "The twelve classics pass the nose." Also, Zhao Xuemin's *Chuan Ya Nei Bian* (*Internal Treatise of Folk Medicine*) and *Chuan Ya Wai Bian* (*External Treatise of Folk Medicine*) extensively collected the experience of folk medical practitioners, among which there are many nasal treatment prescriptions, which were simple and effective and are still used in clinical practice today [1–5]. We organize the above content in Table 5.1.

5.2 The Understanding of Nasal Therapy in Western Natural Medicine

Nasal therapy played an important role in western medicine's development, and the understanding of nasal therapy in western natural medicine also had a long history.

For example, in North America, Indians treated headaches by inhaling a powder from leaves through the nose. In ancient India, Brahman cured some disease by inhaling mandala and cannabis. The *Ebers Papyrus*'s book (the earliest book on pharmacological knowledge in ancient Egypt), circa 1554 BC, described the treatment of dyspnea by inhaling *Hyoscyamus* smoke. At that time, there was no special inhalation device; thus, patients needed to roast *Hyoscyamus* on the block to vaporize the scopolamine and inhale it. As early as 650 BC, the cuneiform scripted the treatment from ancient Assyrians using inhalation of chromone to treat asthma. Around 460 BC in ancient Greece, Hippocrates created a pot-shaped device, herbs

Table 5.1 Records of nasal therapy in classic medical books

Times	Records on nasal therapy
Spring and autumn and the warring states	*Wu Shi Er Bing Fang* (*prescriptions for fifty-two diseases*): "Ming is kind of lava, live in the nose or beside the mouth; newly born fish can treat it"
	Huang Di Nei Jing (*Huangdi's internal classic*): "Open the orifice to the nose, hide the essence in the lungs"; "lung Qi flows through the nose, lungs function well and nose can know the smell"; "using the grass to insert the nostril and induce the sneezing"
Eastern Han dynasty	*Nan Jing* (*classic of difficult issue*): "Lung Qi passes through the nose, nose functions well will know the smell"
Jin dynasty	*Zhou Hou Bei Ji Fang* (*handbook of prescriptions for emergencies*): "To rescue the sudden death, take the yellow core of the green onion and insert it into people's nostril for seven to eight inches, left in male, right in the female; it is better to see the blood in eyes"
Tang dynasty	*Qian Jin Yi Fang* (*supplement to the essential prescriptions worth a thousand gold*): "...if meets the year of pestilence, burn this formula in the dose of 1/10 edge of the knife in every first day's morning of the month, patients will also be smoked"
Song dynasty	*Chuang Yang Jing Yan Quan Su* (*complete manual of experience in the treatment of sores*): "Because the nose is in the middle position of the face, substance through the nose can quickly transfer into blood; nostrils is the orifice of the lung, Qi passes it can go up to the brain and go down to the lung"
	Tai Ping Sheng Hui Fang (*peaceful holy benevolent prescriptions*): "In the treatment of infantile malnutrition, blow the formula into the nose, this also named *Tong Ding San Fang*"
Ming dynasty	*Ben Cao Gang Mu* (*compendium of Materia Medica*): "Zhi Ling Powder: Realgar and asarum are divided into two equal powder parts, each of them blew into the nose with a dose of one-character size on the coins"
	Pu Ji Fang (*formulary of universal relief*): "Chu Bi Shen Xiao Powder:...Regardless of the dosage of vitriolum caeruleum, grind it into powder and then blow them into the nose by the reed, the blood will suddenly stop"
Qing dynasty	*Yi Lin Gai Cuo* (*correction of errors in medical classics*): "The nose passes through the brain, and the smell is attributed to the brain"
	Li Yue Pan Wen (*rhymed discourse for topical remedies*): "The twelve classics pass the nose"; "as the diseases in the upper body, grand the formula into powder. Twitch nostrils until sneeze, sweat out, is the first shortcut"
	Chuan Ya Nei Bian (*internal treatise of folk medicine*): "To treat the wind syndrome of the head, potassium nitrate one tael, Qingdai (*indigo Naturalis*), Chuanxiong (*chuanxiong Rhizoma*), Bohe (*Menthae Haplocalycis Herba*) each one mace"

and resins soaked with vinegar and oil were heated in this device to generate an aerial fog. There was an opening on the lid of the pot, and reed stalks were placed, so the aerosol would then emerge from the rod for patients to inhale. In the second century AD, Galen of Rome advised patients with breathing difficulties to inhale sulfur-containing gases under the volcano. The first book on asthma was written by the doctor, Dr. Maimonides, born in Spain in 1190 AD. *On Asthma*, the book, proposed a variety of measures and methods for treating asthma, including inhaling the gas that was created by herbs after the fire's roast. In 1804, the treatment of nasal rhinitis was nasal irrigation with a mixture of rhatany root and lime after grinding, patients needed to wash their nose with the powder three to four times a day, and sometimes diarrhea drugs could also be given. In the 1860s, it was also reported that bronchial asthma could be treated by inhaling cigarettes containing arsenic. In 1867, French doctor Tosser mentioned *Datura* to prepare cigarette formula for diseases, which added the opium and *atropa belladonna*. When it comes to the new era, in 1984, a symposium on the "nasal route of systemic administration" was held in New Brunswick, New Jersey. Since then, intranasal administration was considered an ideal route of drug administration. Frey first proposed that drugs could be directly transferred from the nasal cavity to the brain in 1989. Many subsequent studies had shown that nasal drug delivery based on the pathway from the nasal cavity to the CNS had the potential to treat CNS diseases. There was also a conference held in France by the European Academic Research Association in 1991 that aimed to discuss "Buccal and Nasal Administration as an Alternative to Intravenous Administration." At the 15th International Congress of Rhinology held in Tokyo, in September 1991, there were several papers devoted to studying the function of nasal mucosa absorption drugs, marking that the research of otolaryngology had entered the field of pharmacology and exerted their unique roles [6–8] (Table 5.2).

5.3 Development in Anatomy

Recently, with the advanced development of natural sciences such as physiology, pathology, and anatomy, extensive elementary knowledge and basic concepts of the structure of nasal cavity have built.

Modern anatomical studies have shown that the nasal cavity can be divided into three areas (Fig. 5.1), the nasal vestibule, the respiratory region, and the olfactory region, according to functions and tissue structures [9–13]. The nasal cavity is both a respiratory organ and an olfactory organ. The nasal septum divides the nasal cavity into two cavities, 12–15 cm in length, and the volume of the unilateral nasal cavity was about 15 mL. The total area of the nasal mucosa is approximately 150 cm^2. Besides, the nasal administration and absorption sites are mainly contributed by the turbinate bone and parts of the nasal septum. In the inner respiratory tract area, the cell surface of the absorption area has a large number of microvilli, thus highly increasing the effective surface area for drug absorption. Meanwhile, the nasal mucosa is about 2–5 mm, so it can also greatly increase the efficacy of drug

Table 5.2 Western history of nasal therapy

Times	History of nasal therapy
Ancient India	Brahman cures illness by inhaling mandala and cannabis
N.A. Indians	Treating headaches by snorting a leaf powder
1554 BC	*Ebers Papyrus*'s book described the treatment of dyspnea by inhaling *Hyoscyamus* smoke
650 BC	Cromones inhalation for asthma
460 BC	Herbs and resins soaked with vinegar and oil were heated in the device to generate an aerosol, and then the aerosol would then emerge from the rod for patients to inhale
Second AD	Galen of Rome advised patients with breathing difficulties to inhale sulfur-containing gases under the volcano
1190	Spanish doctor Maimonides wrote the first book on asthma, *on asthma*, which puts forward a variety of measures and methods for treating asthma, including inhaling the gas produced by fire-roasting herbs
1804	Nasal rinse with a mixture powder of rhatany root and lime for nasal rhinitis
1860	Treatment of bronchial asthma by inhaling cigarettes containing arsenic
1867	French doctor Tosser mentioned *Datura* to prepare cigarette formula for diseases, which added the opium and *atropa belladonna*
1984	A symposium on the "nasal route of systemic administration" was held in New Brunswick, New Jersey. Since then, intranasal administration was considered an ideal route of drug administration
1989	Frey first proposed that drugs could be directly transferred from the nasal cavity to the brain in 1989. Many subsequent studies had shown that nasal drug delivery based on the pathway from the nasal cavity to the CNS had the potential to treat CNS diseases
1991	A conference was held in France by the European academic research association in 1991 that aimed to discuss "buccal and nasal administration as an alternative to intravenous administration"
	At the 15th international congress of rhinology held in Tokyo, there were several papers devoted to studying the function of nasal mucosa absorption drugs, marking that the research of otolaryngology had entered the field of pharmacology and exerted their unique roles

absorption. Nasal mucosa appears on each wall of the nasal cavity, and it is divided into the vestibular area, the respiratory area (which occupies most of the nasal mucosa), and the olfactory area. However, the nasal vestibule has almost no absorption function, and the respiratory region occupies the largest area of the nasal cavity. The olfactory area is located in the upper turbinate, with an area of about 10 cm^2, directly under the sieve plate where drugs can be absorbed into the cerebrospinal fluid and thus enter the central nervous system (CNS).

Respiratory area is the main site for the systemic absorption of drugs after nasal administration. The mucosa of the respiratory area has abundant capillaries for a drug to enter the systemic circulation. In this way, it can avoid the first-pass effect of the liver. The surface of mucosal columnar epithelial cells in the respiratory area is

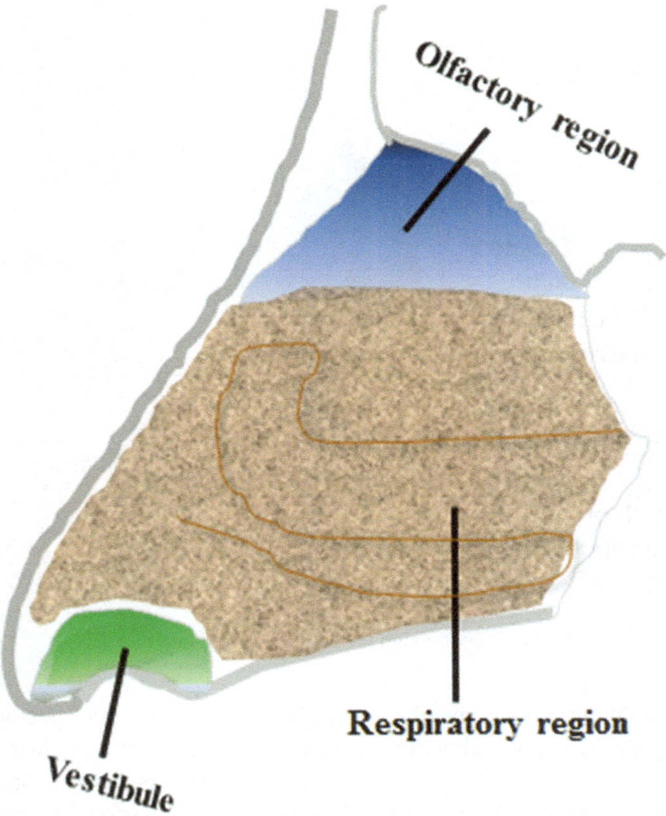

Fig. 5.1 The areas of the nasal cavity: the nasal vestibule, the respiratory region, and the olfactory region

rich in microvilli, which greatly increases the effective area of drug absorption. After the drug passes through the mucous membrane of the respiratory region, some are metabolized, the rest will enter the gastrointestinal tract, the capillaries of the respiratory region, and the trigeminal nerve. Besides, some drugs in the gastrointestinal pathway are metabolized, and some are metabolized by the liver's first-pass effect, and only the left can finally enter the systemic circulation. There is also evidence which suggests that drugs from the capillary pathway of the respiratory region can directly enter the systemic circulation. Drugs from the trigeminal nerve pathway can also directly enter the CNS because they can bypass the blood-brain barrier (BBB) and enter the brain directly.

When giving the drug by the nasal cavity, it will enter the CNS through the olfactory mucosal epithelial pathway and the olfactory nerve pathway, where drug can get away from the BBB and exert their therapeutic effect, as shown in Fig. 5.2. Now, it is gradually accepted that "nasal-brain" delivery is a complicated

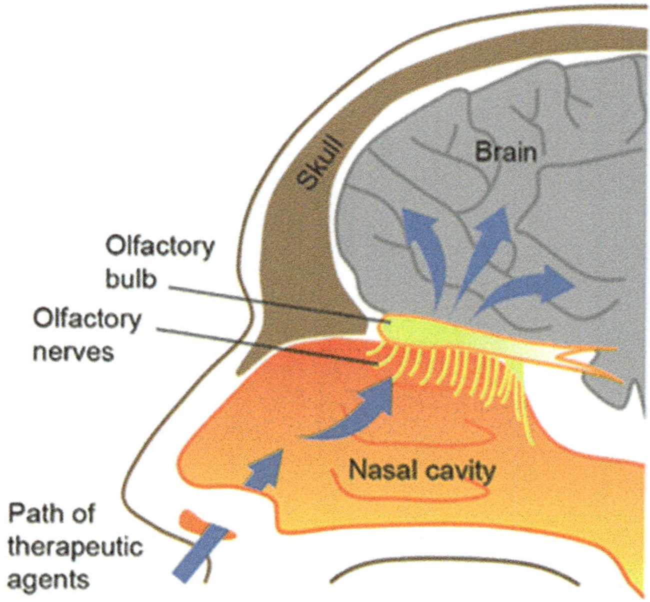

Fig. 5.2 Brain targeted drug delivery through the nasal olfactory route

process. Also, this process is mainly divided into three parts: the olfactory nerve pathway, the olfactory mucosal epithelial pathway, and the blood circulation pathway. In the "nasal-brain" pathway, drugs can enter the brain either through the olfactory mucosal epithelial pathway or in intracellular transport by cell bypass transport. Among them, the axonal transmission of the olfactory nerve can avoid the blood-brain barrier and achieve fast and efficient drug delivery. This process is the most direct pathway for "nasal-brain" delivery and also the key to brain targeting for nasal administration. When it comes to the "nasal-blood-brain" pathway, because the nasal mucosa in the nasal breathing zone is extremely thin, the submembranous blood vessels are rich, so the nasal capillary network can be directly anastomosed with the cerebral blood vessels through the sinus. After nasal medication, blood circulation will cross the blood-brain barrier into brain tissue, which are the main indirect pathways for nasal drug delivery targeting CNS. Furthermore, there are other pathways for administration, such as the trigeminal nerve pathway and lymphatic pathway.

At last, because of the differences in physiological structure of the nasal cavity, it has the unique characteristics of rapid absorption, fast onset, high bioavailability, good brain targeting, and convenient use when compared to others, which also made it gradually become one of the hot spots in preparation areas in recent years. However, it is important to realize that there are still some problems in nasal administration that need further discussion to solve, for example, the low drug dose, unclear related mechanism, etc.

5.4 Development of Modern Preparations

With the development of modern science and technology, various dosage forms such as nasal drops, aerosols and sprays, microemulsions, gels and in situ gels, liposomes, and nanoparticles have emerged.

5.4.1 Nasal Drops

Nasal drops [14, 15] refer to liquid preparations for dripping into the nasal cavity. They are generally made into solutions, suspensions, or emulsions and are one of the most commonly used dosage forms for nasal administration. The commonly used solvents for nasal drops are water, propylene glycol, liquid paraffin, and vegetable oil. Suitable antioxidants, solubilizers, preservatives, or other additives can be added according to the nature of the extract or medicine of the drug, and various additives must not be irritating to the respiratory tract and mucous membranes. To promote absorption and prevent mucosal edema, osmotic pressure, pH value, and viscosity should be adjusted appropriately. Generally, the pH should be 5.5–7.5 and isotonic with nasal mucus. Nasal drops are easy to produce, are low cost, and have certain stability and safety. However, due to the clearance of vibrissa, the time that medicinal solution stays in the nasal cavity is short and is easily lost from the nasal cavity, which affects the absorption and curative effect. Nasal drops also have been used in clinical treatment, such as the treatment of nasal diseases (rhinitis, sinusitis, etc.), cardiovascular and cerebrovascular diseases, cold fever, migraine, acute mastitis, and so on. The efficacy of traditional formula Yizhihao granule in the treatment of acute, chronic rhinitis and allergic rhinitis is not as good as that of nasal drops in the bioavailability. The early compound Yizhihao nasal drops can make up the insufficient but did not choose the optimal extraction process based on its effective ingredients, which caused some loss. Therefore, Chen et al. [16] optimized the extraction process of the compound Yizhihao nasal drops. They used artemisinic acid, chlorogenic acid, pseudoephedrine hydrochloride, total flavonoid content, and cream extraction rate as evaluation indicators. Liquid-to-liquid ratio, material-to-liquid ratio, and extraction time are the influencing factors. Finally, the Box-Behnken response surface method and analytic hierarchy process are used to optimize the extraction process. The results showed that the optimal conditions were 60% ethanol in volume, 1 h extraction time, three times extraction, and a material-to-liquid ratio of 1:12. Artemisinin, chlorogenic acid, pseudoephedrine hydrochloride, and total flavonoid contents were 0.949, 2.606, 0.343, and 20.813 mg/g, and the rate of ointment extraction is 17.57%. The method used to extract the compound scent of compound Yizhihao nasal drop is stable, reproducible, reasonable, feasible, and reliable, which can provide a certain reference for industrial production.

So far, some nasal drops with effects have been listed on the market, such as Bitongdi Nasal Drops produced by Shenyang Shuangding Pharmaceutical Co., Ltd., which is mainly used to treat nasal congestion, runny nose, chronic pharyngitis, and wind colds, but may cause adverse reactions such as a dry nasal cavity.

5.4.2 Aerosols and Sprays

Aerosol [17] refers to medicine with a suitable propellant packaged together in a pressure-resistant sealed container with a special valve system. When in use, the content of the propellant is used to spray the contents into a mist, foam, or other forms of preparation. According to the dispersion system, it can be divided into three types: solution type, emulsion type, or suspension type. However, the aerosol contains a propellant, which will pollute the environment. Also, it uses a pressure-resistant container, which the production process of it is more complicated. Therefore, it is currently not widely used in nasal administration when compared to the spray. Hammurabi et al. [18] had experimented on the acute toxicity, local irritation, and allergies of Cangxin aerosol. They observed the acute toxicity and its degree after nasal administration in guinea pigs with the maximum dose method. The result was that Cangxin aerosol was administered intranasally at a maximum dose of 25.6 g/kg for 14 days, no deaths and obvious acute toxicity were observed; No death and local irritation reaction were found after continuous administration of 8.6g/kg for 7 days, and no abnormal histopathological examination was found. In the active skin allergy experiments of guinea pigs, no allergic symptoms were found. These results indicate that Cangxin aerosol has no acute toxicity, local irritation, and allergic reactions within the dose range of this test, and the results suggest that it is safe for clinical use.

Spray refers to a formulation that contains no propellant and sprays the liquid medicine into a mist with the help of the pressure of a hand pump or other methods. According to the dispersion system, sprays are generally divided into three types: solution type, emulsion type, and suspension type. When compared with nasal drops, sprays have finer droplets, more uniform distribution in the nasal cavity, and faster absorption and thus have a higher bioavailability. However, the spray administration can make the medicinal solution deposited in the front of the nasal cavity and dispersed in small droplets. Its clearance rate is slower than the movement of the vibrissa. If used repeatedly, the spray will have much fewer pathological changes on the mucosa than the nasal drops, but the drug will have a shorter duration in the nasal cavity. Wang et al. [19] studied the pharmacokinetics and brain targeting of headache nasal spray in rats. They divided 84 SD rats into nasal and intravenous dose groups, 42 in each group, with a dose of 1.2 mL/kg, 5, 10, 15, 30, 60, 90, and 120 min in the abdominal aorta 5 mL, and took brain tissue (6 per point in time); high-efficiency liquid chromatography-series mass spectrometry was used to determine the concentration of prim-*o*-glucosylcimifugin and 5-*O*-methylvisammioside (cimicin, 5-*O*-mares amoelione) in each group of rat plasma and brain tissue, and DAS2.0 software was used to calculate pharmacological parameters and brain-targeted index. The results show that after a nasal injection of headache nasal spray, some drugs could be directly transferred to the brain through nasal absorption. Yang et al. [20] prepared a naloxone hydrochloride nasal spray and further investigate its toxicity on vibrissa of isolated toad palate, pharmacokinetic behavior in rats, and stability in pH 3.5–5.5. Also, they studied the promoting effects of different absorption enhancers on the spray. Results indicated that the naloxone hydrochloride solution was stable in pH 3.5–5.5, and Ethylene Diamine Tetraacetic Acid (0.2%, W/V) showed best penetration promoting effect on the nasal spray. They also found that the naloxone hydrochloride nasal spray had a quick therapeutic effect with recoverable and little vibrissa toxicity, and the bioavailability of the spray in rats is equivalent to that of intramuscular injection. According to the evidence, it can be proved that the nasal spray is stable and controllable in vitro and has little toxicity to vibrissa, fast onset of action, and high bioavailability which are proven to have a broad application in the future.

Currently available drugs are GlaxoWellcome, SA (GlaxoSmithKline Group), fluticasone propionate nasal spray, which can be used to prevent and treat seasonal allergic rhinitis and perennial allergic rhinitis. This spray has a high bioavailability and can be fast absorbed and evenly distributed, but may cause adverse reactions such as dry nose and irritation.

5.4.3 Gelling Agent and in Situ Gel

The nasal gel [21–24] refers to a gel-like semi-solid preparation made of a medicament with a suitable excipient. The gel has a large viscosity, which can increase the retention time of the drug in the nasal cavity, improve bioavailability, and reduce the times of drug administration. When the gel is mixed with the mucus in the nasal cavity, the viscosity increases, which is conducive to retaining the drug and prolonging the absorption time. Besides, gels are specifically suitable for heat-sensitive peptide and protein drugs. At present, scholars have developed the polyacrylic acid gel of insulin, calcitonin, and polyacrylic acid sustained-release gel of propranolol hydrochloride by spray drying.

In situ gel, also known as in vivo gel, is a preparation that undergoes a phase change in the nasal cavity after being administered in a solution state and is converted from a liquid to a semi-solid gel, which can extend the residence time of the drug in the nasal cavity and improve bioavailability and prolonged efficacy. According to different principles of phase change, it was divided into temperature-sensitive, pH-sensitive, and ion-sensitive in situ gels. The drug is prepared into an in situ gel preparation, which is formed into a semi-solid after being dripped into the nasal cavity in liquid form and adheres to the nasal mucosa to improve the compliance of patients. He et al. [25] studied the pharmacokinetics and brain targeting of gastrodin nasal gel in rats. The experimental group was administered with gastrodin nasal gel. The control group was intravenously injected with gastrodin. After administration, blood and brain tissues (brain and cerebellum) of two groups of rats were taken respectively, and the content of gastrodin in the blood and gastrodigenin in brain tissue was measured by the HPLC method. Then, the drug-time curve was drawn, the pharmacokinetic parameters such as the area under the curve (AUC) and mean residence time (MRT) were calculated, and the bioavailability F (%) and brain targeting parameter (BTI) between the two groups were also compared. The results showed that, when compared with the intravenous injection of gastrodin, the gastrogenin content in the brain tissue of rats fed with gastrodin temperature-sensitive gel was significantly increased, and the area under the curve of the brain and cerebellum increased significantly. The figures for BTI were 2.83 to 1.93, respectively, and the mean retention time (MRT) of the drug increased almost twofold. Besides, bioavailability *F* (%) also increased significantly. These all proved that the gastrodin nasal temperature-sensitive gel with TMC-P407P188-carbomer as the matrix could play a good role in pharmacodynamics and had certain brain targeting and sustained drug release. To develop a heat-sensitive drug delivery tool for nasal delivery, H. Nazar et al. [26] synthesized a series of systematic *N*-trimethyl chitosan by synthesizing polyethylene glycol and glycerol phosphate with three kinds of chitosan with different average molecular weights, and the chloride polymer was co-formulated as a hydrogel. According to rheological evaluation, *N*-trimethyl chitosan-derived hydrogels have a lower degree of quaternization and a higher or medium average molecular weight and relatively short sol-gels at physiologically relevant temperatures in transition time. Similarly, the same hydrogels show good water retention and strong mucosal adhesion potential, and their mixture with mucus exhibits rheological synergy. Hydrogel formulations derived from *N*-trimethyl chitosan with a medium average molecular weight and a low degree of quaternization appear to be particularly promising because they have the following characteristics: great in rheology and mucoadhesive behavior and the sol-gel transition occurred at 32.5 °C in 7 min. Further research is currently underway to study its absorption-enhancing properties and biocompatibility, and preliminary positive results indicate that this is a promising solution.

5.4.4 Microemulsion

The microemulsion [27] is an anisotropic, transparent or translucent, low-viscosity, thermodynamically stable dispersion system formed by mixing the water phase, oil phase, surfactant, and co-surfactant in proper proportions. Besides, the microemulsion is a new type of ideal drug release carrier, whose characteristics are targeted at drug release to improve the efficacy of drugs and reduce adverse reactions. Oral and nasal experiments in rabbits have shown that puerarin microemulsion in nasal administration is faster in absorption and bioavailability than oral administration. Zhang et al. [28] explored the safety evaluation of huperzine A microemulsion nasal administration on ciliated toads and nasal mucosa of rats. So, they created a toad upper jaw model to investigate the effects of huperzine A microemulsion in nasal administration on the survival time and transportability of toad cilia on toads, and scanning electron microscopy was used to observe the effects of huperzine A microemulsion on nasal mucosal cilia of rats. According to results, when compared with the normal saline group, huperzine A microemulsion had no significant effect on the survival time of toad cilia on toads; when compared with the syndrome before administration, huperzine A microemulsion had no significant change on the toad cilia transport capacity; images from scanning electron microscopy showed that the nasal mucosa ciliated with huperzine A microemulsion had no significant change in morphology during 2 h, but the cilia morphology changed slightly at 4 h after perfusion, indicating that nasal administration of huperzine A microemulsion may stimulate nasal mucosa in a very light level. Also, Rajshree et al. [29] explored the application of docosahexaenoic acid (DHA) in the treatment of cerebral-nasal neurocysticercosis by intranasal microemulsion. They designed a new combination of intranasal microemulsions (MEs) for nasal delivery of albendazole sulfoxide (ABZ-SO) and curcumin (CUR) to the brain for neurocysticercosis (NCC). The DHA microemulsion prepared by simple solution showed good stability and negative ζ potential, and the size was smaller than 20 nm, and the rapid and high permeability of the drug through sheep nasal mucosa in vitro. Compared with the same dose of intravenous DHA microemulsion, intranasal DHA microemulsion indicated high brain concentration, and the brain region under the curve (AUC) increased by 10.76 (ABZ-SO) and 3.24 (CUR) times. Direct nose-to-brain transport (DTP) of both drugs were exceeded 95%. Compared to Capmul microemulsions and drug solutions, high drug-targeting efficiency (DTE) to the brain indicates that DHA is helpful for nasal-brain delivery, and no significant changes have been confirmed by histopathological studies. These indicate that intranasal DHA is a promising nasal-brain targeted delivery system. This study was the first suggesting that this novel combination of ABZ-SO and CUR could improve the treatment of NCC. It is clear that although microemulsions can provide targeted delivery to the brain, DHA microemulsions can provide greater benefits, confirming that DHA in microemulsions can not only enhance nasal-brain delivery but also maintain a 24 h continuous level. It turns out that DHA microemulsion is a targeted intranasal drug delivery system for use from the nose to the brain. In conclusion, microemulsion as a new formulation, in addition to the general characteristics of emulsions, also has the special advantages of small particle size, transparency, stability, and so on. So, microemulsions can be targeted for drug release, can improve the efficacy of drugs, reduce toxic and side effects, and are increasingly used in pharmaceutical preparations and clinical applications. At last, combining microemulsions with nasal administration would show better results.

5.4.5 Liposome

Liposomes [30] refer to tiny vesicles formed by drugs encapsulated in a lipid-like bilayer, composed of phospholipids and cholesterol, and have a bilayer structure similar to the biofilm. Because it is similar in structure to biofilms, liposomes are also known as "artificial biofilms," which can encapsulate water-soluble and fat-soluble drugs. Because the structure is similar to that of biofilm, liposomes are promised to have advantages like reducing drug dose, reducing toxicity and irritation, reducing allergies and immune responses, delaying the release, reducing the rate of elimination in the body, changing the distribution of drugs in the body, and being able to target drug release; besides, they also received extensive attention and in-depth research. This similar structure can also reduce the toxicity and irritation of the drug in the nasal mucosa, prevent the drug from being degraded by enzymes, keep the drug concentration at the site of administration, and continuously release the encapsulated drug with a long-acting slow-release effect. For example, *Cheng et al.* [31] explored the effects of nasal administration of epimedium liposomes on behavior and neurotransmitters in rats with Parkinson's disease (PD). In detail, 16 rats were selected randomly as a sham operation group (sham operation), and other 64 modeled PD rats were divided into 4 groups (n=16), including PD model group (PD/ in-group) and epimedium plastid nasal administration group (ICA-PGL/in-group), epimedium nasal administration group (ICA/in-group), epimedium liposome intravenous administration group (ICA-PGL/i.v.-group). After continuous drug intervention for 2 weeks, the ICA/in-group was observed by detecting changes in apomorphine rotation times, cylinder experiments, TH expression in the striatum, and related neurotransmitter content in rats. The results showed that the motor function of every epimedium treatment group was improved to different extents when compared with the PD/in-group. The TH-positive fiber expression in the striatum area and the concentration of monoamine neurotransmitters like DA, DOPAC, and HVA were increased to varying degrees. Among them, the ICA-PGL/in-group had the most prominent effect. These proved that the nasal administration of epimedium liposomes to motor function and nerves in Parkinson's disease rats had a good repair effect in neurotransmitters. Also, liposomes are highly bio-adhesive, which are not easily cleared by nasal mucosa after nasal administration. They also have a long residence time, which is conducive to drug absorption through the nasal mucosa. At the same time, the drug is slowly released through the liposome phospholipid bilayer, which also extends the drug duration of action in the body.

5.4.6 Nanoparticles

Nanoparticles [32] are solid colloidal particles with a particle size of 10–1000 nm. They are divided into nanospheres and nanocapsules and belong to colloidal solution systems. Lipid nanoparticles have a large specific surface area, long circulation time, good biocompatibility, and good nasal mucosa penetrability and are not easy to be cleared by phagocytes. Also, they have the advantages of slow-release, targeting, and high bioavailability. The bio-carrier prepared by polysaccharide nanoparticles is cross-linked with morphine and can be administered in the nasal cavity, thus prompting the direct transport of morphine from the nasal cavity to the brain but does not increase its transport to the blood. Because the organism has good tolerance to nanoparticles, this dosage form is of great value for nasal administration. To prove this statement, Lu et al. [33]. studied the pharmacokinetics of PEG-PLA-α-asarum nanoparticles in the brain after intranasal and intravenous administration. Using rats as animal models, hemodynamics, cerebral pharmacokinetics, and fluorescent labeling were used to observe the comparative study on the distribution. The results showed that PEG-PLA-α-asarum brain nanoparticles showed more obvious brain target effect than the intravenous injection and PEG-PLA-α-asarum brain nanoparticles were suitable for nasal administration to treat brain diseases. Currently, therapies that reduce gene expression in brain diseases require long-term administration of cerebrospinal fluid (CSF) via intrathecal perfusion or direct intra-brain injection. Although they may well tolerate it in the short term, this approach is not feasible throughout the management life cycle. Vasyl et al. [34] had found nanoparticles rich in shell sugar resistant to HTT siRNA in the nasal-brain pathway in the genetically modified YAC128 mouse model of Huntington's disease (HD). So they designed a series of chitosan-based nanoparticle (NP) preparations, which were coated with anti-HTT small interfering RNA (siRNA) to protect the effective carrying drug from being degraded before reaching the target. Later, through the same animal model, they found the factors that could increase the effective nanocarrier production of anti-HTT siRNA, and four nanocarrier preparations were found to effectively reduce HTT mRNA expression by at least 50%. Therefore, nasal administration of nanoparticles carrying siRNA is a promising, safe, and effective treatment option for reducing mutant HTT expression. siRNA-rich chitosan nanoparticles can effectively reduce Huntington's disease gene expression after nasal administration. In conclusion, because the organism has good tolerance to nanoparticles, this dosage form is of great value for nasal administration.

As a new type of drug carrier, nanoparticles are currently the focus of research. Nanoparticles have high drug loading, high encapsulation efficiency, suitable preparation and purification methods, appropriate particle size, and shape, can control drug release, increase efficacy, and have low or no toxicity. Therefore, nanomedicine has a faster dissolution rate, increased penetrating ability, stable drug effect, controlled release in vivo, enhanced action targeting, and improved oral absorption of poorly soluble drugs and can be used as a special carrier for biological macromolecules. So, it is reasonable to say that using nanoparticles as carriers has overcome many shortcomings and unsolvable problems of traditional drugs and will have broad application prospects in the future.

5.4.7 Summary

After finishing the literature research [35], we found that in terms of preparations, more researched formulations are new formulations such as liposomes, gels, and nano-formulations. These new formulations are mainly designed to prolong the residence time of the drug in the nasal mucosa and reduce the stimulation of the drug on the mucous membranes can improve the bioavailability of the drug. In clinical applications, they are beneficial to the study of the nasal-brain pathway and increase the brain intake of the drug to treat central nervous system diseases such as Alzheimer's disease. Although there have been more in-depth research reports on nasal administration in recent years, the only approved for marketing are sprays that have been widely used clinically, and other new nasal formulations remain at the basic research stage, this situation may be related to the immature in the preparation of new dosage forms and unstable product quality. At the same time, many dosage forms are still far away from industrial production, which severely restricts the development of new formulations for nasal administration. In terms of the development in nasal administration, we should focus more on the basic and applied research on nasal preparations, especially the development of new auxiliaries, new technologies, and new processes for nasal preparations. At the same time, the preclinical pharmacokinetics, pharmacodynamics, nasal mucosal toxicity, and irritation of such preparations are the prominent consideration that needs more attention. At last, we believe that the development and in-depth studies in nasal administration will be potential competition for some traditional administration as they showed a low targeted induction and are not convenient for patients to use on their own.

5.5 The Combination of Traditional Chinese Medicine and Modern Preparations

As an important part of the splendid culture of the Chinese nation, TCM has its own independent and complete theoretical knowledge system. Nowadays, many people choose TCM in their daily lives like acupuncture, massage, and pulses, which proves TCM's unshakable advantages and status.

With the continuous improvement of medical technology, traditional Chinese medicine preparation methods have been unable to meet the development needs of traditional Chinese medicine modernization. We should not focus on the past but also inherit and develop traditional Chinese medicine preparations under the guidance of the theory of traditional Chinese medicine which could combine traditional Chinese medicine with modern preparations to create new Chinese medicine preparations.

5.5.1 Inclusive Compound Preparation Technology

Inclusive compound preparation technology [36] refers to a technology in which one molecule is contained in the hole structure of another molecule to form an inclusion compound. The inclusion compound is composed of a host molecule and a guest molecule. The main molecule refers to an outer molecule having an encapsulation effect, and the minor molecule refers to a small molecule substance contained in a hole of the host molecule. Cyclodextrin (CD) and its derivatives are commonly used inclusion materials.

Wang et al. [37] explored the feasibility of the intranasal release of asarum hydroxypropyl-β-cyclodextrin solution into the brain. The extract of *Asarum chinensis* (also known as α-asarone), a traditional Chinese medicine, is mainly used in pneumonia, asthma, and seizures. Asarum brain has low oral bioavailability, and the injection itself has poor safety and poor applicability and may cause harm to patients. Asarum brain and hydroxypropyl-*n*-*n*-cyclodextrin formed an inclusion compound. After nasal irrigation, the absorption of blood and ethmoid brain was higher than that of a water-saturated solution, and the bioavailability of asarum in the brain was improved.

5.5.2 Solid Dispersion Technology

The solid dispersion system [38] refers to a system in which drugs are dispersed in a suitable carrier material in a molecular, colloidal, microcrystalline, or amorphous state. The method for making a drug into a solid dispersion is called solid dispersion technology. According to the state of the drug's dispersion, solid dispersions can be divided into eutectic mixtures, solid solutions, glass solutions, and coprecipitates.

The study found [39] that menthol has the effect of promoting transdermal drug absorption. Borneol and menthol at room temperature, in a certain percentage of the milling, may form a eutectic mixture, which can promote the percutaneous absorption of tetramethylpyrazine and present better results than using single borneol. Also, the borneol-menthol binary eutectic mixture can be stored for a long time under normal temperature conditions and retain its physical and chemical properties.

5.5.3 Microsphere Preparation Technology

Microspheres refer to tiny spherical entities formed by dissolving or dispersing drugs in excipients, and their particle size is usually at the nanometer level.

Astragalus polysaccharide is one of the main active ingredients of traditional Chinese medicine Huangqi (*Astragali Radix*) [40], which can be obtained through high-tech extraction and separation. Besides, it can increase the expression of cell surface adhesion molecules and promote lymphocyte recycling, thereby exerting immune enhancement and immune regulation effects. Astragalus polysaccharide/chitosan microspheres in nasal administration can make astragalus polysaccharides, which are better than nasal mucosa, and swell on the mucosal surface to form a film-like substance, preventing allergens from contacting the nasal mucosa.

5.5.4 Nanotechnology

Curcumin is an effective drug for the treatment of Alzheimer's disease (AD) [41]. It is a natural active ingredient extracted from Jianghuang (*Curcumae Longae Rhizoma*). However, curcumin has a short half-life in the body, low water solubility, poor stability, fast metabolism, and low oral bioavailability. About 89% of the curcumin is excreted in its original form, and high-dose oral administration of this drug will cause gastrointestinal discomfort, greatly limiting its clinical application. Curcumin polylactic-*co*-glycolic acid copolymer nanoparticles (Cur-PLGA-NPs) were prepared using polylactic-*co*-glycolic acid copolymer (PLGA) as a carrier material by an improved self-emulsifying solvent volatilization method. In the study of pharmacokinetic behavior in rats and its brain tissue distribution, Cur-PLGA-NPs significantly increased the accumulation of curcumin in vivo and brain tissue and delayed elimination after nasal administration.

Traditional Chinese medicine preparations are mainly used as ointments, soup, powders, and pills, while modern Chinese medicine preparations [42] have been comprehensively developed based on soups, powders, and pills. Today, traditional Chinese medicine preparations are almost the same as western medicine preparations, such as tablets, capsules, ointments, gel preparations, and so on. With the development of science and technology, new technologies and new dosage forms of traditional Chinese medicine preparations have appeared, such as clathrate technology, liposome technology, solid dispersion technology, microcapsule and microsphere technology, nanotechnology, etc. They use scientific and reasonable preparation methods to produce safe, effective, and controllable quality preparations and reduce the toxic and side effects of drugs and improve the scientificity, controllability, and advanced nature of drug treatment. In recent years, the safety issues of Chinese medicine injections have occurred frequently. Therefore, the development of Chinese medicine types with good curative effects and high safety such as mucosal administration has become a research hotspot. However, there are still shortcomings in the nasal administration of Chinese medicine. On the one hand, the compound Chinese medicine has a larger dose, and the nasal mucosa dose needs to be increased compared with the injection. However, the nasal cavity's drug-bearing volume is limited, and its unique physiological structure may lead to an inaccurate inhaled dose administered; on the other hand, the composition of traditional Chinese medicine is complex, and the detection in vivo is relatively difficult. It is not easy to select an absorption enhancer based on the absorption metabolism of the representative component and to achieve the efficacy; sometimes, it is necessary to choose a slightly more toxic absorption or accelerators which may cause certain irritation and damage to the nasal cavity.

5.6 Problems and Prospects

5.6.1 Problems

Nasal administration [43] is a drug delivery method that can be efficiently and quickly absorbed, has high bioavailability, can avoid the first-pass effect of the liver, and is convenient to use, non-invasive, and convenient to carry. Besides, it is a non-invasive brain-targeted drug delivery method that can bypass the blood-brain barrier and directly enter the brain. It is especially suitable for the elderly and infants, stroke patients with dysphagia, and patients with brain diseases. Although we have seen the advantages of nasal administration, there are still some problems in nasal administration that we need to solve and overcome.

After collating and analyzing the relevant literature, we found that modern medicine studies focus more on the nasal-brain pathway in nasal administration for the treatment of central nervous system diseases, which has reduced its application value; plus the blood concentration and the complex relationship between brain and drug concentration make it difficult to predict the drug concentration in the brain. At the same time, the dose of drugs administered in the nasal cavity is also limited. To achieve the efficacy, we need to increase the residence time of the drugs in the nasal cavity and pay attention to the drug loading of the preparation. So far, the specific brain-entry mechanism of drugs administered through the nasal cavity is still difficult to figure out. In terms of experimental models in vivo, we often use experimental animals such as rats as research objects, but the mucosa of the olfactory region of rats is much larger than that of humans, which is not convincing. Besides, in the course of administration, the drug may have certain irritation and toxicity to the mucous membranes and cilia in the nasal cavity. Furthermore, some excipients were added for the sake of stability, permeability or bioavailability of drugs, while the potential toxicity of them are not easy to detect in the clinic. In TCM's nasal administration, medicines are mostly some products with strong smell and irritation, which can easily cause damage to the mucosa if used accidentally. The modern research on the mechanism of nasal clearance mostly follows the ideas and methods of chemical drugs and biological drugs. They have not formed their theoretical system, and most of their research objects are aromatic drugs. In conclusion, the existence of these problems has prompted researchers to actively find solutions to problems.

5.6.2 Prospects

With the development of new dosage forms and the continuous improvement of drug delivery devices, the nasal drug delivery system will become a more convenient, effective, and fast drug delivery route and improve the bioavailability of drugs. At the same time, it found another way of drug delivery system that could penetrate the blood-brain barrier, made targeted drug delivery possible, and provided an effective way to treat central nervous system diseases. Besides, some companies are constantly improving nasal drug delivery devices to make the dosage more accurate, a better absorption effect, and a novel method of drug administration that is more in line with the physiological characteristics of the human body. Although most of the current nasal preparations are only focused on the treatment of local and acute conditions such as allergic rhinitis, migraine, epilepsy. They will certainly exert great potential in the treatment of systemic and brain diseases. Traditional Chinese medicine has a long history in clinical nasal administration and clinical experience. Therefore, the nasal administration system of traditional Chinese medicine will have broad development prospects with the advancement in new technology, new auxiliary material, new administrative devices, and new applications. We believed that in the coming future, China will have more Chinese medicine nasal preparations with independent intellectual property rights on the market that meet the needs of clinical disease treatment.

References

1. Rong, L., Honggui, C., Yanshou, H., & Wu, W. (2000). Application of nasal administration of traditional Chinese medicine in emergencies. *Chinese Folk Therapy, 8*(06), 48–49.
2. Guo, X., Jiayong, L., Lin, C., & Yang, F. (2011). Exploration of medicines used for nasal administration of traditional Chinese medicine to treat brain diseases. *Journal of Guangdong College of Pharmacy, 27*(02), 211–214.
3. Wu, W., Haiyan, Z., Wei, S., He, Y., Fang, L., Zheng, Q., & Yang, M. (2011). Study on transnasal administration of Chinese medicine. *Chinese Journal of Experimental Prescriptions, 17*(20), 288–292.
4. Yanru, S. (2011). History of nasal medicine therapy in traditional Chinese medicine. *Clinical Research of Traditional Chinese Medicine, 3*(09), 122.
5. Libin, Z., & Yuan, R. (2007). Research progress of nasal administration of traditional Chinese medicine. *Gansu Chinese Medicine, 20*(12), 66–68.
6. Peng, B., & Yongchang, S. (2013). History of inhalation therapy (1). *Chinese Journal of Tuberculosis and Respiratory Medicine, 36*(07), 555–556.
7. Peng, B., & Yongchang, S. (2013). History of inhalation therapy (2). *Chinese Journal of Tuberculosis and Respiratory Diseases, 36*(11), 876–877.
8. Chinese Medicine Research Promotion Association. (2005). Research progress of new dosage forms for nasal administration. China Association for the promotion of traditional Chinese medicine. In *Compilation of the second National Conference on the Application of New Medicinal Excipients and New Technologies of Traditional Chinese Medicine* (pp. 77–81). Chinese Medicine Research Promotion Association.
9. Zhu Huaxu, Guo Liwei, Lu Jin, et al. (2014). The "particle size" problem in the design of transnasal brain targeted preparations and its solution. In *2014 Annual Meeting of Jiangsu Provincial Particle Society and Jiangsu Environmental Protection Technology Proceedings of the 2014 Symposium* (pp. 339–345).
10. Zhenzhen, W., Xiaoyan, F., Shuike, F., Mengfan, P., Ming, B., & Mingsan, M. (2019). Research progress of Chinese medicine based on "nasal-brain" pathway in preventing and treating cerebral ischemic injury. *Chinese Journal of Traditional Chinese Medicine, 44*(22), 4800.

11. Cheng, Y. (2013). Research progress of transnasal brain targeted drug delivery. Chinese Medicine Preparation Branch of Chinese Society of Chinese Medicine, World Federation of Chinese Medicine Societies Professional Committee of Chinese Medicine Pharmacy. In *"Good Doctor Cup" TCM Preparation Innovation and Development Forum Proceedings (Part 2)* (pp. 405–408).
12. Wang, P., & Xuefeng, X. (2013). Research progress of transnasal brain targeted drug delivery system. *Modern Medicine and Clinic, 28*(01), 96–100.
13. Nan, L., & Tan, Y. (2017). Overview of traditional Chinese medicine customs clearance. *Shi Zhen Guo Yi Guo Yao, 28*(08), 1971–1974.
14. Na, H. (2011). Overview of the application of Chinese medicine nasal drops in the past ten years. In *The General Assembly of the Otolaryngology and Stomatology Professional Committee of WFCMS and the third academic annual meeting and the 17th academic exchange meeting of the Otolaryngology Branch of the Chinese Society of Chinese Medicine and the otolaryngology academic exchange meeting of the Guangdong Society of Traditional Chinese Medicine and Integrative Medicine* (pp. 535–539).
15. Peng, G., & Gao, J. (2014). Research progress of Chinese medicine nasal drops. *Anhui Medicine, 18*(06), 1001–1004.
16. Zhendong, C., Yan, M., Zhengyi, G., Jinhua, H., Xiaocui, C., Xintang, W., & Yan, L. (2018). Optimization of extraction process of compound artemisia annua nasal drops. *Chinese Traditional Patent Medicine, 40*(04), 957–961.
17. Xie, W. (2014). Research progress of nasal administration of traditional Chinese medicine. *Journal of Baotou Medical College, 30*(02), 135–137.
18. Hasmu, H., Xu, L., Hu, M., & Lanlan, Z. (2017). Experimental study on acute toxicity, local irritation and allergy of Cangxin aerosol. *Xinjiang Medicine, 47*(11), 1250–1253.
19. Wang, J., Guo, J., Wang, T., Wang, J., Xiaofeng, C., Zhitao, J., & Yu, H. (2017). Pharmacokinetics and brain targeting study of Toutongning nasal spray in rats. *Chinese Pharmacy, 28*(34), 4804–4807.
20. Yang, P., Wanqing, L., Ying, L., Jianxu, S., Hui, Z., Gao, J., Xiaoxing, Y., & Zheng, A. (2017). Preparation and evaluation of naloxone hydrochloride nasal spray. *International Journal of Pharmaceutical Research, 44*(06), 616–621.
21. Huimin, F., & Fugen, G. (2018). Advances in the research and clinical application of new dosage forms for nasal administration. *West China Journal of Pharmacy, 33*(05), 548–554.
22. Xinfang, L., Xiangui, L., Ma, Z., Yanqiang, Z., Gao, Y., & Yang, F. (2017). Preparation and safety study of menthol nasal gel in situ [J]. *Journal of Pharmaceutical Practice, 35*(04), 321–324, 366.
23. Yu, S., Xiaofang, L., Wu, S., Ling, L., & Yijing, W. (2014). Research progress on the application of in-situ gel delivery system in traditional Chinese medicine preparations. *Journal of Chengdu University of Traditional Chinese Medicine, 37*(03), 120–123.
24. Dong, F., Zhu, H., Li, L., Zhiliang, C., & Qiang, L. (2013). Pharmacokinetics of Zhibing in-situ gel rabbit in vivo. *Chinese Journal of Experimental Prescriptions, 19*(02), 144–147.
25. He, W., Miao, X., & Guo, X. (2017). Pharmacokinetics and brain targeting of gastrodin nasal in situ gel in rats. *Chinese Pharmacist, 20*(01), 68–72.
26. Nazar, H., Fatouros, D. G., van der Merwe, S. M., Bouropoulos, N., Avgouropoulos, G., Tsibouklis, J., & Roldo, M. (2011). Thermosensitive hydrogels for nasal drug delivery: The formulation and characterisation of systems based on N -trimethyl chitosan chloride. *European Journal of Pharmaceutics and Biopharmaceutics, 77*(2), 24–28.
27. Hong, D. (2008). *Research on the key technology of microemulsion drug loading system of traditional Chinese medicine*. Beijing University of Chinese Medicine.
28. Wanggang, Z., Zheng, G., Liangzhong, L., Wang, S., & Guoshen, C. (2014). Nasal administration of huperzine a microemulsion to the palate cilia of the toad and the nasal mucosa of the rat. *China Pharmaceutical Industry Journal, 45*(12), 1160–1162.

29. Shinde, R. L., Bharkad, G. P., & Devarajan, P. V. (2015). Intranasal microemulsion for targeted nose to brain delivery in neurocysticercosis: Role of docosahexaenoic acid. *European Journal of Pharmaceutics and Biopharmaceutics, 96*, 363.
30. Gang, K., Wu, Z., Yang, M., Guilin, R., Jumin, H., Hu, P., & Wang, S. (2015). Analysis and application of liposome technology conversion and key issues. *World Chinese Medicine, 10*(03), 331–336.
31. Cheng, Z., Jianping, H., Zhu, W., Yinghao, Z., & Yingzheng, Z. (2019). Effect of nasal administration of icariin liposomes on ethology and neurotransmitters in Parkinson's disease rats [J]. *Modern Chinese Doctors, 57*(19), 43–47.
32. Kong, X., Guo, M., Ying, F., & Yan, H. (2015). Research progress of nano-targeted preparations. *Journal of Guangxi Medical University, 32*(04), 682–685.
33. Lu, J., Champion, Z., & Guo, L. (2019). Pharmacokinetics of PEG-PLA-α-asarone brain nanoparticles after nasal and intravenous administration. *Modern Chinese Applied Pharmacy, 36*(19), 2411–2416.
34. Sava, V., Fihurka, O., Khvorova, A., & Sanchez-Ramos, J. (2020). Enriched chitosan nanoparticles loaded with siRNA are effective in lowering Huntington's disease gene expression following intranasal administration. *Nanomedicine: Nanotechnology, Biology, and Medicine, 24*, 102119.
35. Yan, X., Yu, L., Tan, Y., & Nan, L. (2020). Application of new dosage forms and new technologies in the transnasal brain targeted drug delivery system of active ingredients of traditional Chinese medicine. *Chinese Patent Medicine, 42*(04), 991–995.
36. Qiuyan, H. (2016). *Cang wormwood oil inclusion compound-in-situ gel preparation and nasal absorption pharmacokinetics study*. Yunnan University of Traditional Chinese Medicine.
37. Wang, G., Pan, Y., Kong, Q., & Jun, T. (2012). The feasibility of intracerebral drug release of asarone hydroxypropyl-β-cyclodextrin solution for nasal administration. *Chinese Journal of Experimental Pharmacology, 18*(03), 16–18.
38. Paudwal, G., Rawat, N., Gupta, R., Baldi, A., Singh, G., & Gupta, P. N. (2019). Recent advances in solid dispersion technology for efficient delivery of poorly water-soluble drugs. *Current Pharmaceutical Design, 25*(13), 1524.
39. Guobao, C., Pan, Y., & Fanzhu, L. (2009). The effect of borneol-menthol eutectic on neurotoxin nanoparticles loaded into the brain by nasal administration. *China Journal of Chinese Materia Medica, 34*(06), 698–701.
40. Yuqing, S., Wentao, L., Kang, L., Limin, Z., & Weifen, Z. (2017). The therapeutic effect of astragalus polysaccharide/chitosan sustained-release microspheres on allergic rhinitis in rats. *Journal of Shandong University (Medical Edition), 55*(09), 60–65.
41. Xiaoli, Y., Wang, F., Qingyu, L., Wang, B., Xinjun, C., Ling, C., Zhu, J., & Wei, Y. (2017). Preparation and curative study of curcumin PLGA nanoparticles. *Chinese Journal of Traditional Chinese Medicine, 35*(03), 728–731.
42. Cheng, L. (2019). Application of new technology of pharmaceutical preparation in modern Chinese medicine. *Electronic Journal of Clinical Medicine Literature, 6*(85), 192.
43. Pingping, Z., & Wenyang, F. (2013). The latest research progress of Chinese medicine preparations for nasal administration. *Chinese Medical Guide, 11*(14), 65–66.

Chapter 6
Brain-Targeting Drug Delivery Systems for Chinese Medicines

Baolin Huang and Zheng Cai

Abstract Many Chinese medicines are used to treat brain diseases. However, due to the blood-brain barrier (BBB), drugs can hardly reach the site of action. In this chapter, the research situation of brain-targeting delivery systems for Chinese medicines in recent years is introduced. The physiological structure characteristics of the BBB and the establishment of a BBB model in vitro are briefly described. The common strategies for promoting Chinese medicines to cross the BBB are comprehensively reviewed. These strategies include intranasal administration, penetration enhancers, prodrugs, and nanoparticle carriers. In addition to modern pharmaceutical technology, some traditional methods are used in brain-targeting drug delivery systems for Chinese medicine.

Keywords Brain targeting · Chinese medicine · Intranasal drug delivery · Penetration enhancer · Prodrug · Nanoparticle carrier

6.1 Introduction

Many Chinese medicines, such as *Danshen* (*Salviae Miltiorrhizae Radix et Rhizoma*), *Huangqin* (*Scutellariae Radix*), and *Tianma* (*Gastrodiae Rhizoma*), are commonly used in the treatment of brain diseases. They have neuroprotective effects that can effectively slow down brain injury. However, due to the physiological blood-brain barrier (BBB), the drug concentration in the brain is insufficient, leading to unsatisfactory effects. Therefore, brain-targeting drug delivery systems for Chinese medicines should be developed. The brain-targeting delivery of Chinese medicine can play an important role in the treatment of brain diseases, such as stroke, Alzheimer's disease (AD), and brain tumors [1].

In ancient China, some brain-targeting drug delivery methods have been developed to treat brain diseases. According to *Pu Ji Fang* (*Formulary of Universal*

B. Huang · Z. Cai (✉)
School of Pharmaceutical Sciences, Southern Medical University, Guangzhou, China
e-mail: caizheng@fimmu.com

N. Feng, Z. Yang (eds.), *Novel Drug Delivery Systems for Chinese Medicines*,
https://doi.org/10.1007/978-981-16-3444-4_6

Relief), garlic juice was dropped into the nose to treat headaches. *Zhou Hou Bei Ji Fang* (*Handbook of Prescriptions for Emergencies*) recorded that washing the nose with raw radish juice could treat migraine [2]. *Ben Cao Gang Mu* (*Compendium of Materia Medica*) recorded that ginger juice was dropped into the nose to treat headaches. *Zhang Zhongjing*, a famous doctor of traditional Chinese medicine (TCM) in the Han Dynasty, said that placing *Xiebai* (*Allii Macrostemonis Bulbus*) juice into the nose could treat delirium [3]. In summary, most of the traditional brain-targeting drug delivery systems were mainly administered through the nose. In addition, some aromatic penetration enhancers were used [4].

Modern medical research shows that the BBB is the biggest obstacle for drugs to enter the brain [5]. Previous studies on brain-targeting strategies are mainly based on intranasal drug delivery, the combination of penetration enhancers, and simple structural modification. With the development of technology, an increasing number of targeting technologies, such as nanotechnology, transporter-mediated, monoclonal antibody-mediated, and focused ultrasound microbubble brain-targeting techniques, have been developed. At present, the brain-targeting drug delivery strategies are mainly divided into invasive and non-invasive strategies [6], while the brain-targeting drug delivery strategies used in Chinese medicines can be divided into five categories, including intranasal administration, penetration enhancers, prodrugs, nanoparticle carriers, and other strategies.

In this chapter, the research situation and progress of brain-targeting drug delivery systems for Chinese medicines are reviewed.

6.2 Physiological Barrier of the Brain for Drug Delivery

Drugs need to pass through the brain's physiological barrier before entering the brain to exert their effects. The brain has five principal barrier interfaces that protect the central nervous system (CNS): (a) the BBB, (b) the arachnoid barrier, (c) the blood-cerebrospinal fluid barrier, (d) the circumventricular organs, and (e) the ependyma (Fig. 6.1) [6]. Among them, the BBB is the most important in the design of brain-targeting drug delivery [7]. The BBB poses a severe challenge to the treatment of CNS diseases and the development of brain-targeting drug delivery systems. At present, 98% of small molecular drugs and recombinant proteins, peptides, antibodies, and viral vectors including adeno-associated virus for macromolecular therapy cannot work because of the physiological barrier of the brain [6]. Therefore, we must fully understand the brain's physiological barrier and design a brain-targeting strategy according to this barrier.

The BBB is a special barrier between the blood and brain tissue, and it is mainly composed of brain capillary endothelial cells (BCECs), pericytes (PCs), astrocytes (ACs), and the extracellular matrix [8]. The tight junction between BCECs is a necessary condition for BBB function formation. BCECs and their tight junction are important barriers to plasma and foreign neurotoxic components [9, 10]. PCs are embedded in the microvascular basement membrane between BCECs and ACs and

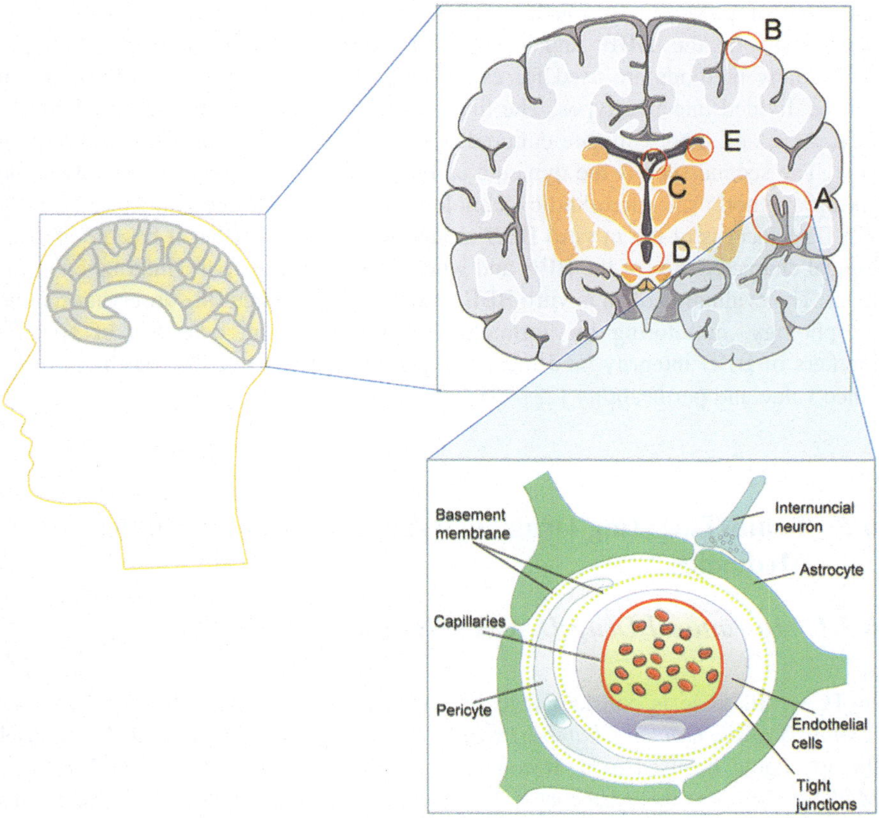

Fig. 6.1 Barriers in the human brain: (*A*) the blood-brain barrier, (*B*) the arachnoid barrier, (*C*) the blood-cerebrospinal fluid barrier, (*D*) the circumventricular organs, and (*E*) the ependyma

extend to all sides. The terminal foot of glial cells formed by ACs is embedded in the outermost matrix membrane and plays an important role in the regulation of CNS homeostasis [11]. Intermediate neurons connect with ACs at the outermost periphery of the BBB to conduct electrical signals [6] (Fig. 6.1).

The cells of the BBB express many functional proteins, including inflammatory proteins, tight junction proteins, and transporters, which mainly affect the permeability of the BBB. The transporters include solute carrier (SLC) and ATP-binding cassette transporters [12]. At present, the brain-targeted delivery strategies of Chinese medicines using functional protein mainly include SLC proteins to transport drugs to the brain [13], downregulation of the expression of tight junction proteins, the temporary opening of the BBB to allow the drugs to enter the brain [14], and inhibition of the activity of efflux proteins to reduce drug efflux [15]. In addition, the expression of inflammatory proteins can affect the permeability of the BBB [16].

The establishment of an in vitro BBB model is important for the development of brain-targeting drug delivery systems. The BBB function of the human brain in vivo should be reproduced as much as possible to enhance the prediction of drug penetration in the BBB and design brain-targeting drug delivery strategies [17]. Many methods are used for establishing an in vitro model of BBB, which can be divided into two types. The first type is the static culture method. BCECs, PCs, ACs, and other cells are cultured or co-cultured in the transwell culture pool [18]. The second type is the dynamic culture method. The representative dynamic culture method uses microfluidic technology to co-culture three kinds of cells [19–22]. The success of the in vitro BBB model depends on whether it has the physiological characteristics of the BBB and whether it can simulate the internal environment. The evaluation of an in vitro BBB model mainly includes the observation of its morphology, monitoring the formation of tight junction, detection of specific markers of BBB integrity, and measurement of the transepithelial electrical resistance value and permeability [23].

6.3 Brain-Targeting Drug Delivery Strategies for Chinese Medicines

6.3.1 Intranasal Drug Delivery Systems

In TCM, the nose is considered to be connected to the brain. *Jin Gui Yao Lue* (*Synopsis of the Golden Chamber*) written by *Zhang Zhongjing* recorded that nasal therapy could be used to treat coma. *Yi Lin Gai Cuo* (*Correction on Errors in Medical Classics*) recorded that "The nose is connected with the brain, and odor smelled by the nose will be transmitted to the brain." Relatively complete and systemic nasal therapy was recorded in *Li Yue Pian Wen* (*Rhymed Discourses on External Therapy*), a classic TCM book published in the Qing Dynasty. Many nasal therapies for the treatment of encephalopathy were recorded in this book [24]. Based on the above literatures, the treatment of encephalopathy by nasal administration has a long history. Nasal administration methods in TCM mainly include dripping, perfusion, and fumigation [25].

Anatomically, a direct pathway exists between the nasal cavity and the brain that bypasses BBB [26]. Modern medicine studies show that the brain-targeting pathways of intranasal administration include the olfactory epithelium, olfactory nerve, and blood circulation pathways. In the olfactory epithelial pathway, the drug passes through the basement membrane into the lamina propria, enters the peripheral olfactory nerve, and then is transported to the CNS [27]. In the olfactory pathway, the drug is absorbed through the olfactory mucosa and enters the olfactory neurons through endocytosis or endocytosis. The intracellular axons transport the drug along the neurons to the olfactory bulb and then further distribute it in the CNS [28]. In the blood circulation pathway, the drug is absorbed directly in the highly vascularized nasal respiratory epithelium and lymphatic system and then transferred to the systemic circulation [29, 30] (Fig. 6.2).

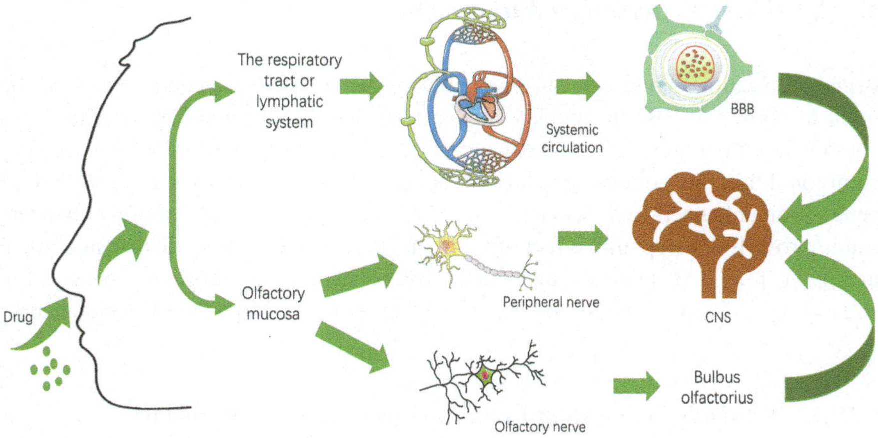

Fig. 6.2 Brain-targeting mechanism of intranasal administration

The olfactory mucosal and olfactory nerve pathways help drugs bypass the BBB to achieve rapid administration and absorption and eliminate the first-pass effect of the liver and kidney to improve the brain transport of Chinese medicine for the treatment of brain diseases. The active components of Chinese medicines, such as resveratrol, baicalin, and quercetin, are carried by nano-liposomes or nano-emulsions for intranasal administration. The brain-targeting efficiency of these drugs has been enhanced [31–33]. Perillyl alcohol (POH), a natural compound with strong anticancer activity, has been developed as a nasal spray by Chen et al. Clinical tests show that POH nasal spray has obvious anticancer activity in patients with recurrent glioma and is well tolerated with almost no side effects. In addition, portable lightweight atomizers lead to very high (> 95%) patient compliance. The therapeutic effect of the intranasal administration of POH shows the brain-targeting capability and feasibility of the intranasal administration strategy [34]. Gastrodin, the main bioactive component of the Chinese medicine "*Tianma* (*Gastrodiae Rhizoma*)," is a hydrophilic small molecular compound. Therefore, it cannot cross the BBB easily. Cai et al. developed a novel ion-activated in situ gelling system for the nasal delivery of gastrodin, which can effectively improve the analgesic and sedative effects of gastrodin [35]. *Xingnaojing* Injection, a TCM compound injection containing gardenia-borneol co-compound, is widely used in the treatment of stroke. Lu et al. found that the bioavailability of the drug administered intranasally is almost equal to that administered intravenously. Compared with intravenous administration, intranasal drug delivery has the advantages of safety, convenience, and low cost, thus making the development of nasal drug delivery systems for brain-targeting delivery of Chinese medicines important [36].

6.3.2 Brain Penetration Enhancers

Brain penetration enhancers can reversibly open the BBB in specific areas of the brain to allow the BBB to quickly increase transient permeability [37]. The drugs combined with brain penetration enhancers can successfully enter into the brain. The common brain penetration enhancers include aromatic and non-aromatic TCM penetration enhancers and vasoactive substances. Using brain penetration enhancers can improve the therapeutic effect of brain diseases and has a long history in clinical treatment [38]. At present, the most widely used brain-targeting penetration enhancers for Chinese medicines are mainly aromatic TCM penetration enhancers.

6.3.2.1 Aromatic Penetration Enhancers from Chinese Medicines

Aromatic TCM penetration enhancers are called "aromatic resuscitation drugs" (Fig. 6.3) in TCM. Aromatic resuscitation drugs are a kind of messenger drug that guides the movement of drugs toward the brain [39]. Most of the aromatic resuscitation drugs are lipophilic small molecular compounds, which not only pass through the BBB easily but also have strong neuropharmacological effects [4]. Borneol is a simple bicyclic monoterpene extracted from borneol resin and volatile oil. As a representative of aromatic resuscitation drugs, borneol has been widely used in brain-targeted administration [40].

When some Chinese medicines or their active ingredients are used in combination with aromatic resuscitation drugs, they increase the brain transport of the drug and

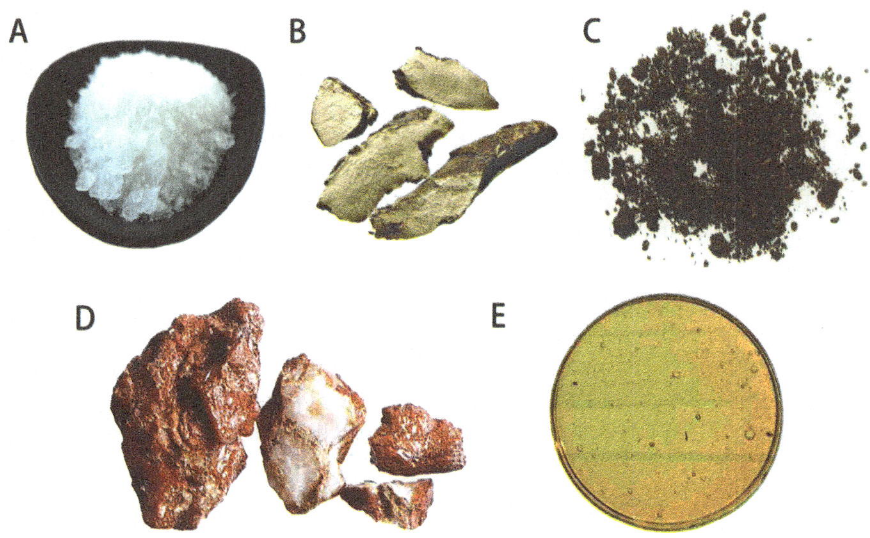

Fig. 6.3 Aromatic resuscitation drugs: (**a**) borneol, (**b**) *Rhizoma acori graminei*, (**c**) musk, (**d**) benzoin, and (**e**) styrax (*Liquidambar orientalis* Mill extract)

Table 6.1 Mechanism of BBB penetration enhancers

Penetration enhancer	Main effective components	Mechanism	References
Borneol	Borneol and isoborneol	Adenosine receptor is activated to downregulate the expression of ZO-1	[42]
Rhizoma acori graminei	Asarone	Adenosine receptor is activated to downregulate the expression of ZO-1	[42]
Musk	Muscone	The expression of P-gp and MMP-9 is downregulated	[43]
Styrax	Volatile oil of salicylic acid	Inhibit the efflux function of P-gp	[44]
Benzoin	Volatile oil of benzoin	Inhibit the efflux function of P-gp	[44]
Quercetin	Quercetin	Inhibit the efflux function of P-gp	[45]
Ginkgo biloba	Ginkgolide and ginkgo flavonoids	Ginkgolide activates the A1AR pathway and phosphorylates ERM/MLC protein, and ginkgo flavonoids downregulate P-gp expression	[46, 47]
BK	–	B1 and B2 are activated, and claudin-5 expression is downregulated	[48, 49]
RMP-7	–	B2 is activated, and claudin-5 expression is downregulated	[50]
RI-BK	–	B2 is activated, and claudin-5 expression is downregulated	[51]

avoid the risk of systemic toxicity. Considering that aromatic resuscitation drugs have the excellent penetration-promoting ability, the penetration enhancers of aromatic resuscitation drugs have become a research hotspot. Cai et al. investigate the effect of borneol on the distribution of gastrodin to the brain via oral administration. The results indicate that borneol can accelerate the absorption of gastrodin in the gastrointestinal tract and promote its distribution to the brain [41]. In a study on the penetration mechanism of aromatic resuscitation drugs, Wu et al. found that borneol and asarone (the main component of *Acorus calamus*) could promote the penetration of puerarin and tetramethylpyrazine through the BBB by activating the adenosine receptor (AR) pathway (including A1AR and A2AAR pathway) and downregulating the expression of tight junction protein zonula occludens-1 (ZO-1) [42]. Wang et al. proved that muscone, the main component of musk, could increase BBB permeability by downregulating the expression of P-glycoprotein (P-gp) and matrix metalloproteinases [43]. Yang et al. found that vanillin and benzoin, the active components of storesin and benzoin, could increase the permeability of P-gp by inhibiting the efflux function of the BBB [44] (Table 6.1).

6.3.2.2 Non-aromatic Penetration Enhancers from Chinese Medicines

In addition to aromatic resuscitation drugs, some non-aromatic Chinese medicines can increase BBB permeability. Quercetin is a classical flavonoid P-gp inhibitor. In the study of Youdim et al., the interaction between quercetin and P-gp inhibited the activity of P-gp, thus increasing BBB permeability [45]. Ginkgolides in *Ginkgo biloba* extract could induce ezrin/radixin/moesin and myosin light chain phosphorylation by activating the A1AR pathway. Phosphorylation causes actin filaments to contract at tight junctions and increases the intercellular gap, which results in a reversible increase in BBB permeability. In addition, the total glycosides of *Ginkgo biloba* flavonoids could downregulate the expression of P-gp and reduce the drug efflux [46, 47] (Table 6.1).

6.3.2.3 Vasoactive Substances

Vasoactive substances such as bradykinin (BK) and its active analogs (e.g., retro-inverso bradykinin (RI-BK) and RMP-7) can also temporarily open the BBB to allow the drugs to pass through the BBB [52–54]. BK is a component of the kallikrein-kinin system in the blood and brain parenchyma and acts through its BK type 1 receptor (B1R) and BK type 2 receptor (B2R) [55]. BK receptors on brain endothelial cells can downregulate the expression of claudin-5 and increase the permeability of BBB [48, 49]. RI-BK showed resistance to proteolysis and high binding activity to the B2R [50]. RMP-7 is a BK analog with a molecular weight of 1096 Da. Compared with BK, RMP-7 has a more selective binding ability to the BBB, and RMP-7 can stimulate the expression of the B2R in nerve tissue [54].

Kuo and Tsao et al. linked quercetin with RMP-7 and lactoferrin and encapsulated them with liposomes to transfer quercetin to human neuroepithelioma cells to prevent cell apoptosis and treat AD [51] (Table 6.1).

Metalloproteinase-9 (MMP-9) belongs to matrix metalloproteinase family and is a specific serum marker for degradation of the extracellular matrix after brain injury; ezrin/radixin/moesin (ERM)/myosin light chain (MLC) protein is an important actin-binding molecule and a target for threonine phosphorylation in various signal pathways to induce actin remodeling and control vascular permeability.

6.3.3 Prodrug Delivery Systems

The prodrug was first introduced by Adrien Albert in 1958. At that time, the concept of prodrug means that a compound becomes a compound with pharmacological action after biotransformation [56]. At present, prodrugs are derivatives or precursors of molecules with therapeutic activity. In vivo, prodrugs can be bioconverted into therapeutic molecules through spontaneous processes such as hydrolytic degradation or biocatalytic mechanisms [57].

In targeting research, prodrug design is an important strategy. For Chinese medicine brain-targeting delivery, the current prodrug strategy mainly includes ligand and chemical structure modification strategies.

6.3.3.1 Ligand Modification

The ligand modification strategy aims to modify the drug with ligands and transport the drug into the brain by using the affinity of the receptor and specific ligand in the brain [58, 59]. Considering the specific recognition of endogenous receptors on the surface of the BBB, the ligands of the receptors are used to construct brain-targeting drug delivery systems. The affinity binding between the receptors and ligands in the brain is used to transport drugs to the brain. The receptors commonly used in brain-targeting drug delivery systems include transferrin receptor (TfR), B2R, organic cation transporter, organic anion transporter, nutrients such as glucose transporter, amino acid transporter, low-density lipoprotein receptor, and related protein, *N*-acetylcholine receptor, insulin receptor, scavenger receptor class B type I, and diphtheria toxin receptor [60–62].

In brain-targeting research, the application prospect of ligand modification strategy is highly recognized. At present, it has been used in the targeting design of drugs for the treatment of neurodegenerative diseases and cerebral ischemia-reperfusion injury. In many application instances, the brain-targeting delivery of drugs modified by ligands has been enhanced. For example, Montaser et al. modified the natural phenolic compound ferulic acid with L-type amino acid transporter ligand (LAT1) to transport it to the BBB and treat neuroinflammation and neurodegenerative diseases [63]. Besides LAT1, other expression transporters in the BBB such as TfR also have the potential to become brain-targeting modified ligands for drugs [60]. To deliver salvianolic acid B and baicalin to brain tissue to repair the neuronal injury and improve cerebral ischemia-reperfusion injury, Wu constructed a nano-lipid carrier containing baicalin and salvianolic acid B modified with the TfR monoclonal antibody (OX26) [64].

6.3.3.2 Chemical Modification

Because the drugs that easily pass through the BBB generally have the characteristics of low molecular weight and high-fat solubility, the chemical modification strategy mainly aims to improve the affinity between the drug and biofilm by changing the physical and chemical properties, such as logP or pH, so that it can pass through the BBB smoothly. In addition, reducing the sensitivity of efflux protein to the drug by chemical modification can avoid the drug from being pumped out of the BBB [65, 66].

The chemically modified prodrug design strategy is widely used in the drug-targeting design of effective components of Chinese medicine. Gastrodin is derived from *Tianma*, a famous traditional Chinese herbal medicine. It is used to treat headaches, neurasthenia, and other brain diseases. Gastrodin is a highly water-soluble phenolic glucoside with poor liposolubility. In 1982, the Kunming Pharmaceutical Factory developed the tetrahydroxyacetylation product of gastrodin (acetylgastrodin) to increase its fat solubility and BBB permeability [67]. Resveratrol can improve lipid solubility and BBB permeability through alkylation [68]. The antitumor drug paclitaxel (PTX) was covalently linked with conjugated linoleic acid (CLA). CLA-PTX could be distributed into the brain tissue and maintained at a high concentration for 360 h. The antitumor effect of the CLA-PTX group was obviously higher than that of the PTX group [69]. In addition, another prodrug delivery strategy involves the modification of active groups that inhibit efflux proteins. Tanshinone was modified with tetramethylpyrazine, a P-gp inhibitor, to improve its brain-targeting capability [66].

6.3.4 Nanoparticle Drug Delivery Systems

Nanoparticle drug delivery systems are submicron drug carrier delivery systems belonging to the nanoscale category. Drug encapsulation in the submicron scale can adjust the release rate, increase the permeability of biofilm, change the distribution in vivo, and improve the bioavailability. Compared with common drug delivery systems, nanoparticle drug delivery systems have significant advantages in targeting drug delivery. Some nanoparticles can adhere to the olfactory epithelium and allow the drug to be transported by the cell side or within the cell, while in rare cases, particles smaller than 200 nm can be directly transported through olfactory and trigeminal pathways [29]. In addition, nanoparticle delivery systems can help drugs cross the BBB by using smaller size or functionalized surfaces.

In recent years, several brain-targeting nanoparticle drug delivery systems for Chinese medicines have been developed. Ahmad et al. used a double emulsion solvent evaporation method to develop chitosan-coated glycyrrhizic acid nanoparticles and found that the bioavailability of glycyrrhizic acid in the brain was obviously improved [70]. Mursaleen et al. developed a nano-carrier delivery system of antioxidant curcumin iron chelator deferoxamine and proved that the preparation effectively inhibited brain oxidative stress and cell damage [71]. Zheng et al. prepared nano-liposomes loaded with *Ginkgo biloba* extract by spray drying. This material could prolong the time of action, increase the distribution of drugs in the brain, and improve the poor bioavailability of *Ginkgo biloba* extract and had a good control effect on AD [72].

In addition, ginsenoside liposomes are used for the treatment of cerebral ischemia, and hyaluronic acid-modified PTX liposomes are used for the inhibition of brain tumor stem cells. The development of nanoparticle delivery drug systems can enhance the treatment of brain diseases with Chinese medicines [73–75].

6.3.5 Other Drug Delivery Systems

Besides the above brain-targeting delivery strategies, some other Chinese medicine brain-targeting strategies include intrathecal injection and focused ultrasound microbubbles. Intrathecal injection is an invasive drug delivery system, which has a certain risk of drug delivery, but it has good targeting. Focused ultrasound microbubbles temporarily open the BBB through physical technology to assist the drug to pass through the BBB to achieve brain targeting [76, 77].

At present, intrathecal injection is mainly used in the analgesic treatment of cancer patients. Morphine is commonly used for analgesia through intrathecal injection [78]. Kim et al. administered Korean red ginseng to the brain by intrathecal injection, which reduced the neuropathic pain induced by chemotherapy [79].

Focused ultrasound microbubbles are still in the early stage of development and are currently applied in the treatment of cancer and neurodegenerative diseases. According to the literature, ultrasound microbubbles loaded with PTX and doxorubicin trigger the targeted delivery in the brain, resulting in the targeted and continuous drug delivery for tumor therapy [80].

6.4 Conclusion

At present, the research strategies of brain-targeting drug delivery systems for Chinese medicines include nasal drug delivery, penetration enhancer, prodrug delivery, nanoparticle drug delivery, intrathecal injection, and focused ultrasound microbubble targeting strategies. Among them, intranasal administration is the most widely used in brain-targeting drug delivery design for Chinese medicine. However, the compliance of nasal administration is not ideal. Penetration enhancers are easy to use, but some of them can cause mucosal irritation. The research and development of safe and efficient penetration enhancers are of great significance. In recent years, nanoparticle drug delivery systems have become a research hotspot. Nanotechnology can achieve better targeting, but druggability and industrialization of the nanoparticle drug delivery systems need to be developed.

Overall, the current brain-targeting drug delivery strategies for Chinese medicine have their advantages and disadvantages. In the follow-up research and development, the mechanism should be studied to determine exact targets and targeted molecules, further improve the targeting efficiency, and simplify the production process, which will promote the use of more brain-targeting drug delivery systems for Chinese medicines in the clinic.

References

1. Yu, S., Fu, L., Lu, J., Wang, Z., & Fu, W. (2020). Xiao-Yao-San reduces blood-brain barrier injury induced by chronic stress in vitro and vivo via glucocorticoid receptor-mediated upregulation of Occludin. *Journal of Ethnopharmacology, 246*, 112–165.
2. Wei, Z. Z., Fang, X. Y., Fan, S. K., Peng, M. F., Bai, M., & Miao, M. S. (2019). Research progress on traditional Chinese medicine in preventing and treating cerebral ischemia injury based on "nose-brain" pathway. *China Journal of Chinese Material Medicine, 44*(22), 4800–4805. (Chinese).
3. Dong, Y., Di, L. Q., Zhao, X. L., Bi, X. L., Li, J. S., & Cai, B. C. (2019). Pharmaceutical research progress in the design of brain drug delivery system for intranasal administration. *Chinese Pharmacological Journal, 21*(3), 271–273. (Chinese).
4. Zhang, Q. L., Fu, B. M., & Zhang, Z. J. (2017). Borneol, a novel agent that improves central nervous system drug delivery by enhancing blood-brain barrier permeability. *Drug Delivery, 24*(1), 1037–1044.
5. Dufès, C., Al Robaian, M., & Somani, S. (2013). Transferrin and the transferrin receptor for the targeted delivery of therapeutic agents to the brain and cancer cells. *Drug Delivery and Translational Research, 4*(5), 629–640.
6. Pandit, R., Chen, L., & Gotz, J. (2019). The blood-brain barrier: Physiology and strategies for drug delivery. *Advanced Drug Delivery Reviews*. https://doi.org/10.1016/j.addr.2019.11.009
7. Zhou, Y., Peng, Z., Seven, E. S., & Leblanc, R. M. (2018). Crossing the blood-brain barrier with nanoparticles. *Journal of Controlled Release, 270*, 290–303.
8. Park, T. E., Mustafaoglu, N., Herland, A., Hasselkus, R., Mannix, R., FitzGerald, E. A., & Prantil-Baun, R. (2019). Hypoxia-enhanced blood-brain barrier chip recapitulates human barrier function and shuttling of drugs and antibodies. *Nature Communications, 10*(1), 2621.
9. Rustenhoven, J., & Kipnis, J. (2019). Bypassing the blood-brain barrier. *Science, 366*(6472), 1448–1449.
10. Abdulkadir, R. R., Alwjwaj, M., Othman, O. A., Rakkar, K., & Bayraktutan, U. (2020). Outgrowth endothelial cells form a functional cerebral barrier and restore its integrity after damage. *Neural Regeneration Research, 15*(6), 1071–1078.
11. Ma, F., Zhang, X., & Yin, K. J. (2020). MicroRNAs in central nervous system diseases: A prospective role in regulating blood-brain barrier integrity. *Experimental Neurology, 323*, 1130–1194.
12. Arvanitis, C. D., Ferraro, G. B., & Jain, R. K. (2020). The blood-brain barrier and blood-tumour barrier in brain tumours and metastases. *Nature Reviews. Cancer, 20*(1), 26–41.
13. Liu, H., Yu, N., Lu, S., Ito, S., Zhang, X., Prasad, B., He, E., Lu, X., Li, Y., Wang, F., Xu, H., An, G., Unadkat, J. D., Kusuhara, H., Sugiyama, Y., & Sahi, J. (2015). Solute carrier family of the organic anion-transporting polypeptides 1A2- Madin-Darby Canine Kidney II: A promising in vitro system to understand the role of organic anion-transporting polypeptide 1A2 in blood-brain barrier drug penetration. *Drug Metabolism and Disposition, 43*(7), 1008–1018.
14. Lochhead, J. J., Ronaldson, P. T., & Davis, T. P. (2017). Hypoxic stress and inflammatory pain disrupt blood-brain barrier tight junctions: Implications for drug delivery to the central nervous system. *The AAPS Journal, 19*(4), 910–920.
15. Puech, C., Hodin, S., Forest, V., He, Z., Mismetti, P., Delavenne, X., & Perek, N. (2018). Assessment of HBEC-5i endothelial cell line cultivated in astrocyte conditioned medium as a human blood-brain barrier model for ABC drug transport studies. *International Journal of Pharmaceutics, 551*, 281–289.
16. Oddo, A., Peng, B., Tong, Z., Wei, Y., Tong, W. Y., Thissen, H., & Voelcker, N. H. (2019). Advances in microfluidic blood-brain barrier (BBB) models. *Trends in Biotechnology, 37*(12), 1295–1314.
17. Cucullo, L., Aumayr, B., Rapp, E., & Janigro, D. (2005). Drug delivery and in vitro models of the blood-brain barrier. *Current Opinion in Drug Discovery & Development, 8*(1), 89–99.

18. Stone, N. L., England, T. J., & O'Sullivan, S. E. (2019). A novel transwell blood brain barrier model using primary human cells. *Frontiers in Cellular Neuroscience, 13*, 230.
19. Santaguida, S., Janigro, D., Hossain, M., Oby, E., Rapp, E., & Cucullo, L. (2006). Side by side comparison between dynamic versus static models of blood-brain barrier in vitro: A permeability study. *Brain Research, 1109*(1), 1–13.
20. Cucullo, L., McAllister, M. S., Kight, K., Krizanac-Bengez, L., Marroni, M., Mayberg, M. R., et al. (2002). A new dynamic in vitro model for the multidimensional study of astrocyte-endothelial cell interactions at the blood-brain barrier. *Brain Research, 951*(2), 243–254.
21. Modarres, H. P., Janmaleki, M., Novin, M., Saliba, J., El-Hajj, F., RezayatiCharan, M., Seyfoori, A., Sadabadi, H., Vandal, M., Nguyen, M. D., Hasan, A., & Sanati-Nezhad, A. (2018). In vitro models and systems for evaluating the dynamics of drug delivery to the healthy and diseased brain. *Journal of Controlled Release, 273*, 108–130.
22. Herland, A., VanderMeer, A. D., FitzGerald, E. A., Park, T. E., Sleeboom, J. J., & Ingber, D. E. (2016). Distinct contributions of astrocytes and pericytes to neuroinflammation identified in a 3D human blood-brain barrier on a chip. *PLoS One, 11*(3), e0150360.
23. Jiang, L., Li, S., Zheng, J., Li, Y., & Huang, H. (2019). Recent progress in microfluidic models of the blood-brain barrier. *Micromachines, 10*(6), 375.
24. Lei, X. (2009). Application of nasal therapy in acute Chinese medicine. *Journal of Emergency Traditional Chinese Medicine, 18*(11), 1824–1825; 1853 (Chinese).
25. Gao, T. S. (2011). The present situation of the application of traditional Chinese medicine nasal delivery system in the treatment of brain diseases. *Journal of Traditional Chinese Medical Research, 24*(10), 76–79. (Chinese).
26. Akel, H., Ismail, R., & Csoka, I. (2020). Progress and perspectives of brain-targeting lipid-based nanosystems via the nasal route in Alzheimer's disease. *European Journal of Pharmaceutics and Biopharmaceutics, 148*, 38–53.
27. Xie, J., Shen, Z., Anraku, Y., Kataoka, K., & Chen, X. (2019). Nanomaterial-based blood-brain-barrier (BBB) crossing strategies. *Biomaterials, 224*, 119491.
28. Lochhead, J. J., & Davis, T. P. (2019). Perivascular and perineural pathways involved in brain delivery and distribution of drugs after intranasal administration. *Pharmaceutics., 11*(11), 598.
29. Bourganis, V., Kammona, O., Alexopoulos, A., & Kiparissides, C. (2018). Recent advances in carrier mediated nose-to-brain delivery of pharmaceutics. *European Journal of Pharmaceutics and Biopharmaceutics, 128*, 337–362.
30. Zhou, M. Y., & Qin. X. Y. (2016). "The golden phoenix" flying out of Dayaoshan mountain. *TCM Healthy Life Nurturing, 7*, 68–70.
31. Salem, H. F., Kharshoum, R. M., Abou-Taleb, H. A., & Naguib, D. M. (2019). Nanosized transferosome-based intranasal in situ gel for brain targeting of resveratrol: Formulation, optimization, in vitro evaluation, and in vivo pharmacokinetic study. *AAPS PharmSciTech, 20*(5), 181.
32. Xiang, Y., Long, Y., Yang, Q., Zheng, C., Cui, M., Ci, Z., Lv, X., Li, N., & Zhang, R. (2020). Pharmacokinetics, pharmacodynamics and toxicity of Baicalin liposome on cerebral ischemia reperfusion injury rats via intranasal administration. *Brain Research, 1726*, 146503.
33. Ahmad, N., Ahmad, R., Naqvi, A. A., Alam, M. A., Ashafaq, M., Abdur Rub, R., & Ahmad, F. J. (2018). Intranasal delivery of quercetin-loaded mucoadhesive nanoemulsion for treatment of cerebral ischaemia. *Artificial Cells, Nanomedicine Biotechnology, 46*(4), 717–729.
34. Chen, T. C., da Fonseca, C. O., & Schonthal, A. H. (2018). Intranasal perillyl alcohol for glioma therapy: Molecular mechanisms and clinical development. *International Journal of Molecular Science, 19*(12), 3905.
35. Cai, Z., Song, X., Sun, F., Yang, Z., Hou, S., & Liu, Z. (2011). Formulation and evaluation of in situ gelling systems for intranasal administration of gastrodin. *AAPS PharmSciTech, 12*(4), 1102–1109.
36. Lu, Y., Du, S., Bai, J., Li, P., Wen, R., & Zhao, X. (2012). Bioavailability and brain-targeting of geniposide in gardenia-borneol co-compound by different administration routes in mice. *International Journal of Molecular Sciences, 13*(11), 14127–14135.

37. Gao, C., Liang, J., Zhu, Y., Ling, C., Cheng, Z., Li, R., Qin, J., Lu, W., & Wang, J. (2019). Menthol-modified casein nanoparticles loading 10-hydroxycamptothecin for glioma targeting therapy. *Acta Pharmaceutica Sinica B, 9*(4), 843–857.
38. Wang, L. P., Feng, J. F., & Hu, K. L. (2014). Progress in regulation effect of aromatic refreshing traditional Chinese medicine on BBB permeability and its mechanism. *China Journal of Chinese Material Medicine, 39*(6), 949–954. (Chinese).
39. Liang, J., Gao, C., Zhu, Y., Ling, C., Wang, Q., Huang, Y., Qin, J., Wang, J., Lu, W., & Wang, J. (2018). Natural brain penetration enhancer-modified albumin nanoparticles for glioma targeting delivery. *ACS Applied Materials & Interfaces, 10*(36), 30201–30213.
40. Cai, Z., Lei, X. L., Lin, Z. F., Zhao, J., Wu, F. Z., Yang, Z. X., Pu, J., & Liu, Z. (2014). Preparation and evaluation of sustained-release solid dispersions co-loading gastrodin with borneol as an oral brain-targeting enhancer. *Acta Pharmaceutica Sinica B, 4*, 86–93.
41. Wu, J. Y., Li, Y. J., Yang, L., Hu, Y. Y., Hu, X. B., Tang, T. T., Wang, J. M., Liu, X. Y., & Xiang, D. X. (2018). Borneol and Alpha-asarone as adjuvant agents for improving blood-brain barrier permeability of puerarin and tetramethylpyrazine by activating adenosine receptors. *Drug Delivery, 25*(1), 1858–1864.
42. Cai, Z., Hou, S., Li, Y., Zhao, B., Yang, Z., Xu, S., & Pu, J. (2008). Effect of borneol on the distribution of gastrodin to the brain in mice via oral administration. *Journal of Drug Targeting, 16*(2), 178–184.
43. Wang, G. Y., Wang, N., & Liao, H. N. (2015). Effects of muscone on the expression of P-gp, MMP-9 on blood-brain barrier model in vitro. *Cellular and Molecular Neurobiology, 35*(8), 1105–1115.
44. Yang, Y. (2012). Effects of benzoin aldehyde, vanillin and β-asarone on the function of P-glycoprotein. *Chinese Traditional Patent Medicine, 34*(7), 1364–1366. (Chinese).
45. Youdim, K. A., Qaiser, M. Z., Begley, D. J., Rice-Evans, C. A., & Abbott, N. J. (2004). Flavonoid permeability across an in situ model of the blood-brain barrier. *Free Radical Biology & Medicine, 36*(5), 592–604.
46. Liang, W., Xu, W., Zhu, J., Zhu, Y., Gu, Q., Li, Y., Guo, C., Huang, Y., Yu, J., Wang, W., Hu, Y., Zhao, Y., Han, B., Bei, W., & Guo, J. (2020). Ginkgo biloba extract improves brain uptake of ginsenosides by increasing blood-brain barrier permeability via activating A1 adenosine receptor signaling pathway. *Journal of Ethnopharmacology, 246*, 112243.
47. Zhang, C., Fan, Q., Chen, S. L., & Ma, H. (2015). Reversal of P-glycoprotein overexpression by Ginkgo biloba extract in the brains of pentylenetetrazole-kindled and phenytoin-treated mice. *The Kaohsiung Journal of Medical Sciences, 31*(8), 398–404.
48. Marcos-Contreras, O. A., Martinez de Lizarrondo, S., Bardou, I., Orset, C., Pruvost, M., Anfray, A., Frigout, Y., Hommet, Y., Lebouvier, L., Montaner, J., Vivien, D., & Gauberti, M. (2016). Hyperfibrinolysis increases blood-brain barrier permeability by a plasmin- and bradykinin-dependent mechanism. *Blood, 128*(20), 2423–2434.
49. Zhou, L., Yang, B., Wang, Y., Zhang, H. L., Chen, R. W., & Wang, Y. B. (2014). Bradykinin regulates the expression of claudin-5 in brain microvascular endothelial cells via calcium-induced calcium release. *Journal of Neuroscience Research, 92*(5), 597–606.
50. Xie, Z., Shen, Q., Xie, C., Lu, W., Peng, C., Wei, X., Li, X., Su, B., Gao, C., & Liu, M. (2015). Retro-inverso bradykinin opens the door of blood-brain tumor barrier for nanocarriers in glioma treatment. *Cancer Letters, 369*(1), 144–151.
51. Kuo, Y. C., & Tsao, C. W. (2017). Neuroprotection against apoptosis of SK-N-MC cells using RMP-7- and lactoferrin-grafted liposomes carrying quercetin. *International Journal of Nanomedicine, 12*, 2857–2869.
52. Chen, J. T., Lin, Y. L., Chen, T. L., Tai, Y. T., Chen, C. Y., & Chen, R. M. (2016). Ketamine alleviates bradykinin-induced disruption of the mouse cerebrovascular endothelial cell-constructed tight junction barrier via a calcium-mediated redistribution of occludin polymerization. *Toxicology, 368–369*, 142–151.

53. Su, B., Wang, R., Xie, Z., Ruan, H., Li, J., Xie, C., Lu, W., Wang, J., Wang, D., & Liu, M. (2018). Effect of retro-inverso isomer of bradykinin on size-dependent penetration of blood-brain tumor barrier. *Small, 14*(7), 331.
54. Packer, R. J., Krailo, M., Mehta, M., Warren, K., Allen, J., Jakacki, R., Villablanca, J. G., Chiba, A., & Reaman, G. (2005). A Phase I study of concurrent RMP-7 and carboplatin with radiation therapy for children with newly diagnosed brainstem gliomas. *Cancer, 104*(9), 1968–1974.
55. Mugisho, O. O., Robilliard, L. D., Nicholson, L. F. B., Graham, E. S., & O'Carroll, S. J. (2020). Bradykinin receptor-1 activation induces inflammation and increases the permeability of human brain microvascular endothelial cells. *Cell Biology International, 44*(1), 343–351.
56. Zhang, Y., Yang, Y., & Zhou, H. L. (2015). Research progress of brain-targeted prodrugs based on "Lock-in" chemical delivery system. *Journal of Jilin Institute of Chemical Technology, 32*(6), 31–39. (Chinese).
57. Walther, R., Rautio, J., & Zelikin, A. N. (2017). Prodrugs in medicinal chemistry and enzyme prodrug therapies. *Advanced Drug Delivery Reviews, 118*, 65–77.
58. Zhang, Y., Wu, X. Y., Ren, Y., & Hai, L. (2013). Synthesis of brain-targeted venlafaxine prodrugs with affinity for glucose transporters. *West China Journal of Pharmaceutical Science, 28*(3), 226–228. (Chinese).
59. Beard, R., Gaboriau, D. C. A., Gee, A. D., & Tate, E. W. (2019). Chemical biology tools for probing transcytosis at the blood-brain barrier. *Chemical Science, 10*(46), 10772–10778.
60. Kou, L., Sun, R., Ganapathy, V., Yao, Q., & Chen, R. (2018). Recent advances in drug delivery via the organic cation/carnitine transporter 2 (OCTN2/SLC22A5). *Expert Opinion on Therapeutic Targets, 22*(8), 715–726.
61. Omori, K., Tachikawa, M., Hirose, S., Taii, A., Akanuma, S. I., Hosoya, K. I., & Terasaki, T. (2020). Developmental changes in transporter and receptor protein expression levels at the rat blood-brain barrier based on quantitative targeted absolute proteomics. *Drug Metabolism and Pharmacokinetics, 35*(1), 117–123.
62. Sonali, Singh, R. P., Singh, N., Sharma, G., Vijayakumar, M. R., Koch, B., Singh, U., Dash, D., Pandey, B. L., & Muthu, M. S. (2016). Transferrin liposomes of docetaxel for brain-targeted cancer applications: Formulation and brain theranostics. *Drug Delivery, 23*(4), 1261–1271.
63. Montaser, A., Huttunen, J., Ibrahim, S. A., & Huttunen, K. M. (2019). Astrocyte-targeted transporter-utilizing derivatives of ferulic acid can have multifunctional effects ameliorating inflammation and oxidative stress in the brain. *Oxidative Medicine and Cellular Longevity*. https://doi.org/10.1155/2019/3528148
64. Wu, Y., Song, X., Kebebe, D., Li, X., Xue, Z., Li, J., Du, S., Pi, J., & Liu, Z. (2019). Brain targeting of Baicalin and Salvianolic acid B combination by OX26 functionalized nanostructured lipid carriers. *International Journal of Pharmaceutics, 571*, 118754.
65. Wang, X., Liu, G., Chen, N., Wu, J., Zhang, J., Qian, Y., Zhang, L., Zhou, D., & Yu, Y. (2020). Angiopep2-conjugated star-shaped polyprodrug amphiphiles for simultaneous glioma-targeting therapy and MR imaging. *ACS Applied Materials & Interfaces, 12*(10), 12143–12154.
66. Hui, A., Yin, H., Zhang, Z., Zhou, A., Chen, J., Yang, L., Wu, Z., & Zhang, W. (2018). Enhancement of brain-targeting delivery of danshensu in rat through conjugation with pyrazine moiety to form danshensu-pyrazine ester. *Drug Delivery and Translational Research, 8*(3), 787–796.
67. Zhang, Q., Huang, J., Xue, H. J., Bao, H., Yang, Z. X., & Cai, Z. (2017). Determination of equilibrium solubility, apparent oil/water partition coefficient and stability of acetyl gastrodin. *Chinese Journal of Hospital Pharmacy, 37*(9), 819–821. (Chinese).
68. Penalver, P., Belmonte-Reche, E., Adan, N., Caro, M., Mateos-Martin, M. L., Delgado, M., González-Rey, E., & Morales, J. C. (2018). Alkylated resveratrol prodrugs and metabolites as potential therapeutics for neurodegenerative diseases. *European Journal of Medicinal Chemistry, 146*, 123–138.

69. Ke, X. Y., Zhao, B. J., Zhao, X., Wang, Y., Huang, Y., Chen, X. M., Zhao, B. X., Zhao, S. S., Zhang, X., & Zhang, Q. (2010). The therapeutic efficacy of conjugated linoleic acid - paclitaxel on glioma in the rat. *Biomaterials, 31*(22), 5855–5864.
70. Ahmad, N., Al-Subaiec, A. M., Ahmad, R., Sharma, S., Alam, M. A., Ashafaq, M., Abdur Rub, R., & Ahmad, F. J. (2019). Brain-targeted glycyrrhizic-acid-loaded surface decorated nanoparticles for treatment of cerebral ischaemia and its toxicity assessment. *Artificial Cells, Nanomedicine and Biotechnology, 47*(1), 475–490.
71. Mursaleen, L., Somavarapu, S., & Zariwala, M. G. (2020). Deferoxamine and curcumin loaded nanocarriers protect against rotenone-induced neurotoxicity. *Journal of Parkinson's Disease, 10*(1), 99–111.
72. Zheng, B., Teng, L., Xing, G., Bi, Y., Yang, S., Hao, F., Yan, G., Wang, X., Lee, R. J., Teng, L., & Xie, J. (2015). Proliposomes containing a bile salt for oral delivery of Ginkgo biloba extract: Formulation optimization, characterization, oral bioavailability and tissue distribution in rats. *European Journal of Pharmaceutical Sciences, 77*, 254–264.
73. Zhou, H. W., Wu, R. G., Wu, F. G., Luo, J. J., Hu, Y. Y., & Wang, Y. R. (2012). Research on interaction between Ginsenoside Rg1 and liposomes. *China Journal of Traditional Chinese Medicine and Pharmacy, 27*(4), 1140–1143. (Chinese).
74. Han, L. J., Guo, W., Liu, W., Du, J., & Wei, D. D. (2015). Primary evaluation on inhibiting effects of hyaluronic acid-modified paclitaxel loaded liposome against brain tumor stem cells. *Chinese Journal of Hospital Pharmacy, 35*(9), 773–776. (Chinese).
75. Yang, W. Y., Jiang, C. Y., Yan, D., & Yang, X. Y. (2011). Development of resveratrol nasal gel using Tibetan Hulless Barley β-glucan as a matrix. *Chinese Journal of Experimental Traditional Medical Formulare, 17*(12), 6–11. (Chinese).
76. El-Yahchouchi, C. A., Willard, F. H., Kaufmann, T. J., Wald, J. T., Diehn, F. E., Geske, J. R., & Maus, T. P. (2020). Synovial cysts confounding access to the dorsal S1 neural foramen in transforaminal epidural steroid injections. *Pain Medicine, 21*(3), 570–575.
77. Alli, S., Figueiredo, C. A., Golbourn, B., Sabha, N., Wu, M. Y., Bondoc, A., Luck, A., Coluccia, D., Maslink, C., Mith, C., Wurdak, H., Hynynen, K., O'Reilly, M., & Rutka, J. T. (2018). Brainstem blood brain barrier disruption using focused ultrasound: A demonstration of feasibility and enhanced doxorubicin delivery. *Journal of Control Release, 281*, 29–41.
78. Liu, W., Liu, H., Zhang, Z., & Huang, J. (2019). Effects of intraperitoneal and intrathecal morphine analgesia on the expression of μ-opioid receptors in bone cancer pain rats. *Dose-Response, 17*(4), 1–7.
79. Kim, Y. O., Song, J. A., Kim, W. M., & Yoon, M. H. (2020). Antiallodynic effect of intrathecal korean red ginseng in cisplatin-induced neuropathic pain rats. *Pharmacology, 105*(3–4), 173–180.
80. Cochran, M. C., Eisenbrey, J., Ouma, R. O., Soulen, M., & Wheatley, M. A. (2011). Doxorubicin and paclitaxel loaded microbubbles for ultrasound triggered drug delivery. *International Journal of Pharmaceutics, 414*(1–2), 161–170.

Chapter 7
Chinese Herbal Medicine and Targeted Delivery Strategy for the Treatment of Kidney Disease

Lei Zhang, Lina Gao, and Hongzhi Qiao

Abstract Chronic kidney disease (CKD) is a worldwide public health issue with poor treatment outcomes and high medical costs. Current treatment options for CKD are limited. A large part of the world's population has been using Chinese herbal medicine (CHM) for kidney disease treatment, and many active compounds have been identified as useful for CKD. Besides, several well-designed kidney-targeted drug delivery systems have been developed to improve drug efficacy and safety in CKD therapy. In this chapter, the structure and physiological function of the kidney are reviewed. The efficacy of several CHMs, supported by either clinical evidence or experimental studies, and renal targeting delivery strategies are presented. Current challenges for further research are also discussed.

Keywords Chronic kidney disease · Chinese herbal medicine · Kidney-targeted delivery · Renal proximal tubular cells · Nanomedicine · Inflammation

7.1 Introduction

Kidney is an important organ of the urinary system. It is responsible for the excretion of metabolites, maintenance of acid-base balance, and a homeostatic function in regulating water and electrolytes to maintain blood pressure. Any disorder in renal physiological function may cause serious problems such as urinary tract infection, inflammation, and hypertension. If there is no effective treatment, it will eventually lead to chronic kidney disease (CKD).

In the past 20 years, CKD has received increasing attention around the world due to poor prognosis and high medical costs. It affects more than 500 million people worldwide, with 80% of those patients living in low- and middle-income countries

L. Zhang · L. Gao · H. Qiao (✉)
Jiangsu Key Laboratory for Functional Substance of Chinese Medicine, Jiangsu Engineering Research Center for Efficient Delivery System of TCM, School of Pharmacy, Nanjing University of Chinese Medicine, Nanjing, P. R. China
e-mail: qiaohz@njucm.edu.cn

N. Feng, Z. Yang (eds.), *Novel Drug Delivery Systems for Chinese Medicines*,
https://doi.org/10.1007/978-981-16-3444-4_7

[1, 2]. Therefore, to address the growing burden of CKD, it is critical to understand the prevention and treatment of CKD. Different types of CKD usually share a progressive process to develop glomerular sclerosis, tubular atrophy, and/or renal interstitial fibrosis, which possibly induce the final kidney failure. The pathogenesis is quite complex, and current therapy remains limited on the protection of renal function. Angiotensin II-converting enzyme inhibitors or angiotensin II receptor blockers are the mainstay of CKD treatment. But many patients still progress to end-stage renal disease (ESRD). Treatment of glomerular disease with corticosteroid and immunosuppressive medications is often associated with serious adverse effects [3]. Furthermore, resistance to therapy and relapse of disease after discontinuation of medication are difficult to manage. Therefore, the lack of therapeutic options for CKD has prompted people to seek out more potent and safer treatments.

Over the centuries, Chinese herbal medicine (CHM) has been a major complementary and alternative branch of CKD therapy in China [4]. The practice of CHM is based on the cumulative empirical experience of previous practitioners, which was summarized in history textbooks. Nowadays, scientists have made efforts to understand the cellular and molecular mechanisms of these CHMs by using modern techniques and identify active ingredients from them. Furthermore, to achieve greater curative effects and avoid systemic toxicity and side effects in treating kidney disease, kidney-targeted delivery strategies for these active ingredients have been developed constantly due to their features including site-targeted accumulation, controlled release of drugs, and protection of the loaded therapeutic agents.

In this chapter, we will review the structure and physiological function of the kidney and then introduce several CHMs in CKD, which are supported by either clinical evidence or experimental studies. Besides, renal targeting delivery strategies will be described. We hope that our review will not only update the knowledge of CHM in CKD but also help researchers in this field to design and implement better nephropathy treatments in the future.

7.2 Structure and Physiological Function of the Kidney

7.2.1 Structure

Under microscopic observation, the kidney mainly consists of about one million nephrons and a small amount of connective tissues, with abundant blood vessels and nerve fibers between them. Nephrons are composed of a renal corpuscle and its associated tubules along which substances can be exchanged between the bloodstream and urine.

7.2.1.1 Renal Corpuscle

The renal corpuscle is mainly composed of blood vessels and has the function of filtering blood to form urine. The renal corpuscle is approximately spherical, with a diameter of about 200 μm. The center of the renal corpuscle is a glomerulus made up of capillaries, which is surrounded by Bowman capsule. The structure of the renal corpuscle is shown in Fig. 7.1.

Glomerular capillaries are composed of endothelial cells, basement membrane, and epithelial cells. The endothelial cells are flattened to be covered in the side of the capillary wall and directly in contact with the bloodstream. The endothelium contains fenestrations, which have a diameter of approximately 80–100 nm [5, 6]. So blood cells and some macromolecules are blocked and not filtered out, forming the first barrier of the capillary wall of the glomerulus. The next barrier, the basement membrane, is the primary filtration barrier of the glomerulus to ensure the integrity of the capillary wall and a certain permeability. The basement membrane is negatively charged because of abundant heparan sulfate and charged proteoglycans presenting on it, which strongly favor the passage of anionic molecules [7, 8]. Epithelial cells attached to the lateral basement membrane are the largest cells in the glomerulus. They have special morphology and foot-like protrusions of varying sizes. So they are called podocytes, which form the last barrier of the glomerulus. The space between the foot process of podocytes is called a hiatus, with a diameter of about 5–7 nm [8], which is bridged by the slit diaphragms. These diaphragms determine the upper size limit of macromolecules and particles that pass through the glomerulus. Mesangium, located between capillaries and adjacent to the endothelium or basement membrane, is mainly composed of mesangial cells and mesangial matrix. Mesangial cells constitute 30–40% of the total glomerular cell population. They function as microvascular pericytes and maintain the structural architecture of the capillaries tuft [5, 9]. Mesangial cells are primarily responsible for

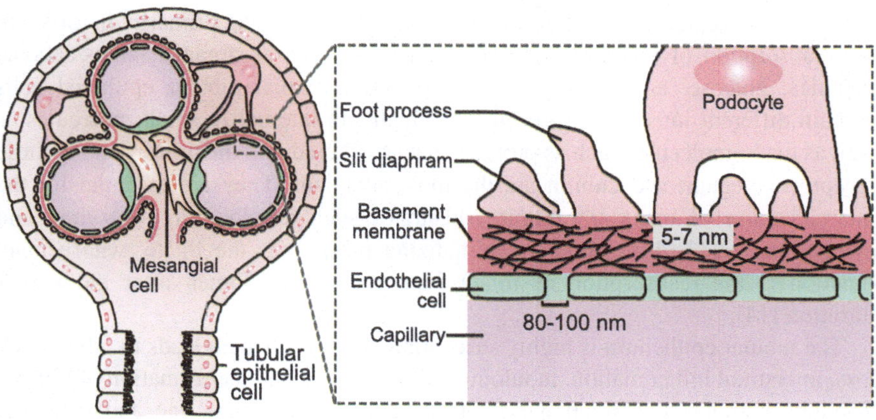

Fig. 7.1 The kidney glomerulus and the glomerular filtration barrier

glomerular matrix growth and homeostasis, regulation of filtration surface area, and clearance of apoptotic cells or immune complexes near glomerular capillaries.

Glomerular pathology is complex and involves many glomerular cell types, including mesangial cells, podocytes, and endothelial cells [8]. Mesangial cell proliferation and matrix expansion are hallmarks of glomerular diseases such as IgA nephropathy, and mesangial cell dysfunction is an important feature of diabetic nephropathy. Podocytopathy is the main mechanism of glomerular proteinuria, which is closely associated with membranous nephropathy, glomerulosclerosis, and diabetic nephropathy. The consequence of podocyte injury includes actin cytoskeleton derangement, loss of slit diaphragm proteins, and the structural integrity, leading to eventual inevitable foot processes effacement and podocyte detachment or apoptosis. Ultimately, the podocyte loses its functional capacity to maintain the glomerular filtration barrier, leading to progressive kidney disease [10, 11]. Impairment of the endothelial cells leads to albuminuria and vascular disease, and damage to this layer can lead to scarring and glomerulosclerosis. Preclinical and clinical studies have shown that damage to the endothelial surface layer strongly correlates with diabetes-induced proteinuria [5].

7.2.1.2 Renal Tubules

The renal tubule is another important component of the nephron and responsible for the maintenance of fluid and electrolyte homeostasis. The tubules are usually divided into three segments, the proximal tubules, the loop of Henle (LoH), and the distal tubules. Among these segments, proximal tubules constitute the biggest part of the renal tubules anatomically and functionally, which play a prominent role in urine filtration. Besides, the proximal tubule, consisting of a monolayer of the epithelium, is the main location for secretion and reabsorption of components into and from the urine and contains a variety of transporters and receptors to perform this role (Fig. 7.2) [12]. Based on the preferential substrate selectivity, the renal transporters are classified as either organic anion or cation transporters and primarily involved in the reabsorption of endogenous small molecules, such as organic anions/cations, peptides, glucose, and nucleosides. Moreover, proximal tubular epithelial cells contain different internalizing receptors, which can internalize small molecules as well as macromolecules such as proteins that are filtered into the urine. Among these receptors, megalin and cubilin are the most abundant. They are essential for the internalization of many ultrafiltrate substrates such as albumin, lysozyme, and cytochrome c [13, 14]. Another internalizing receptor is the folate, whose main function is the reabsorption of folate from the tubular lumen after glomerular filtration [14].

The tubular epithelium is highly susceptible to injury, which leads to tubular cell loss, interstitial inflammation, tubulointerstitial lesions, and the formation of fibrosis through chemotaxis, antigen presentation, and cytokine autocrine and paracrine modes.

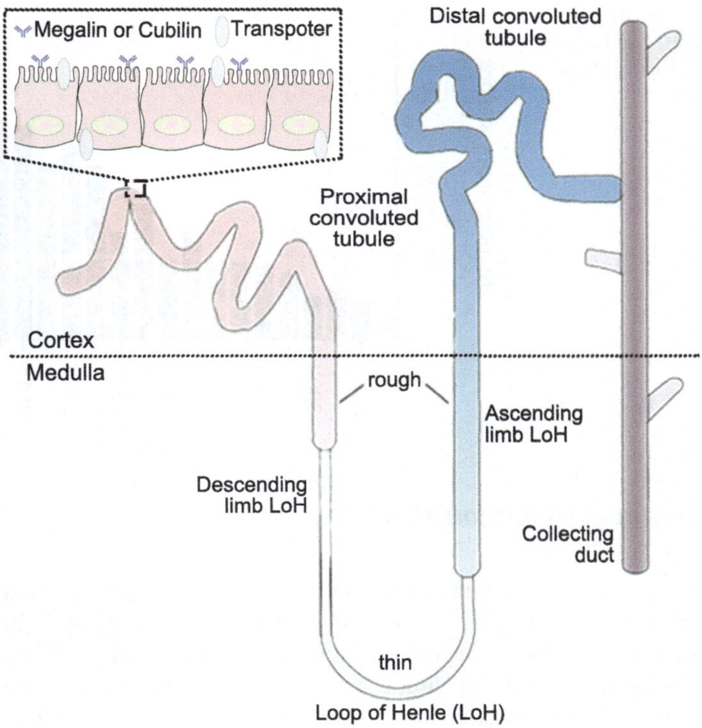

Fig. 7.2 The structure of renal tubule and proximal tubule epithelium

7.3 Chinese Herbal Medicine in the Treatment of CKD

The efficacy of CHM in the treatment of kidney diseases has been widely confirmed in long-term clinical practice with its advantages. It has fewer side effects in comparison with hormones and cytotoxic drugs. It makes the immune system from hyperactivity or depressed state back to a balanced state. It can simultaneously improve symptoms, prevent complications, and delay the progression of renal failure.

Recently, peer-reviewed articles in this field have significantly increased based on data from PubMed (Fig. 7.3). We searched PubMed using the search terms CHM, herbal medicine, and kidney, within a time frame between 2000 and 2019. We only selected articles published in peer-reviewed English-language journals. By analyzing the research field, we found that researchers focused on the mechanisms of CHM for the treatment of kidney disease before 2013. Recent studies have more concentrated on active compounds purified from herbal medicines. These data help us understand structure-function relationships and the molecular mechanisms of CHM and represent important progress in this field. These studies indicated that the main effects of CHM are connected with antioxidative, anti-inflammatory, antifibrotic, and immunomodulatory pathways, as listed in Table 7.1.

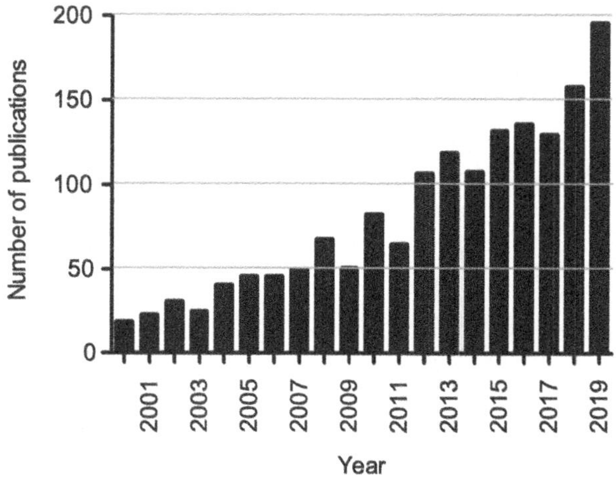

Fig. 7.3 The number of articles on CHM and kidney published in English from 2000 to 2019

7.3.1 Huangqi (Astragali Radix)

Huangqi (*Astragali Radix*) is the dried root of *Astragalus membranaceus* (Fisch.) Bge. var. *mongholicus* (Bge.) Hsiao or *Astragalus membranaceus* (Fisch.) Bge. It contains over 60 ingredients including glycosides (astragalosides I–VII), polysaccharides (astroglucans A–C), palmitic acid, sitosterol, amino acids, and various microelements [17]. Pharmacological studies have confirmed that different ingredients of *Huangqi* have multiple beneficial effects on the promotion of diuretic activity, stimulation of the immune system, antioxidation, anti-inflammation, and antifibrotic effects through regulation of expression of HSP70, Nrf2/HO-1, NF-kB, p38 MAPK, TGF-β1, and Toll-like receptor-mediated pathways [36–38]. On the bases of these benefits on the kidney, *Huangqi* has been used by itself or as one of the ruler drugs in CHM decoctions to treat CKD. Modern studies have shown that *Huangqi* can effectively reduce urinary protein leakage, which may be related to the trace element selenium. Selenium can protect the body from oxidative damage and enhance the antioxidant effect of some free radical scavengers. *Huangqi* can protect the charge and mechanical barrier of the glomerular basement membrane and reduce proteinuria through the above actions. Besides, *Huangqi* has the functions of slowing down the thickening of the glomerular basement membrane, improving platelet function, protecting glomerular podocytes, and regulating plasma endothelin levels [25, 39]. Okuda M [40] found that after the administration of *Huangqi* in patients with CKD, the glomerular filtration rate could be increased and the renal replacement therapy could be delayed for at least 1 year.

Table 7.1 Summary of the mechanisms of action and indications of CHM

Name	Main active compounds	Mechanisms	Indications
Huangqi (*Astragali Radix*)	Astragalosides I–VII, polysaccharides, flavonoids	Anti-inflammatory, antioxidative, antifibrotic, immunomodulation	Glomerular disease [15], membranous nephropathy [16], diabetic nephropathy [17]
Dahuang (*Rhei Radix et Rhizoma*)	Emodin, rhein	Anti-inflammatory, antioxidative, antifibrotic, immunomodulation	CKD [18], chronic allograft nephropathy [19], diabetic nephropathy [20]
Danshen (*Salviae Miltiorrhizae Radix et Rhizoma*)	Tanshinone II A, salvianolic acid	Anti-inflammatory, antioxidative, antifibrotic, immunomodulation	CKD [21], diabetic nephropathy [21, 22]
Leigongteng (*Radix et Rhizoma Tripterygii*)	Triptolide, celastrol	Anti-inflammatory, antifibrotic, immunomodulation	Glomerular disease [23], diabetic nephropathy [24]
Danggui (*Angelicae Sinensis Radix*)	Polysaccharide, ligustilide, ferulic acid	Anti-inflammatory, antioxidative, antifibrotic, immunomodulation	CKD [25]
Chaihu (*Bupleuri Radix*)	Saikosaponins A, B2, and D	Anti-inflammatory, antioxidative, antifibrotic	CKD [26], IgA nephropathy [3]
Mudanpi (*Moutan Cortex*)	Paeonol, paeoniflorin	Anti-inflammatory, antioxidative	CKD [27], diabetic nephropathy [27, 28]
Dongchongxiacao (*Cordyceps*)	Cyclic peptides, H1-A	Anti-inflammatory, antioxidative	CKD [29], chronic allograft nephropathy [30]
Gegen (*Puerariae Lobatae Radix*)	Puerarin	Anti-inflammatory, antioxidative	Diabetic nephropathy [3]
Dihuang (*Rehmanniae Radix*)	Catalpol	Anti-inflammatory	Diabetic nephropathy [31]
Niubangzi (*Fructus Arctii*)	Arctigenin	Anti-inflammatory, antioxidative	Diabetic nephropathy [32]
Shanzhuyu (*Corni Fructus*)	Loganin	Anti-inflammatory, antioxidative	Diabetic nephropathy [31]
Huanglian (*Coptidis rhizome*)	Berberine	Anti-inflammatory, antioxidative	Diabetic nephropathy [33]
Chuanxiong (*Chuanxiong Rhizoma*)	Ferulic acid, ligustrazine	Anti-inflammatory, antioxidative, immunomodulation	CKD [34], glomerular disease [35]

CKD chronic kidney disease, *PKD* polycystic kidney disease

7.3.2 Dahuang (Rhei Radix et Rhizoma)

Dahuang (*Rhei Radix et Rhizoma*) is the dried root and rhizomes of *Rheum palmatum L.*, *Rheum tanguticum Maxim. ex* Balf., or *Rheum officinale* Baill. It is known to contain free, reduced, combined, or dimer forms of anthraquinone derivatives, in which emodin and rhein have been extensively studied. Emodin has various biochemical activities including antioxidant, anti-inflammation, antifibrotic, anti-diuretic, anti-diabetic, and immunosuppressive activities [41]. Previous studies have illustrated that emodin could suppress the expression of fibronectin by inhibiting the MAPK signal pathway in glomerular mesangial cells and efficiently ameliorate renal fibrosis in diabetic rats [42]. Other reports suggested that the dendritic cell maturation inhibition and an increase in the number of regulatory T cells were likely involved in the immune system modulation of emodin. Besides, studies have demonstrated that emodin can reduce endothelial cell damage, which may be related to the inhibition of CCL5 expression and subsequent cellular stress/inflammatory events. Likewise, rhein is a monomer of anthraquinone derivatives and exhibits strong renal protective properties, as exemplified by the treatment of glomerulosclerosis and renal tubular injury [43]. Further clinical and animal studies suggest that rhein affects many cellular processes such as glucose metabolism, inflammation, oxidative stress, and tissue fibrogenesis [19, 44]. However, the cellular targets of rhein are not identified, and the underlying molecular mechanisms remain to be fully understood. Zhang Q [18] found that rhein could reverse Klotho repression via promoting demethylation and protecting against kidney injury in mice with CKD, which brought new insights into Klotho-targeted treatment of rhein for kidney disease.

7.3.3 Danshen (Salviae Miltiorrhizae Radix et Rhizoma)

Danshen (*Salviae Miltiorrhizae Radix et Rhizoma*) is the dried root and rhizomes of *Salvia miltiorrhiza* Bge. and has been used in treating CKD for more than 2000 years in China. Pharmacological activity evaluation shows that *Danshen* can dilate blood vessels, improve hemorheology, reduce renal cell apoptosis, remove oxygen free radicals, inhibit fibroblast proliferation, and reduce urinary protein excretion. *Danshen* extracts contain several ingredients, including water-soluble phenolic acids such as salvianolic acid B, and lipophilic diterpene compounds like tanshinone IIA [22]. Tanshinone IIA has been shown to ameliorate blood pressure via endothelial nitric oxide synthase stimulation in renovascular hypertension model hamsters and has renoprotective effects against the progression of CKD [45]. It has been reported that tanshinone IIA reduced oxidative stress damage and attenuated inflammation and renal fibrosis via regulating the expression of NF-κB and TGF-β/Smad signaling pathways [21]. Xu YM [46] found that in the rats with kidney injury induced by ischemia-reperfusion, tanshinone II A could reduce the activities of myeloperoxidase, macrophage migration inhibitory factor MIF, TNF-α, and IL-6. Besides, tanshinone II A could stabilize the cytoskeleton, protect the damaged podocytes by improving the rearrangement of the cytoskeleton protein, and reduce the formation of podocyte filiform and layered pseudopodia.

7.3.4 *Leigongteng (Radix et Rhizoma Tripterygii)*

Leigongteng (*Radix et Rhizoma Tripterygii*) has been widely used in the treatment of glomerulonephritis. It has been found to alleviate glomerulosclerosis by decreasing the extracellular matrix synthesis and suppression of the TGF-β1/Smad signaling pathway [47]. Triptolide, the major bioactive component of *Leigongteng*, possesses various promising pharmacological effects of *Leigongteng* like anti-inflammatory, antifibrotic, and immunosuppressive activities. Lu Y [48] found that TAB1 was a binding target of triptolide in macrophages. Triptolide could inhibit the activity of TAK1 kinase by interfering with the formation of the TAB1-TAK1 complex, and the binding affinity between triptolide and TAB1 was highly correlated with the activity of triptolide to inhibit the activation of MAPK pathway. These studies provided a potential molecular mechanism for the anti-inflammatory effects of triptolide [24]. In the human mesangial cells, triptolide has been shown to attenuate renal fibrosis by restoring autophagy through the miR-141-3p/PTEN/Akt/mTOR pathway. Furthermore, dendritic cells treated with triptolide have been shown to induce T-cell regulation and prolong the survival of kidney transplant recipients. Besides, triptolide has been reported to effectively alleviate proteinuria and foot process effacement in several podocyte injury model [49]. Celastrol, another biologically active component in *Leigongteng*, has a potent immunosuppressive and anti-inflammatory effect. Research has been shown that celastrol is effective in treating both reversible and irreversible mesangioproliferative glomerulonephritis in rat models [23].

7.3.5 *Danggui (Angelica Sinensis Radix)*

Danggui (*Angelicae Sinensis Radix*) is the dried root of *Angelica sinensis* (Oliv.) Diels. It can effectively alleviate renal anemia. Wang KP [50] found that *Angelica* polysaccharide could restore the production of erythropoietin and effectively increase the iron content. *Angelica* has been shown to reduce the production of pro-inflammatory cytokines IL-12, IL-17, and IL-18 in the renal ischemia-reperfusion model, which can help reduce the cascade reaction of inflammatory cytokines and improve renal ischemia-reperfusion injury. Furthermore, *Danggui* can inhibit the mesangial cell proliferation, decrease the mesangial matrix accumulation, and reduce tubulointerstitial lesion. In the practical application, *Danggui* and *Huangqi* are the classic medicine pair. A mixture of *Danggui* and *Huangqi* was demonstrated to retard the progression of renal fibrosis and deteriorate the renal function by inhibiting the expression of TGF-β1 and promoting the degradation of the extracellular matrix [51]. Besides, the decoction of the combination of two herbs can improve renal interstitial fibrosis in rats with unilateral ureteral obstruction. This combination is also shown to improve renal blood flow and morphology [52].

7.3.6 Others

Among other kinds of Chinese herbs medicine applied to treat CKD, saikosaponin A and its epimer saikosaponin D are obtained from *Chaihu* (*Bupleuri Radix*), the dried root of *Bupleurum chinense* DC. or *Bupleurum scorzonerifolium* Willd. Their anti-inflammatory and antioxidative effects have been identified in kidney cells [53]. Besides, saikosaponin B2 has been reported to attenuate kidney fibrosis via inhibiting the Hedgehog Pathway [26]. *Mudanpi* (*Moutan Cortex*), the root bark of *Paeonia suffruticosa Andr.*, has been shown to have an anti-inflammation effect on mesangial cell dysfunction in diabetic rats [28]. Its bioactive component, paeonol, has been observed to effectively inhibit renal oxidative stress and inflammation by regulating NF-κB activation [27]. Ferulic acid is commonly found in *Chuanxiong* (*Chuanxiong Rhizoma*), which can effectively inhibit the proliferation of glomerular mesangial cells, suppress inflammation and immune responses, and reduce urinary protein. Ligustrazine is an alkaloid monomer isolated from the rhizome of *Chuanxiong*. In a study, 50 patients with CKD were treated with ligustrazine, and the results showed that the urinary protein was reduced significantly. Berberine is an isoquinoline alkaloid isolated from *Huanglian* (*Coptidis rhizome*). Research has shown that berberine exerts renoprotective effects by regulating the AGEs-RAGE signaling pathway in mesangial cells during diabetic nephropathy [54]. Catalpol and loganin, as the principal active components of *Dihuang* (*Rehmanniae Radix*) and *Shanzhuyu* (*Corni Fructus*), respectively, are effective for exerting cooperative ameliorating effects on podocyte apoptosis upon diabetic nephropathy [31]. Arctigenin, a major component of *Niubangzi* (*Arctii Fructus*), has been reported to attenuate proteinuria and podocyte injury in mice with diabetes [32].

7.4 Kidney-Targeted Delivery Strategy

It is corroborant that long-term administration of enzyme inhibitors and non-steroidal anti-inflammatory drugs can increase the risk of renal diseases. Moreover, under pathological conditions such as abnormal glomerular filtration and proteinuria, even a high dose of drugs might not reach sufficient concentrations in the kidney cells, blocking the curative effect. In consequence, the renal targeted drug delivery is investigated to improve the therapeutic effect of nephropathy due to the

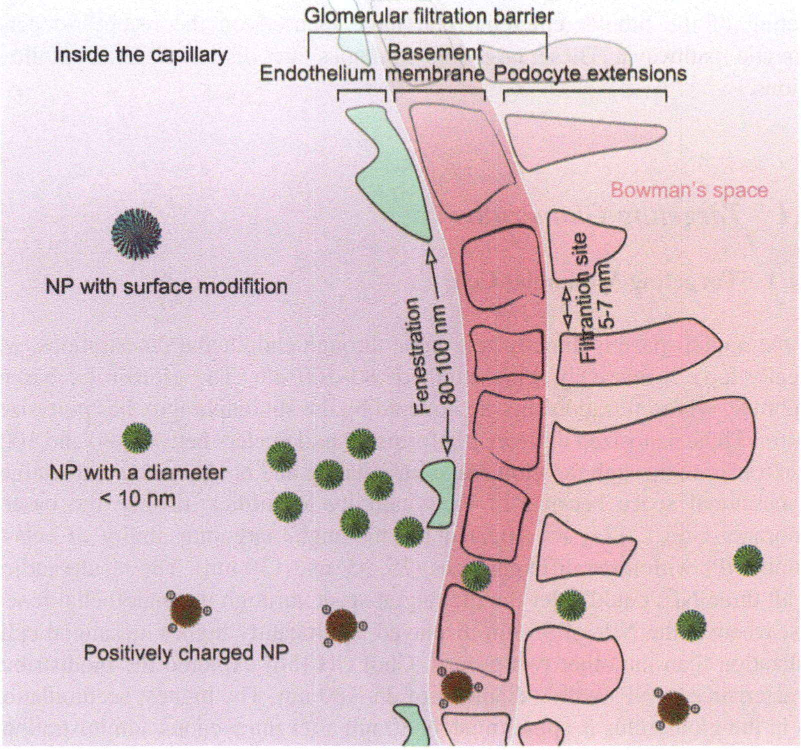

Fig. 7.4 Kidney-targeted NP transport in glomeruli

specialties of accumulation of target sites, controlled drug release, and protection of loaded therapeutic agents. Recently, a series of nanotechnology-based drug delivery strategies including macromolecular carriers, prodrugs, antibody fragments, low-molecular-weight peptide-drug conjugates, and small molecule-drug conjugates have been developed. Many of these delivery systems are applied in the loading of active ingredients of CHM for kidney-targeted delivery and treatment [55].

Since the kidney nephron is composed of various compartments, any drug or nanocarrier should be targeted to the specific cells for better treatment efficacy. The final destination of nanoparticles (NPs) within the kidney is determined by their physical features including their size, shape, charge, and surface targeting ligands (Fig. 7.4). For instance, NPs with a hydrodynamic diameter smaller than 10 nm fall below the kidney filtration threshold, pass through the glomerulus, and are excreted, while nanoparticles with a size larger than 150 nm cannot pass through the glomerular filtration barrier to accumulate in diseased areas [56]. Positively charged NPs are more likely to pass through the renal filtration barrier because of charge interaction. The targeting ligands such as bioactive-penetrating molecules and stimulus-responsive moieties were introduced to enhance the NP localization to the kidney. Furthermore, tubular cell-targeted delivery needs a carrier that can reach the target and subsequently be internalized by these cells. Most studies concerning the targeting of the tubular epithelial cell have focused on the receptor-dependent endocytic pathways. These targeting strategies are discussed in the following sections.

7.4.1 Targeting Glomerulus

7.4.1.1 Targeting Mesangial Cell

The mesangial space is directly accessible through endothelial fenestrations, which typically have a relatively wide width of 80–100 nm. The glomerular basement membrane, whose filtration slits are covered by the slit diaphragm, has pore sizes of 5–7 nm. Thus, nanosized delivery platforms with diameters between 80 and 100 nm can extravasate through the glomerular vasculature and be deposited and retained in the mesangial space because of their inability to further traverse the basement membrane. Guo L [23] investigated the mesangial-targeting ability of celastrol-albumin NPs with three different sizes (75, 95, and 130 nm). The results indicated that all three NPs could enter the mesangial space through the endothelial fenestrations, whereas the NPs of 95 nm displayed significantly higher mesangial cellular localization than the other two groups. Choi CH [56] explored the biodistribution characteristics of NPs with a diameter of 25–180 nm. The highest accumulation of NPs in the glomerulus is approximately 80 nm after intravenous administration.

The surface charge of NPs is another important factor affecting their distribution in the glomerulus. The glomerular capillary wall is negatively charged because of abundantly negative-charged proteoglycans (such as heparan sulfate) presenting on the glomerular basement membrane. Positively charged NPs with a size slightly larger than the renal filtration threshold can pass through the kidney filtration barrier because of charge interactions, while filtration through the kidney is difficult for negatively charged or neutral NPs with the same hydrodynamic diameter. Wang YF [57] constructed size- and surface charge-dependent liposomal nanoparticles with a size of ~110 nm and surface charge of 6.64 ± 0.83 mV, which are loaded with both p38α MAPK and p65 siRNA. Due to the filtration and electrostatic action, the NPs successfully crossed fenestrated endothelium, accumulated in mesangial cells, efficiently silenced p38α MAPK and p65 genes, and eventually alleviated proteinuria.

Except for passive targeting through promoting permeability and retention effect, active targeting strategies have been investigated along with certain ligands such as proteins, peptides, antibodies, or aptamers. For example, TRX-20, a cationic moiety, has a strong and selective binding ability to certain surface chondroitin sulfate proteoglycans expressed on the mesangial cells. Z. X. Yuan [58] applied pegylated TRX-20-modified liposomes loaded with triptolide in the membranous nephropathic rats. The system could effectively achieve cytoplasmic accumulation in the mesangial cells and improve biochemical markers including proteinuria, serum cholesterol, and albumin. Moreover, actinomycin D-modified NPs were prepared and showed up to five times higher uptake by the mesangial cells than by epithelial cells. The NP uptake was considered to be mediated by uncertain receptors through an active process involving the cytoskeletal mobilization [8].

7.4.1.2 Targeting Podocytes

Podocyte is a highly specialized cell and an essential component of the glomerular filtration barrier. Between adjacent foot processes of podocytes are slit diaphragms with a diameter of about 10–70 nm. Particle size and charge characteristics of NPs could be tailored to optimize their interactions with the podocytes. It has been reported that NPs with the size of 5–30 nm can cross the glomerular filtration barrier to target podocytes in kidney glomerulus [59]. However, in glomerular diseases, the integrity of the size and the charge-selective barrier is compromised, and larger particles may also be able to reach the podocyte. To prove this hypothesis, Chiang WC [60] synthesized lipid carriers with a larger and broader particle size range of 125–1700 nm. They can be effectively uptake by podocytes which associated with their strong endocytosis capability.

7.4.2 Targeting Proximal Tubules

7.4.2.1 Targeting Megalin and Cubilin Receptors

Megalin is a member of the low-density lipoprotein receptor family and expressed on several cell types, which triggers the endocytic trafficking of ligands. The complex of megalin with cubilin, located on the membrane of proximal tubule cells, can bind and promote the endocytosis of small molecules and proteins (iron carriers, hormones, vitamins, and enzymes). They are essential for the internalization of many ultrafiltrate substrates to prevent their loss in urine. Megalin-mediated drug delivery takes advantage of differential expression of the megalin and cubilin receptors between the kidney and other tissues. Accumulating data indicated lysozyme, chitosan, and polymyxin B can bind to the megalin receptor, mediating the endocytosis of diverse drugs for kidney disorders, such as renal interstitial fibrosis.

Lysozyme has some advantages as a macromolecular carrier for drug delivery to proximal tubule cells, including specific renal uptake, biodegradability, non-immunogenicity, and ease of conjugation to drugs. For instance, 14-succinyl triptolide-lysozyme conjugate was developed for targeted delivery of triptolide to the tubular epithelial cell [61]. The renal triptolide concentration was found to be up to eightfold higher than triptolide itself. Similarly, imatinib-lysozyme conjugate rapidly accumulated in the proximal tubular cells upon intravenous and intraperitoneal administration, showing the improved renal targeting effect.

Chitosan is a natural copolymer of glucosamine and *N*-acetyl-glucosamine derived from chitin. Because of its excellent biocompatibility and biodegradability, chitosan has been widely used in drug delivery systems. Chitosan can be specifically taken up by renal tubular cells via megalin and cleared from the kidneys more rapidly compared to lysozyme. A nano-complex constructed from catechol conjugated to chitosan, plus metal ions and emodin, was used to treat antifibrosis in the UUO model [62]. When emodin incorporated in the HCA-Ch-Cu complex and intravenously administered to UUO mice, the NPs were taken up by the tubular epithelial cell through the megalin receptor, and the attenuation of fibrosis was observed. Salvianolic acid B incorporated in the HCA-Ch-Ca complex in like manner also showed the effective uptake in the kidney by the megalin receptor-mediated endocytosis [63].

Many investigations have confirmed the strong affinity of polymyxin B toward megalin. The polymyxin B-polyethylenimine (PEI) conjugate was shown to significantly improve gene transfection to renal proximal tubular cells by megalin receptor-mediated mechanism [64]. Besides, some endogenous enzymes such as those involved in amino acid L-decarboxylation and γ-glutamyltranspeptidase have relatively high concentrations in the kidney. Based on this, the aminoglycoside-functionalized PEI was successfully constructed to deliver gene drugs and reach the renal site [65]. Oroojalian F [65] revealed that aminoglycoside-carboxyalkyl-PEI NPs could target megalin-expressing tubular epithelial cells, resulting in improved transfection efficiency.

7.4.2.2 Targeting Folate Receptor

High expression of the folate receptor has been confirmed in the kidney, particularly on the membrane of renal proximal tubule cells. Although designated for targeting cancer cells, low-molecular-weight folate conjugates accumulated substantially in the kidneys when intravenously administered. Particularly in non-cancerous disease, folate-drug conjugates showed successful targeting and therapeutic efficacy in renal disease models. For instance, Shi HL [66] successfully prepared the folate-dactolisib conjugates. They were accumulated in a target-specific manner in kidney tubular epithelial cells after intraperitoneal administration. Trump DP [67] prepared the folate-receptor-targeted DTPA-folate conjugates, which could accumulate rapidly in the kidney and clear rapidly from folate-negative tissues.

7.5 Conclusions

Safe, effective, accurate, and low-cost drugs and treatment strategies are urgently needed for kidney disease. With thousands of years of clinical practice, CHM provides a rich pool of new drug candidates for the treatment of nephropathy. Not only anticancer drugs paclitaxel and camptothecin but also the famous antimalarial drug artemisinin are all inspired by the active ingredients of CHM. It is encouraging to note that current experimental and clinical studies have found and confirmed many compounds with obvious efficacy and low toxicity, which have the potential to be developed as drugs for the treatment of kidney disease. Besides, with the elucidation of the pharmacological mechanism, drug delivery to specific target sites can effectively increase the drug concentration at the lesion site and improve the therapeutic efficiency, which has been confirmed in preclinical animal studies. And further clinical trials need to be promoted. In conclusion, the history of human development is a history of mankind's struggle against diseases. Fortunately, the precious medical experience left by our predecessors always enables us to keep winning the battle against diseases.

References

1. Stanifer, J. W., Kilonzo, K., Wang, D., Su, G., Mao, W., Zhang, L., Zhang, L., Nayak-Rao, S., & Miranda, J. J. (2017). Traditional medicines and kidney disease in low-and middle-income countries: Opportunities and challenges. *Seminars in Nephrology, 37*, 245–259.
2. Hole, B., Hemmelgarn, B., Brown, E., Brown, M., McCulloch, M. I., Zuniga, C., Andreoli, S. P., Blake, P. G., Couchoud, C., Cueto-Manzano, A. M., Dreyer, G., Garcia Garcia, G., Jager, K. J., McKnight, M., Morton, R. L., Murtagh, F. E. M., Naicker, S., Obrador, G. T., Perl, J., ... Caskey, F. J. (2020). Supportive care for end-stage kidney disease: An integral part of kidney services across a range of income settings around the world. *Kidney International. Supplement, 10*, 86–94.
3. Zhong, Y. F., Menon, M. C., Deng, Y. Y., Chen, Y. P., & He, C. J. (2015). Recent advances in Traditional Chinese Medicine for kidney disease. *American Journal of Kidney Diseases: The Official Journal of the National Kidney Foundation, 66*, 513–522.
4. Li, X., & Wang, H. (2005). Chinese herbal medicine in the treatment of chronic kidney disease. *Advances in Chronic Kidney Disease, 12*, 276–281.
5. Kamaly, N., He, J. C., Ausiello, D. A., & Farokhzad, O. C. (2016). Nanomedicines for renal disease: Current status and future applications. *Nature Reviews. Nephrology, 12*, 738–753.
6. Choi, C. H., Zuckerman, J. E., Webster, P., & Davis, M. E. (2011). Targeting kidney mesangium by nanoparticles of defined size. *The Proceedings of the National Academy of Sciences United States of America, 108*, 6656–6661.
7. Miner, J. H. (2012). The glomerular basement membrane. *Experimental Cell Research, 318*, 973–978.
8. Liu, C. P., Hu, Y., Lin, J. C., Fu, H. L., Lim, L. Y., & Yuan, Z. X. (2019). Targeting strategies for drug delivery to the kidney: From renal glomeruli to tubules. *Medicinal Research Reviews, 39*, 561–578.
9. Schlondorff, D., & Banas, B. (2009). The mesangial cell revisited: No cell is an island. *Journal of the American Society of Nephrology, 20*, 1179–1187.
10. Mallipattu, S. K., & He, J. C. (2016). The podocyte as a direct target for treatment of glomerular disease? *American Journal of Physiology. Renal Physiology, 311*, 46–51.
11. Lemley, K. V. (2016). Glomerular pathology and the progression of chronic kidney disease. *American Journal of Physiology. Renal Physiology, 310*, F1385–F1388.
12. Lee, W., & Kim, R. B. (2004). Transporters and renal drug elimination. *Annual Review of Pharmacology and Toxicology, 44*, 137–166.
13. Christensen, E. I., Birn, H., Storm, T., Weyer, K., & Nielsen, R. (2012). Endocytic receptors in the renal proximal tubule. *Physiology, 27*, 223–236.
14. Dolman, M. E., Harmsen, S., Storm, G., Hennink, W. E., & Kok, R. J. (2010). Drug targeting to the kidney: Advances in the active targeting of therapeutics to proximal tubular cells. *Advanced Drug Delivery Reviews, 62*, 1344–1357.

15. Shen, P. C., Yang, X. J., & He, L. Q. (2016). Effect of Astragali and Angelica particle on proteinuria in Chinese patients with primary glomerulonephritis. *Journal of Traditional Chinese Medicine, 36*, 299–306.
16. Lai, W. L., Yeh, T. H., Chen, P. M., Chan, C. K., Chiang, W. C., Chen, Y. M., Wu, K. D., & Tsai, T. J. (2015). Membranous nephropathy: A review on the pathogenesis, diagnosis, and treatment. *Journal of the Formosan Medical Association, 114*, 102–111.
17. Zhang, L., Shergis, J. L., Yang, L., Zhang, A. L., Guo, X., Zhang, L., Zhou, S., Zeng, L., Mao, W., & Xue, C. C. (2019). Astragalus membranaceus (Huang Qi) as adjunctive therapy for diabetic kidney disease: An updated systematic review and meta-analysis. *Journal of Ethnopharmacology, 239*, 111921.
18. Zhang, Q., Liu, L., Lin, W., Yin, S., Duan, A., Liu, Z., & Cao, W. (2017). Rhein reverses Klotho repression via promoter demethylation and protects against kidney and bone injuries in mice with chronic kidney disease. *Kidney International, 91*, 144–156.
19. Su, J., Yin, L. P., Zhang, X., Li, B. B., Liu, L., & Li, H. (2013). Chronic allograft nephropathy in rats is improved by the intervention of rhein. *Transplantation Proceedings, 45*, 2546–2552.
20. He, Y., Meng, F., Zhang, X., Yang, L., Xiang, R., Wang, D., Zhang, Z., Zhang, C., Bai, H., Wang, J., & Zhang, H. (2019). Effect of emodin on Ang II/βig-h3 signaling pathway in diabetic nephropathy rats kidney. *Advances in Integrative Medicine, 6*, S99.
21. Wang, D. T., Huang, R. H., Cheng, X., Zhang, Z. H., Yang, Y. J., & Lin, X. (2015). Tanshinone IIA attenuates renal fibrosis and inflammation via altering expression of TGF-beta/Smad and NF-kappaB signaling pathway in 5/6 nephrectomized rats. *International Immunopharmacology, 26*, 4–12.
22. Jia, Q., Zhu, R., Tian, Y., Chen, B., Li, R., Li, L., Wang, L., Che, Y., Zhao, D., Mo, F., Gao, S., & Zhang, D. (2019). Salvia miltiorrhiza in diabetes: A review of its pharmacology, phytochemistry, and safety. *Phytomedicine: International Journal of Phytotherapy and Phytopharmacology, 58*, 152871.
23. Guo, L., Luo, S., Du, Z., Zhou, M., Li, P., Fu, Y., Sun, X., Huang, Y., & Zhang, Z. (2017). Targeted delivery of celastrol to mesangial cells is effective against mesangioproliferative glomerulonephritis. *Nature Communications, 8*, 878.
24. Li, X. Y., Wang, S. S., Han, Z., Han, F., Chang, Y. P., Yang, Y., Xue, M., Sun, B., & Chen, L. M. (2017). Triptolide restores autophagy to alleviate diabetic renal fibrosis through the miR-141-3p/PTEN/Akt/mTOR pathway. *Molecular Therapy--Nucleic Acids, 9*, 48–56.
25. Shahzad, M., Small, D. M., Morais, C., Wojcikowski, K., Shabbir, A., & Gobe, G. C. (2016). Protection against oxidative stress-induced apoptosis in kidney epithelium by Angelica and Astragalus. *Journal of Ethnopharmacology, 179*, 412–419.
26. Ren, D., Luo, J., Li, Y., Zhang, J., Yang, J., Liu, J., Zhang, X., Cheng, N., & Xin, H. (2020). Saikosaponin B2 attenuates kidney fibrosis via inhibiting the Hedgehog Pathway. *Phytomedicine: International Journal of Phytotherapy and Phytopharmacology, 67*, 153163.
27. Liu, C. M., Yang, H. X., Ma, J. Q., Yang, W., Feng, Z. J., Sun, J. M., Cheng, C., Li, J., & Jiang, H. (2018). Role of AMPK pathway in lead-induced endoplasmic reticulum stress in kidney and in paeonol-induced protection in mice. *Food and Chemical Toxicology: An International Journal Published for the British Industrial Biological Research Association, 122*, 87–94.
28. Chen, J., Hou, X. F., Wang, G., Zhong, Q. X., Liu, Y., Qiu, H. H., Yang, N., Gu, J. F., Wang, C. F., Zhang, L., Song, J., Huang, L. Q., Jia, X. B., Zhang, M. H., & Feng, L. (2016). Terpene glycoside component from Moutan Cortex ameliorates diabetic nephropathy by regulating endoplasmic reticulum stress-related inflammatory responses. *Journal of Ethnopharmacology, 193*, 433–444.
29. Zhang, H. W., Lin, Z. X., Tung, Y. S., Kwan, T. H., Mok, C. K., Leung, C., & Chan, L. S. (2014). Cordyceps sinensis (a traditional Chinese medicine) for treating chronic kidney disease. *Cochrane Database of Systematic Reviews*, (12), CD008353.
30. Li, Y., Xue, W. J., Tian, P. X., Ding, X. M., Yan, H., Pan, X. M., & Feng, X. S. (2009). Clinical application of Cordyceps sinensis on immunosuppressive therapy in renal transplantation. *Transplantation Proceedings, 41*, 1565–1569.

31. Chen, Y. P., Chen, J., Jiang, M., Fu, Y. X., Zhu, Y. H., Jiao, N., Liu, L. P., Du, Q., Wu, H. G., Xu, H. Q., & Sun, J. H. (2020). Loganin and catalpol exert cooperative ameliorating effects on podocyte apoptosis upon diabetic nephropathy by targeting AGEs-RAGE signaling. *Life Sciences, 252*, 117653.
32. Zhong, Y. F., Lee, K., Deng, Y. Y., Ma, Y. M., Chen, Y. P., Li, X. L., & Wei, C. G. (2019). Arctigenin attenuates diabetic kidney disease through the activation of PP2A in podocytes. *Nature Communications, 10*, 4523.
33. Zhang, M. S., Zhang, Y. N., Xiao, D., Zhang, J., Wang, X. X., Guan, F. Y., Zhang, M., & Chen, L. (2020). Highly bioavailable berberine formulation ameliorates diabetic nephropathy through the inhibition of glomerular mesangial matrix expansion and the activation of autophagy. *European Journal of Pharmacology, 873*, 172955.
34. Chen, D. Q., Hu, H. H., Wang, Y. N., Feng, Y. L., Cao, G., & Zhao, Y. Y. (2018). Natural products for the prevention and treatment of kidney disease. *Phytomedicine: International Journal of Phytotherapy and Phytopharmacology, 50*, 50–60.
35. Zhuang, Z., Wang, Z. H., Huang, Y. Y., Zheng, Q., & Pan, X. D. (2020). Protective effect and possible mechanisms of ligustrazine isolated from Ligusticum wallichii on nephropathy in rats with diabetes: A preclinical systematic review and meta-analysis. *Journal of Ethnopharmacology, 252*, 112568.
36. Han, R., Tang, F., Lu, M., Xu, C., Hu, J., Mei, M., & Wang, H. (2016). Protective effects of Astragalus polysaccharides against endothelial dysfunction in hypertrophic rats induced by isoproterenol. *International Immunopharmacology, 38*, 306–312.
37. Liu, B., Miao, J., Peng, M., Liu, T., & Miao, M. (2019). Effect of 3:7 ratio of Astragalus total saponins and Curcumin on the diabetic nephropathy rats model. *Saudi Journal of Biological Sciences, 26*, 188–194.
38. Farag, M. R., Elhady, W. M., Ahmed, S. Y. A., Taha, H. S. A., & Alagawany, M. (2019). Astragalus polysaccharides alleviate tilmicosin-induced toxicity in rats by inhibiting oxidative damage and modulating the expressions of HSP70, NF-kB and Nrf2/HO-1 pathway. *Research in Veterinary Science, 124*, 137–148.
39. Gui, D., Huang, J., Guo, Y., Chen, J., Chen, Y., Xiao, W., Liu, X., & Wang, N. (2013). Astragaloside IV ameliorates renal injury in streptozotocin-induced diabetic rats through inhibiting NF-κB-mediated inflammatory genes expression. *Cytokine, 61*, 970–977.
40. Okuda, M., Horikoshi, S., Matsumoto, M., Tanimoto, M., Yasui, H., & Tomino, Y. (2012). Beneficial effect of Astragalus membranaceus on estimated glomerular filtration rate in patients with progressive chronic kidney disease. *Hong Kong Journal of Nephrology, 14*, 17–23.
41. Gao, Y., Zhang, J., Li, G., Xu, H., Yi, Y., Wu, Q., Song, M., Bee, Y. M., Huang, L., Tan, M., Liang, S., & Li, G. (2015). Protection of vascular endothelial cells from high glucose-induced cytotoxicity by emodin. *Biochemical Pharmacology, 94*, 39–45.
42. Huang, J., Gong, W., Chen, Z., Huang, J., Chen, Q., Huang, H., & Zhao, C. (2017). Emodin self-emulsifying platform ameliorates the expression of FN, ICAM-1 and TGF-beta1 in AGEs-induced glomerular mesangial cells by promoting absorption. *European Journal of Pharmaceutical Sciences, 99*, 128–136.
43. Li, W., Gao, K., & Sun, W. (2019). MON-209 Rhein attenuated palmitic acid-induced renal tubular cell injury by regulating AMPK-mTOR-autophagy pathway. *Kidney International Reports, 4*, S387.
44. Sun, H., Luo, G., Xiang, Z., Cai, X., & Chen, D. (2016). Pharmacokinetics and pharmacodynamics study of rhein treating renal fibrosis based on metabonomics approach. *Phytomedicine: International Journal of Phytotherapy and Phytopharmacology, 23*, 1661–1670.
45. Lee, S. H., Kim, Y. S., Lee, S. J., & Lee, B. C. (2011). The protective effect of Salvia miltiorrhiza in an animal model of early experimentally induced diabetic nephropathy. *Journal of Ethnopharmacology, 137*, 1409–1414.
46. Xu, Y. M., Ding, G. H., Huang, J., & Xiong, Y. (2016). Tanshinone IIA pretreatment attenuates ischemia/reperfusion-induced renal injury. *Experimental and Therapeutic Medicine, 12*, 2741–2746.

47. Wan, Y. G., Che, X. Y., Sun, W., Huang, Y. R., Meng, X. J., Chen, H. L., Shi, X. M., Tu, Y., Wu, W., & Liu, Y. L. (2014). Low-dose of multi-glycoside of Tripterygium wilfordii Hook. f., a natural regulator of TGF-beta1/Smad signaling activity improves adriamycin-induced glomerulosclerosis in vivo. *Journal of Ethnopharmacology, 151*, 1079–1089.
48. Lu, Y., Zhang, Y., Li, L., Feng, X., Ding, S., Zheng, W., Li, J., & Shen, P. (2014). TAB1: A target of triptolide in macrophages. *Chemistry & Biology, 21*, 246–256.
49. Sun, M., Song, H., Ye, Y., Yang, Q., Xu, X., Zhu, X., Zhang, J., Shi, S., Wang, J., & Liu, Z. (2019). Differential toxicities of triptolide to immortalized podocytes and the podocytes in vivo. *Biomedicine & Pharmacotherapy = Biomedecine & Pharmacotherapie, 109*, 2375–2386.
50. Wang, K., Wu, J., Xu, J., Gu, S., Li, Q., Cao, P., Li, M., Zhang, Y., & Zeng, F. (2018). Correction of anemia in chronic kidney disease with Angelica sinensis polysaccharide via restoring EPO production and improving iron availability. *Frontiers in Pharmacology, 9*, 803.
51. Fang, L., Xiao, X. F., Liu, C. X., & He, X. (2012). Recent advance in studies on Angelica sinensis. *Chinese Herbal Medicines, 4*, 12–25.
52. Song, J., Meng, L., Li, S., Qu, L., & Li, X. (2009). A combination of Chinese herbs, Astragalus membranaceus var. mongholicus and Angelica sinensis, improved renal microvascular insufficiency in 5/6 nephrectomized rats. *Vascular Pharmacology, 50*, 185–193.
53. Ma, X., Dang, C., Kang, H., Dai, Z., Lin, S., Guan, H., Liu, X., Wang, X., & Hui, W. (2015). Saikosaponin-D reduces cisplatin-induced nephrotoxicity by repressing ROS-mediated activation of MAPK and NF-kappaB signalling pathways. *International Immunopharmacology, 28*, 399–408.
54. Qiu, Y. Y., Tang, L. Q., & Wei, W. (2017). Berberine exerts renoprotective effects by regulating the AGEs-RAGE signaling pathway in mesangial cells during diabetic nephropathy. *Molecular and Cellular Endocrinology, 443*, 89–105.
55. Zhou, P., Sun, X., & Zhang, Z. (2014). Kidney–targeted drug delivery systems. *Acta Pharmaceutica Sinica B, 4*, 37–42.
56. Oroojalian, F., Charbgoo, F., Hashemi, M., Amani, A., Yazdian-Robati, R., Mokhtarzadeh, A., Ramezani, M., & Hamblin, M. R. (2020). Recent advances in nanotechnology-based drug delivery systems for the kidney. *Journal of Controlled Release: Official Journal of the Controlled Release Society, 321*, 442–462.
57. Wang, Y., Wu, Q., Wang, J., Li, L., Sun, X., Zhang, Z., & Zhang, L. (2020). Co-delivery of p38alpha MAPK and p65 siRNA by novel liposomal glomerulus-targeting nano carriers for effective immunoglobulin a nephropathy treatment. *Journal of Controlled Release: Official Journal of the Controlled Release Society, 320*, 457–468.
58. Yuan, Z. X., Jia, L., Lim, L. Y., Lin, J. C., Shu, G., Zhao, L., Ye, G., Liang, X. X., Ji, H. M., & Fu, H. L. (2017). Renal-targeted delivery of triptolide by entrapment in pegylated TRX-20-modified liposomes. *International Journal of Nanomedicine, 12*, 5673–5686.
59. Chen, D., Han, S., Zhu, Y., Hu, F., Wei, Y., & Wang, G. (2018). Kidney-targeted drug delivery via rhein-loaded polyethyleneglycol-co-polycaprolactone-co-polyethyleneimine nanoparticles for diabetic nephropathy therapy. *International Journal of Nanomedicine, 13*, 3507–3527.
60. Chiang, W. C., Gee, T. M., Altintas, M. M., Sever, S., Ruiters, M. H. J., & Reiser, J. (2010). Establishment of protein delivery systems targeting podocytes. *PLoS One, 5*, e11837.
61. Zhang, Z., Zheng, Q., Han, J., Gao, G. P., Liu, J., Gong, T., Gu, Z. W., Huang, Y., Sun, X., & He, Q. (2009). The targeting of 14-succinate triptolide-lysozyme conjugate to proximal renal tubular epithelial cells. *Biomaterials, 30*, 1372–1381.
62. Qiao, H. Z., Sun, M. J., Su, Z. G., Xie, Y., Chen, M. L., Zong, L., Gao, Y. H., Li, H. P., Qi, J. P., Zhao, Q., Gu, X. C., & Ping, Q. N. (2014). Kidney-specific drug delivery system for renal fibrosis based on coordination-driven assembly of catechol-derived chitosan. *Biomaterials, 35*, 7157–7171.
63. Lia, J., Zhang, C. T., He, W. M., Qiao, H. Z., Chen, J. H., Wang, K. K., Oupický, D., & Sun, M. J. (2017). Coordination-driven assembly of catechol-modified chitosan for kidney-specific delivery of salvianolic acid B to treat renal fibrosis. *Biomaterials Science, 6*, 179–188.

64. Oroojalian, F., Rezayan, A. H., Shier, W. T., Abnous, K., Ramezani, M., Mehrnejad, F., & Ni, A. H. (2017). Efficient megalin targeted delivery to renal proximal tubular cells mediated by modified-polymyxin B-polyethylenimine based nano-gene-carriers. *Materials Science and Engineering: C, 79*, 770–782.
65. Oroojalian, F., Rezayana, A. H., Shier, W. T., Abnous, K., & Ramezani, M. (2017). Megalin-targeted enhanced transfection efficiency in cultured human HK-2 renal tubular proximal cells using aminoglycoside-carboxyalkyl polyethylenimine-containing nanoplexes. *International Journal of Pharmaceutics, 523*, 102–120.
66. Shi, H., Leonhard, W. N., Sijbrandi, N. J., van Steenbergen, M. J., Fens, M. H. A. M., van de Dikkenberg, J. B., Toraño, J. S., Peters, D. J. M., Hennink, W. E., & Kok, R. J. (2019). Folate-dactolisib conjugates for targeting tubular cells in polycystic kidneys. *Journal of Controlled Release, 293*, 113–125.
67. Trump, D. P., Mathias, C. J., Yang, Z. F., Low, P. S., Marmion, M., & Green, M. A. (2002). Synthesis and evaluation of 99mTc(CO)3-DTPA-folate as a folate receptor-targeted radiopharmaceutical. *Nuclear Medicine and Biology, 29*, 569–573.

Chapter 8
Liposomes and Their Application in the Delivery of Herbal Active Ingredients

Zhijun Yang

Abstract This chapter aims to illustrate the application of liposomes in pharmaceutical science and Chinese Materia Medica. It reviews the history and development of liposomes and introduces the composition and formulation of liposomes, including the application of aptamers, antibodies, and other biomaterials. This chapter also describes some important aspects of the preparation of liposomes, including stability and entrapment efficiency, and surface modification for targeted deliveries. The improvement of the qualities of liposomes is discussed, emphatically, such as the surface charges, the morphology, and the size distribution.

Keywords Liposomes · Preparation · Modification · Quality control · Application on Chinese medicine

8.1 History of Liposomes

Liposomes were firstly introduced in China in 1977. They have now been developed as transfersomes, ethosomes, glycerosome, invasomes, etc., by adding other materials to the lipids. In 1982, the liposomes were first applied to the extracted active pharmaceutical ingredients (API) from Chinese medicines [1, 2]. Since then, many research papers on the applications of liposomes to deliver the API of Chinese medicines have been published in Chinese. However, there are few systemic reviews, especially in English, of this literature. Therefore, this chapter describes the basic details of the liposomal system for drug delivery in TCM, including the developments, the composition, preparation, characterization, and application onto Chinese medicines of liposomes.

The history of liposomes begins in the early 1960s. At that time, the British hematologist Alec D Bangham first described phospholipid bilayer vesicles in [3–6]

Z. Yang (✉)
School of Chinese Medicine, Hong Kong Baptist University, Kowloon Tong, Hong kong, China
e-mail: yzhijun@hkbu.edu.hk

N. Feng, Z. Yang (eds.), *Novel Drug Delivery Systems for Chinese Medicines*,
https://doi.org/10.1007/978-981-16-3444-4_8

when using the new electronic microscope to examine dry phospholipids with negative staining at the Babraham Institute, Cambridge. The microscope photos showed the cell membrane with bilayer lipids. Bangham named the lipid bilayers as Banghasomes or multilamellar smectic mesophases. Bangham and his team accurately depicted liposomes as closed bilayer vesicles with the latent release of encapsulated substances when treated with abstergent [7]. The term "liposomes" was coined by Weissmann and published in 1965 [8, 9]. The term liposome comes from the Greek words "lipo" (fat) and "soma" (body) because the main chemical components are phospholipids. Weissmann initially came up with the name during a pub discussion with Bangham in Cambridge. In the 1970s and 1980s, many in vivo studies explored the possibilities of using liposomes to enhance the absorption of the API and deliver drugs to target specific cells or organ tissues. This generated some controversy. Some researches claim that the delivery is limited, and that stability of the liposomal system is a problem. Nevertheless, many scientists continue to study liposomes as nanoscale drug carriers for targeting chemotherapies.

One benefit of using liposomes, i.e., the combination of a ligand in a liposomal vesicle, is that the drugs are delivered unchanged to the target. Furthermore, the drugs are delivered only to the targeted tissues. Therefore, the therapeutic effects are maximized while the side effects can be expected to be minimized.

8.2 The Composition of Liposomes

8.2.1 Liposomal Vesicles (Lipid Vesicles)

Liposomes consist of vesicles composed of bilayers or multilayers that contain phospholipids and cholesterol surrounding an aqueous compartment. Liposomes are defined uniquely by three key characteristics: the closed vesicles, the encapsulated internal aqueous phases, and the compartments separated by the bilayer membrane of lipid molecules. The liposomal vesicles encapsulate and release the drug to the intestinal surface membrane for absorption. Liposomes can be negatively stained and simply identified from micelles and hexagonal lipid phases using transmission electron microscopy [10]. In pharmaceutics, liposomes are defined as spherical vesicles shaped by lipid-water lamellar systems. They are comprised of a sealed water phase inside a lipid bilayer; the lipid bilayer can be prepared with unilocular (small unilamellar vesicles, SUV, and large unilamellar vesicles, LUV) or multilocular vesicles (MLV).

Liposomal vesicles are artificial vesicles enclosed by a lipid membrane, which is similar to the biological membrane depicted by Singer-Nicolson's fluid mosaic prototype. The lipid membrane automatically aggregates to form a bilayer in aqueous media [11]. The aggregation arises from hydrophobic interaction; the lipids' lipophilic group congregate as they disconnect from the water molecules [12]. The reorientation maximizes the effect of hydrogen bonding of the hydrophilic groups and water and minimizes the disadvantageous connection of lipophilic tails and water. The system's entropy is increased by the strengthening of hydrogen bonding, ultimately leading to the spontaneous formation of liposomal vesicles.

8.2.2 The Composition of Liposomes

Lipids are the main components of liposomes. There are eight classes of phospholipids based on their component chemical groups: glycerophospholipids, glycerolipids, polyketides, prenols, saccharolipids, sphingolipids, sterols, and fatty acids [13]. Figure 8.1 shows the schematic molecular structures of the main lipids including the eight phospholipids found in the biological membrane.

The most basic groups are the fatty acid groups biologically, and the carbon numbers (from 4 to 24) determine the length of the chain of the fatty acid [14]. In the carbon chains, there may be several unsaturated carbon bonds; and special functional groups, which may contain oxygen, halogens, nitrogen, and sulfur, could be attached to the chain. The fatty acid chain may be bent by cis-double bonds. The more double bonds the greater the mobility of the lipid membranes at lower temperatures [15]. Mobility is very important to the function of biological membranes [16]. There are three kinds of amphipathic lipids in the cell membrane, which are phospholipids, glycolipids, and sterols. Phospholipids normally account for over 50% of all lipids in an organism [17, 18], while the rest is made up of glycolipids and sterols with about 2%. The membrane of erythrocytes (red blood cells, RBC) is deformable and flexible, and its lipids are mainly phospholipids and cholesterol (phosphatidylserine) [19] in equal proportions by weight [20]. Cholesterol plays a modulatory role in the flexibility of the entire membrane in that the movement of the cell membrane, which may consist of different components, depends on the concentration of cholesterol [21]. Temperature also plays a role. At higher temperatures, cholesterol reduces the mobility of the phospholipid fatty acid chains, reducing permeability to small molecules as well as the flexibility of the membrane. Cholesterol concentration may be upregulated (increased) by decreasing the temperature. At lower temperatures, cholesterol enhances the interactions of fatty acid chains. Cholesterol plays the role of antifreeze to maintain the fluidity of the membrane [21].

As artificial lipid vesicles, liposomes are mainly constructed from phospholipids extracted from biological membranes because of their minimal toxicity. The phospholipid first extracted from biological tissues—the egg yolk of chickens—was determined to be lecithin or phosphatidylcholine (PC) in 1947 by Theodore Nicolas Gobley, a French chemist and pharmacist. In eukaryotes, there is another kind of lipid, sterol, dispersed together with the phospholipids in the biological membranes. Sterols also give membrane flexibility and strength. A phospholipid molecule comprises two fatty acid tails, which are the hydrophobic groups, and a phosphate group with high hydrophilic properties; the three groups are linked by a glycerol molecule. The phosphate groups can incorporate other small organic chemical groups, such as serine, ethanolamine, choline, etc. There are two big species of phospholipids, distinguished by chemical structure. The first species has the

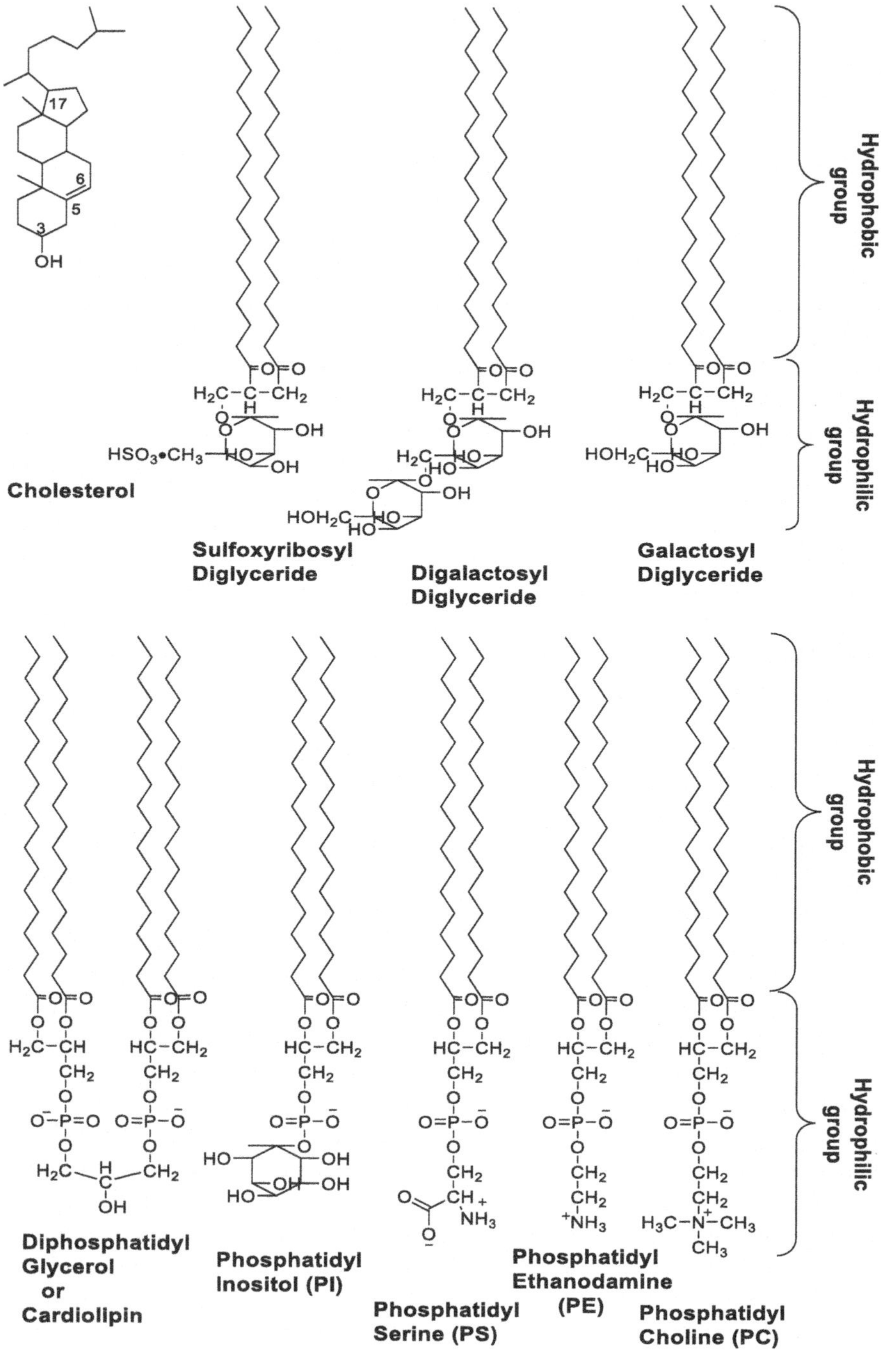

Fig. 8.1 The schematic structures of lipids

structure of diacylglycerol; examples include cephalin (phosphatidylethanolamine, PE), lecithin (phosphatidylcholine, PC), phosphatidate (phosphatidic acid, PA), phosphatidylserine (PS), and phosphoinositides. Phosphoinositides can in turn be subdivided into phosphatidylinositol (PI), phosphatidylinositol phosphate (PIP), phosphatidylinositol bisphosphate (PIP2), and phosphatidylinositol trisphosphate (PIP3). The second species includes phosphosphingolipids including ceramide phosphorylcholine (SPH) or sphingomyelin (SM). Pure phospholipids are commercialized products to be applied to develop nanotechnologies for drug delivery and special biomaterials [22]. Phospholipids auto-assemble the vesicles with lipid bilayers membrane in water by their amphiphilic property. However, this bilayer pattern can be replaced by the pattern of polymorphism lipid because the behavior of lipids is not simple under physiological and other conditions. Today, phospholipids have been widely used in the preparation of liposomes, ethosomes, and other nanosystems for topical, oral, and parenteral drug delivery to improve the bioavailability of drugs, to reduce the toxicity, and increase the membrane permeability of the drugs.

The decision as to what lipids to use can be taken sequentially. Liposome membrane can be made up of a single neutral phospholipid as the structural buttress of the bilayer, while a handful of other lipids scantling of lipids may be overcoating to impart specific characters that may adjust the behavior for special function necessary. The most used lipids are neutral basic lipids because the safety and the robustness of the membrane are concerned. Attachment of PEG and polysaccharides or other biomaterials to the surface of phospholipid vesicles has not yet become a common practice. The choice of phospholipids for pharmaceutical applications depends on the availability, cost, regulatory, and other favorable conditions.

The phospholipid of the first choice is phosphatidylcholine (PC) because it is the most readily available and the predominant lipid in most biological cell membranes. The immutable positive charge of the head group choline neutralizes the negative charge of the phosphate making the head group strongly lipophobic neutral. The tertiary ammonium group interacting with phosphates of the adjacent molecules donates the tightness of encapsulation and expends the dispersion of partial fractions of the charge density. To prepare liposomes, the most commonly used pure PCs are 1-α-dimyristoylphosphatidylcholine (DMPC), 1,2-dioleoyl-sn-glycero-3-phosphocholine (DOPC), dipalmitoylphosphatidylcholine (DPPC), distearoylphosphatidylcholine (DSPC), hydrogenated soy PC (HSPC), and monostearoylphosphatidylcholine (MSPC). PC has a phosphodiester and a choline residue. It has a neutral charge. The size of the polar group is balanced with the size of the hydrophobic group so that it easily assumes a bilayer structure, and thus the liposomes will be formed. Even in the case of PC that forms such "stable" liposomes, observing the morphology of the molecular assembly reveals that liposomes with a carbon number of 10 or more have a morphology of 6–8 carbon atoms. In spherical micelles or liposomes, molecular aggregates can no longer be formed with carbon atoms of 4 or less, and they exist only as monomers in an aqueous solution. PC having two alkyl or acyl groups with a certain minimal chain length forms liposomes morphologically. However, the interaction between hydrophobic groups is incomplete at C10 to C12 and the molecular transfers between monomer and bilayer.

Lauryl PC has a shorter fatty acid chain of 12 carbons that are reported to be severely toxic, and lauryl PC can be inferred from measurements of critical micelle concentration (CMC) and transmembrane transfer. When dimyristoylphosphatidylcholine having 14 carbon atoms is used, the intermembrane translocation ability becomes small, the CMC cannot be measured, and the barrier effect against ions is still insufficient for the encapsulating ingredients. However, dipalmidylphosphatidylcholine having 16 carbon atoms almost makes the barrier impermeable [23]. The structure of the aggregates formed is affected by many parameters, e.g. pH, ionic strength, temperature, divalent cations, etc. A typical phospholipid that is hardly affected by these parameters is PC. Liposomes made from substantiated phospholipid may also have strong surfactant properties due to the phosphoryl group and fatty acid chains.

In a pH 7.4 aqueous environment, other neutral phospholipids used to prepare liposomes are sphingomyelins (SM). SM is a neutral molecule with the same head group of phosphoethanolamine and phosphocholine, which links to the 1-hydroxy group of a ceramide. SM exists in nervous tissue and the erythrocyte plasma membranes of many mammalian species, and it replaced PC in sheep erythrocytes to varying degrees. The hydrocarbon chains have a significant number of carbon atoms with unsaturation to elevate the transition temperature from 20 to 40 °C. The SM membrane is tighter than that of PC because of the hydrogen bonding in the connection region by the amid hydrogen, which strengthens the interaction of the molecules similar to cholesterol. When the temperature is above the phase temperature, the mobility of the membrane can be decreased by cholesterol, and the permeability to solutes in aqueous media may decline, and consequently increasing the stability of the liposomes by the incorporation up to a ratio at 1:1 of PC: cholesterol, which has the strongest stabilizing effect in vitro and in vivo.

Charged phospholipids can denature and can compose liposomal vesicles. There are a large number of reasons to include charged lipids in the liposomes. One reason is to increase the surface charge density to prevent the close approach of liposomal vesicles and hence inhibit aggregation, fusion. Pushing adjacent membranes apart within a multilamellar vesicle increases the internal aqueous volume. For this purpose, the most suitable phospholipids are negatively charged phosphatidylglycerol (PG). PG possesses a constant negative charge when the pH is above the physiological range. PG may be readily synthesized via phospholipase D adopting different lipids together with glycerine, and PG may be isolated from a natural source, e.g. 1-α-dimyristoylphosphatidylglycerol (DMPG), dipalmitoylphosphatidylglycerol (DPPG), distearoyl-sn-phosphatidylglycerol (DSPG). A molar ratio of 10% of PG to total lipids is sufficient to reduce intermembrane interactions. Organizing the negatively charged phosphatidylethanolamine (PE), especially with the unsaturated fatty acyl chains in the membrane may introduce controlled instability of liposomal vesicles. The head group of PE is smaller than PC, and the hydrogen directly connected to ethanolamine's nitrogen provides hydrogen bonding interactions to the neighboring molecules in the membrane. PE tends to be more highly unsaturated than average and has fatty acids of longer and more asymmetric chains. PE has a partial negative charge at or above pH

7 and forms non-bilayer aggregates at low pH. PE membrane converts from stable lamellar to non-lamellar with a change of pH. Dioleoylphosphatidylethanolamine (DOPE), distearoylphosphatidylethanolamine (DSPE), and polyethylene glycol-2000-distearoylphosphatidylethanolamine (PEG2000-DSPE) are the PE commonly used to prepare the liposomes. In acidic or neutral aqueous solutions, when the temperature is higher than the main phase transition temperature (Tc), the ionized amino group gives a neutral molecule which tends to form the second phase of hexagonal transformed micelles to lamellar structures. Other lipids can stabilize the membrane, and the ratio of lipids can be carefully adjusted if the membrane desires to be stabilization. A ratio of between 5% and 10% of PE or their derivatives to total lipids is good for conjugating them with proteins or other molecules; their functional groups may work as anchors for binding the biomolecules to the surface of the liposome.

Other negatively charged phospholipids like phosphatidic acid (PA) and phosphatidylserine (PS) may cause aggregation in the presence of calcium. The naked phosphate groups of PA, e.g. DOPA (1,2-dioleoyl-*sn*-glycerol-3-phosphate), provide strong negative charges. Under the influence of electrostatic effects, PA can produce unilamellar vesicles. Via the hydroxyl, the serine group of PS links with the phosphate, and the free amino links with carboxyl forming a neutral amphoteric ion; the net negative charge of the PS head group comes from the phosphate. Like PA, PS is sensitive to calcium, which causes its molecules to aggregate within the lipid membrane. The aggregation of the liposomes can also be led by a calcium bridge between PS on the membranes of different liposomal vesicles. However, PS can stabilize the lipid membranes during lyophilization in the presence of sugars.

Table 8.1 lists several physical properties of lipids used for liposome formation. Tc is the temperature at which a lipid transitions between the two phases, the gel phase and the fluid or liquid-crystal phase; it is typically higher for phospholipids with long chain of saturated fatty acids. The liposome membrane can be changed from gel state to fluid or liquid-crystal state according to the phase of the lipid by raising or lowering the temperature.

These data provide basic information for using them to prepare liposomes encapsulated with a specific drug to ensure the stable, controlled release of the encapsulated drug.

Cationic lipids bear a net positive charge. 1,2-dioleoyl-3-trimethylammonium-propane (DOTAP) and dioleyl oxypropyl trimethy ammonium chloride (DOPMA) are typically cationic lipids that are possibly cooperated with other lipids into liposomal membranes to deliver biomolecules to cells. Those liposomal vesicles are named ufasomes; they have bilayer membranes formed by single-chain zwitter-ions like non-ionic surfactants. The mechanism of preparation and physicochemical properties of ufasomes resembles those of conventional liposomes.

Apart from lipids, biomolecules, such as monoclonal antibodies, antibody derivatives, peptides, aptamers, floats, lectins, etc., are also composited onto the surface of liposomal vesicles as the ligands for active targeted delivery of the drugs. The therapeutic effect of the ligand-targeted delivery drug system relies on the encapsulated potential drugs and the affinity of the ligand for receptors. The varier patterns

Table 8.1 Physical properties of the lipids used for liposomes [24, 25]

Name	Carbons: unsaturation	Transition/pretransition temperature (Tc, °C)	Net charge at pH 7.4
DLPC	12:0	−1	0
DMPC	14:0	23–23.9/14	0
DPPC	16:0	41–41.5/35	0
DSPC	18:0	54.1–58/56	0
DOPC	18:1	−14 to 22	0
DLPE	12:0	29–30.6	0
DMPE	14:0	47.5–49.6	0
DPPE	16:0	60–63.2	0
DOPE	18:1	−16	0
DPPA-Na	16:0	67	−1.3
DOPA-Na	18:1	−8	−1.3
DMPG-Na	14:0	23	−1
DPPG-Na	16:0	41	−1
DOPG-Na	18:1	−18	−1
DMPS-Na	14:0	35	−1
DPPS-Na	16:0	54	−1
DOPE-Glutaryl-$(Na)_2$	18:1	~−10	−2
Tetra Myristoyl Cardiolipin-$(Na)_2$	14:0	59	−2
DPPE-mPEG-2000-Na	16:0	N/A	−1
DPPE-Carboxy PEG-2000-Na	16:0	N/A	−2
DOTAP · Cl	18:1	~−0	+1
EPC	Mixture	−15 to −7	0
EPE	Mixture	11.3–19.3	0
ESM	Mixture	40	0

formed by ligands are a challenge in the development of targeting drug delivery systems. The strength of the ligand's affinity for the payload is more important than the number of the molecules as the ligand. By the way, the general ligands not only can be conjugated to the surface of liposomes but also can be directly conjugated to the drugs for the delivery or distribution of the drugs actively targeting the diseased tissue or disordered cells, simultaneously decreasing the drug concentration in the normal tissues and cells.

The particular immunological ligands, monoclonal antibodies, that have been applied to carry the drugs also demonstrate the sustaining effects. It has been reported that the cytotoxic anticancer agent doxorubicin has been combined with monoclonal antibodies, and the immunogenetic nanosensor can specially target glioblastoma that was confirmed by using the imaging biomaterials [26]. A human monoclonal antibody, m826, conjugates H7 hemagglutinin (HA); therefore it can prevent H7N9 infection [27]. Cetuximab (C-225), an EGFR inhibitor, has been

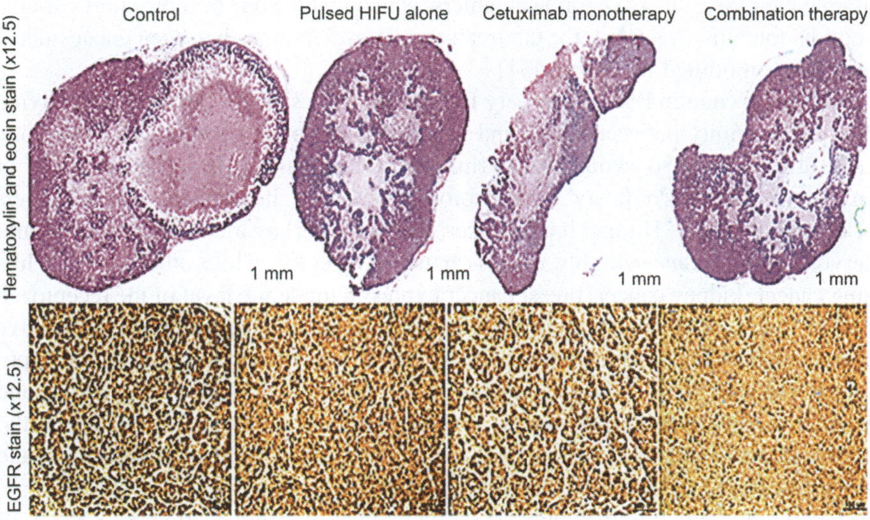

Fig. 8.2 Histopathological sections of HT-29 human colon cancer xenograft models in mice treated with EGFR-targeted cetuximab. The upper row shows hematoxylin and eosin-stained sections. In all specimens, central necrosis is obvious to various extents. The lower row shows a qualitative conversion of the EGFR abundance corresponding to the immunohistochemically stained specimens' in the upper row [28]

shown to affect head and neck cancer, metastatic non-small cell lung cancer, and metastatic colorectal cancer.

Figure 8.2 shows, in histopathological sections, that the effect of EGFR-targeted cetuximab on human colon cancer xenograft models in mice can be improved by pulsed HIFU [28]. In clinical trials, monoclonal antibodies, e.g. panitumumab (ABX-EGF), matuzumab (EMD72000), biciromab, trastuzumab, elotuzumab, vedolizumab, and ruplizumab (but not cetuximab (C-225)), have been developed as the ligand for cancer-targeted formulations. CA9, an antibody, has been combined onto the surface of the liposomes to deliver triptolide to try to treat lung cancer [29].

The fastest developing category of molecules being used for liposomes is antibody derivatives. These derivatives must be attached to specific places on the surface of specific antigens, therefore the length of the antibody derivatives is particularly correlated to the targeting effectiveness and carrier availability for the targeting drug delivery of the antibody derivatives particularly with the full length [29].

Peptide molecules are easily synthesized today if their sequences of amino acids are clear. Some tumor cells highly express peptide receptors that may combine the specific peptides, e.g. aviptadil, somatostatin, gastrin, etc. The liposomes conjugated with peptides delivering the drugs to the targets are based on the molecular interaction between the peptide and corresponding receptor [30].

Aptamers may be the peptide molecules or oligonucleotide molecules that can attach to specific target molecules. Aptamers could be classified into two categories: (1) DNA or RNA or XNA aptamers, which generally have short strands of oligonucleotides; and (2) peptide aptamers, which include one or more short variable peptide domains. A siRNA for the treatment of osteoporosis has been encapsulated in aptamer-modified liposomes [31].

Folate, or vitamin B9, is necessary for the biosynthesis of nucleotides in all living cells. The affinity between folate and its cellular receptor is very high. Eukaryotic cells utilize folate to synthesize pyrimidine and purines. The folate receptor of epithelial cancer has α, β, γ/γ′, and δ isoforms which are the most calculable markers of epithelial cancer. Human brain cancer, uterus cancer, ovarian cancer, and central nervous system cancer highly express α folate receptor, while other cancers, like lung cancer, kidney cancer, breast cancer express a moderate level of the receptor. It can be seen in 4T1 breast tumor cells in vitro that neutral liposomes with positive charges and/or neutral liposomes without charge can conjugate with folate. Liposomes carrying tumor imaging agents show a threefold increase in uptake and brighter fluorescence in microscopic images than those without folate [32]. Lastly, liposomes modified with folate have been prepared for delivering prednisolone and methotrexate for targeting rheumatoid arthritis [33].

Lectins are proteins that bind to carbohydrates existing in diverse species of biodomes including viruses and humans. The liposomes made from galactose-conjugated lipids loaded with silibinin, a hepatoprotective, were able to effectively target the lectin receptor and deliver the drug, and the liposomes can fully converge in the hepatic cells [34].

On the other hand, some other special liposome vesicles are developed by using the lipids plus other materials, such as the so-called transfersomes, invasomes, and ethosomes. Transfersomes are applied transdermally [35]. Non-ionic surfactant Span 80, carbopol 940, and lecithin extracted from soya bean have also been used as pharmaceutical additives in the transfersomes [36]. Invasomes are composed of phospholipids with unsaturated fatty acidic groups, and ethanol and terpenes are marginally added in the aqueous solution as the enhancers for penetration [37]. Ethosomes are composed of multiple bilayers of phospholipids suspended in a high concentration of ethanol (20–45%) aqueous solution; glycols are added in the aqueous solution [38]. And the organelles glycerosome composed of glycogen and proteins may also be used for the delivery of drugs [39].

8.3 Preparation

8.3.1 Relationship Between the Type and the Preparation Method

Liposomes are easily formed by shearing amphipathic lipids in water. Micromixing [40] and the Mozafari method [41] are newer methods employed to produce liposomes. When lipids are dispersed in an aqueous solution at a suitable concentration, the lipids gradually hydrate and swell to form multiple fluid bilayers as liquid-crystal phases, and eventually auto-assemble the liposomal vesicles. The sheets of the hydrous lipids can be isolated by appropriate agitation, and by auto-closure become MLV (multilamellar vesicles) with a wide range in size. The size of vesicles can be reduced by intensive sonication, extrusion, or ethanol injection (techniques of Batzri and Korn), to form small unilamellar vesicles (SUV), i.e., single-shelled vesicles. All lipid vesicles regardless of the composition can be prepared by all these methods. According to the requirement of the functions, size is the first feature and principal criterion of liposomal vesicles, because the size was easily manipulable and control giving out significantly different behaviors.

SUV have many properties; generally, people try to control the diameter and produce those homogenous in size. Large unilamellar vesicles (LUV) denote exceptionally large lipid vesicles, but opinions differ as to the specific dimensions. LUV can be prepared by calcium-induced fusion of SUV. Slow injection of a lipid-ether solution into a thermal enhydrous buffer causes a bilayer membrane to form in large flat sheets. The sheets are generally on the order of 0.5μm in diameter but may vary through several orders of magnitude from 25 nm to 25μm. The liposomes with cell-size (measured in micrometers) diameters are called giant liposomes. Intermediate-sized unilamellar vesicles (IUV) have been produced but not widely adopted. They help to identify the lipid vesicles between 100 and 200 nm in the region of 25 nm (SUV) to 500 nm (LUV). Liposomes with these diameters can be simply fabricated by using an extruder with proper pressurization or by dialysis with detergent. In pharmaceutical science, for IUV to be used as a drug delivery system, the size is controlled to ensure that it is stable, can be maintained in circulation for a long time, and membrane filtrating sterilization. MLV of any size are composed of more than one bilayer membrane and formed most easily by shaking PC in water. The lamellarity of MLV can be with 5–20 lipid bilayer membranes hinge on the lipid composition.

8.3.2 Method of Preparation

Extrusion technology has been developed to prepare LUV [42]. Extrusion of liposomes through porous membranes in an extruder (Fig. 8.3) can modify their size. Lipid vesicles are broken down as they pass through the membrane, and then reorganize as vesicles with sizes approximately the same as the membrane pores. Repetition of the process makes more vesicles; the size of the membrane pores determines the size of the vesicles formed.

Reverse-phase evaporation is another method for preparing liposomes. After the organic phase (ether) is evaporated from the W/O (aqueous in oil) emulsion, a single monolayer of lipids forms as a boundary around the small water balls in the gel. The vesicles can be destroyed by agitation. The optional lipids build the single lipid layer outside and then transforming the rest of the monolayer vesicles to LUV.

Dehydration-rehydration is a two-part process, which is a measure that can prolong the shelf life of liposome-entrapped drugs. Dehydration is the first process

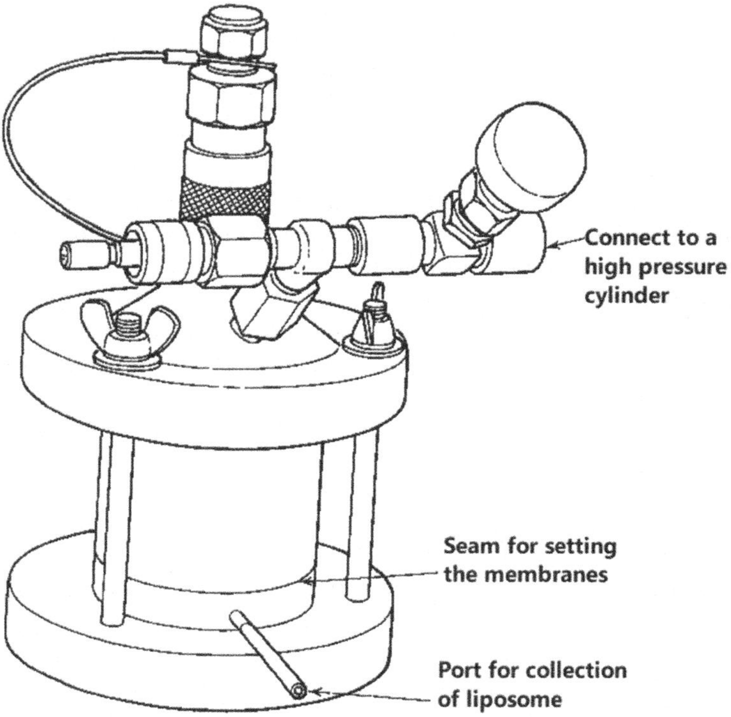

Fig. 8.3 Extruder for liposome preparation. Extruders may be designed and prepared with different sizes and shapes based on the scales of liposomal products

of evaporation or sublimation of the water continuous phase of the liposomal colloid-solution or suspension which should manage to keep the individual wholeness of the liposomal vesicles without water. The rehydration is the second process to recover the water continue phase for suspending the lipid vesicles. It is difficult to maintain the size of the original SUV before dehydration in the rehydrated vesicles. Entrapments greater than 50% can be achieved. Unstable molecules like proteins are suitable for being encapsulated in liposomes using this technique.

8.3.3 Surface Modification

Liposome surface may be modified by conjugating with immunoglobulins by using the coupling of the groups of functional lipids. Immunological molecules, especially, immunoglobulins and any other protein are also used to be the surface modification materials. During the formation of liposomes, the free immunoglobulins coupling lipids may also be incorporated into the liposome membrane. Liposomes can be coated with PEG to increase circulation time in the blood. The linkage of ligands appears to be the terminal of PEG chains; this maximizes exposure of the ligand and access to its target. Proteasome is the name of lipid vesicles with proteins incorporated into the membrane.

Surface modifications are particularly used for prolonging the life of liposomes in vivo. There are two approaches. One is to directly incorporate sphingomyelin linked with gangliosides such as oligosaccharide-ceramides into the membrane. The second is to conjugate polyethylene glycol (PEG) to the surface; the optimal molecular weight for such a PEG chain is 2000 Da. The PEG technology has been trademarked technology and is being applied on liposomes to avoid the uptake of the reticuloendothelial system (RES) and prolong the circulation in the bloodstream.

Transfersomes are those liposomes that are composed of special molecules that exhibit to efficiently transfer the aqueous drug phase across the skin. This liposomal membrane contains bile salt with phospholipid, which increases membrane flexibility. The liposomes are moderate in stimulation and lightly transmutable. These liposomes can be lightly squeezed passing across the incommodious exits integrally and through the dermis block by the effect of the feasible and diverse osmoses.

8.3.4 Loading or Entrapment of Drugs

Loading or entrapment relates to the liposome suspension at any time during manufacture, purification, or further processing. Liposomes load water-soluble API within the inner phase of the aqueous medium. Conventional separation procedures are used to remove unentrapped material. Lipid-soluble compounds may be incorporated within the membrane of the phospholipid mixture; 100% incorporation may be achieved if the ratio relative to phospholipid is not excessive. API may be introduced into the preformed empty liposomes' closed membranes by irreversible passage across the membrane, driven by pH, by osmotic or chemical potential gradients (remote loading), by freeze-drying, or by extrusion to rupture and reform the vesicles.

Liposomes may be passed through a 200 nm sterile filter without damage. This represents an aseptic technique as the sterilization avoids the elevated leakage rates of API from the liposomes by autoclave. Chemical damage or alteration of membrane characteristics is negligible during the process.

8.4 The Qualities of Liposomes

8.4.1 Liposomes Membrane

The thinness of the lipid bilayer may be from 4.5 to 4 nm for distearyl PC at the phase transition from gel to liquid. The area of the membrane surface membrane in the gel phase entirely depends on the lipid headgroup and has almost no relation to the fatty acids or the temperature. In the gel phase, lipid hydrocarbon chains' cross-sectional area is smaller than that of the lipid headgroup. When the headgroups approach closely, the chains incline to the tangential plane of the membrane. PE's headgroup is very small without tilt even below the main transition. One lipid molecule occupies 0.4–0.6 nm^2 of the surface area of the gel phase membrane and 0.75 nm^2 of that of the fluid phase membrane.

Flaws may materialize in lipid lamellae. In the gel phase, phospholipid molecules rotate and laterally mobilize furiously; the flaws persist in membranes for long periods. In the fluid state, such flaws form and settle more easily in short periods because of their mobility. Chemical degradation of lipids introduces species into the membrane to fill non-bilayer states and disrupts the padding within the lipid matrix.

Liposome membranes are often asymmetrical due to the phospholipids of different headgroups on the inner and outer surfaces. For liposomes with high curvature, phospholipids with large headgroups readily remain on the outer surface, while those with smaller headgroups are accommodated internally. As an example, the liposomes prepared with the mixture of PE and PC or PE with hydrophilic polymers such as PEG, the PC, or PE with hydrophilic polymers, the additive remains external. PE is more linked to the surface of the lipid bilayer toward the inner phase. Modifying the outer part of liposomes by chemical reaction alone also results in membrane asymmetry. Alternatively, double emulsion with the inner and outer leaflets of unilamellar lipid vesicles provides asymmetry of acyl chains. Asymmetries arise during further phase separation of membranes with PS by the presence of calcium, thereby inducing a change from a fluid to a condensed phase. Calcium has access to the outer leaflet only; different phases normally present in different halves of the membrane at the same time.

Large, uncharged PC liposomes exhibit aggregation because of the neutral planar phospholipid membranes. The surface curvature and the membrane charges increase the repulsion of the vesicles to prevent liposomes from closely approaching thereby minimizing aggregation. Aggregation occurs over some time, even with small vesicles.

Fusion means two or more separate vesicles combine to form a single vesicle sharing all lipids of the original vesicles. The propensity of membranes to fuse is related to phase discontinuities and irregularities. Liposomes designed especially for fusion usually contain high proportions of unsaturated PE to form inverted hexagonal structures or PS to condense the headgroups in the presence of calcium.

8.4.2 Entrapped Volume and Capture Efficiency

Entrapped or captured volume expresses the total volume of liquid entrapped within a certain quantity and size of liposomes. It is generally quoted in terms of the weight of lipids (μL/mg or L/mol). The entrapped volume of liposomes, which is made from mixed lipids (PG/PC/Chol = 1/4/5), is about 0.5μL/mg of SUV (20–50 nm), and over 10μL/mg of LUV (200–1000 nm) [43].

Capture efficiency expresses the proportion of starting material that ends up inside liposomes after manufacture. Efficiency is related to a process; therefore, it has no meaning for entrapment within liposomes after processing.

The entrapped percentage represents the quantity of solute inside liposomes compared to the total solute present in the solution at any given time. It is identical to capture efficiency immediately after liposomal fabrication. At other times, it is an indicative of leakage of the entrapped API from the liposomes and their stability during other processes and storage periods.

8.4.3 The Morphology and Size of Liposomes

The liposomal structure can be observed and photographed using a Cryo-TEM (Cryogenic transmission electron microscopy) with a virtually artifact-free depiction (Fig. 8.4). The liposome sample dropped on a grid forms a thin film in a liquid phase when the temperature is immediately reduced to 90 K; as a result, the water film

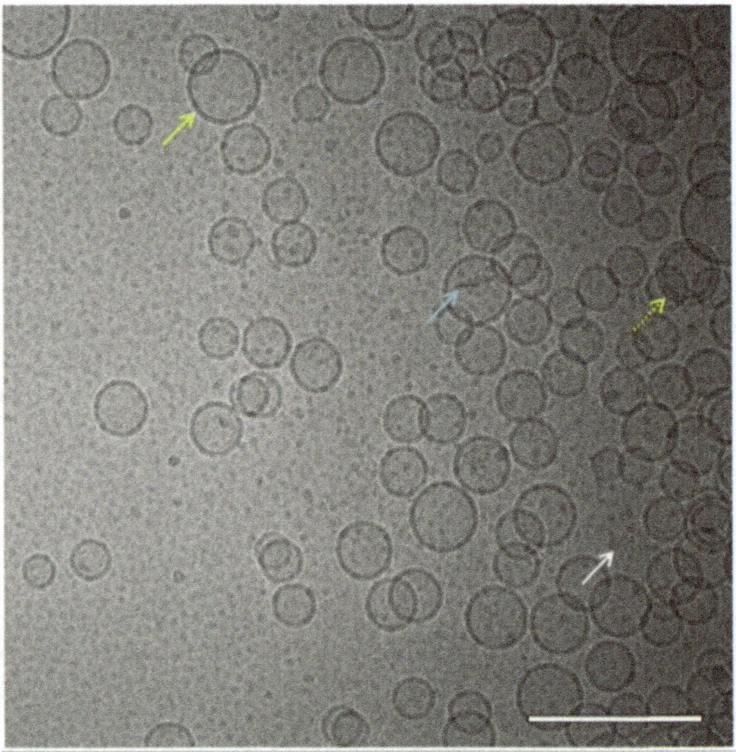

Fig. 8.4 Photograph of liposomes with 8 mg/mL lipids in PBS token by Cryo-TEM. The arrows in yellow, white, and blue, respectively, indicate the unilamellar, multilamellar vesicle, small micelle particles, rod-like particles, Scale bar = 200 nm [44]

freeze into a transparent, formless phase. Different liposome vesicles, such as SUV, LUV, MLV, etc., have been described in terms of size and morphology. Mechanical methods, such as extrusion, micro fluidization, etc., can reduce the size of liposomes, while fusion exposure to calcium, pH, freeze-thawing, etc., may increase the size of liposomes. Loss of aqueous content is a risk with these procedures.

8.4.3.1 Selective Permeability and Fluidity Permeability

Selective permeability is a property of liposome membranes that describes how easily they allow water and some other particular small molecules to pass through. The liposomes maintain their internal API and give selective permeability which allows the liposomes to control the quantum, timing, and rate of movement of these API.

The permeability of membranes increases with rising temperature. This means that encapsulated carbohydrates and/or proteins on the liposomal bilayer can shift their positions. However, the fluidity is not pliability. For example, cholesterol can shift along with a single lipid layer, but strictly restricts deformation of the liposomal bilayer.

8.4.4 Charges, pH, and Calcium

The cooperation of charged phospholipids assists intermembrane repulsion to increase the volume of internal compartments of MLVs and reduce the propensity of vesicles to aggregate. In liposome membranes, ionizable lipids are capable of forming hexagonal phases (e.g. PE) that are unstable at certain pH values, leading to leakage, fusion, or rupture of liposome contents. The stability of such membranes can be modulated by the presence of other components such as proteins. Liposomes made from ionizable negatively charged lipids (e.g., PA or PS) undergo aggregation and/or fusion in the presence of calcium and other divalent cations.

8.4.5 Stability and Storage

The leakage of encapsulated API from liposomes happens normally. Retention is greater for high molecular weight and water-soluble API with charges. Hydrophobic molecules incorporated into the membrane will remain entrapped indefinitely. Both hydrophilic and lipophilic APIs may pass through membranes.

The proximity of liposome membranes leads to aggregate and fuse. Introducing charges into the membranes and reducing the size of the liposomes can prevent irregularities, fluidity, and the tendency for interaction between vesicles, thereby inhibiting aggregation and fusion.

Phase disengagement is the phenomenon in which a unitary phase, such as a solid or a liquid, turns into two or more phases by forming fresh phases at the Tc. The irregularities in the phospholipid membrane arise from the co-existence of domains of the two phases within the same membrane. Also, phase separation increases membrane permeability and susceptibility to intermembrane fusion, vesicle aggregation, and so on. Cholesterol incorporated in the membrane (up to 50 mol%) decreases fluidity above the Tc, increases it below the Tc, and reduces the enthalpy of the phase transition.

As a result of the free radicals working on unsaturated hydrocarbons, the oxidation of lipids generates toxicities and membrane changes. Antioxidants (e.g. tocopherol) and metal ion chelators inhibit the possibility of oxidation. Hydrolysis of phospholipid releases free fatty acids and lyso-derivatives, making the membrane unstable. Hydrolysis easily occurs in aqueous solutions by buffer ions at the extremely high pH and/or extremely low pH and cholesterol-free membranes. Lyophilization (freeze-drying) stabilizes the liposomes in the presence of sugars such as trehalose or sucrose at high concentrations, which inhibit fusion and leakage.

8.5 The Application of Liposomes in Chinese Medicine

At present, the application value of liposomes to Chinese medicines cannot be overstated. Most Chinese medicines are compound prescriptions of many species of herbs with unclear pharmacological ingredients. This makes it difficult for the application of liposomes to deliver the APIs of Chinese Materia Medica. On the other hand, once the API is extracted from the Chinese herbs, it is not normally regarded as Chine medicine. Table 8.2 listed some liposomal API as examples to inspire the way of application of liposomes in Chinese Medicine.

Liposomal delivery has three important advantages. First, it is excellent at delivering API directly into the cells. Second, because lipids are biodegradable, they are essentially non-toxic in nature. Third, liposomes provide a feasible way to improve the API's treatment indices. The liposomes can be applied in pharmaceutics for both therapeutic and diagnostic API. For research on identification, the interaction of cells, and some substances' movements, liposomes can serve as reactants, models, or vehicles [48]. Liposomes may be an adjuvant for enhancing the infiltration of multifarious materials in cosmetics. They can solubilize insoluble API and increase the effect of a vaccine, diagnostic, or therapeutic (Table 8.2).

In Chinese medicine, the use of liposomes is a frontier. Nevertheless, there is intense research on the preparation and characterization of liposomes, particularly combining Western pharmaceuticals with active ingredients from herbs. Taking the anticancer compounds mitoxantrone and vincristine (VCR) extract of *Changchunhua (Catharanthus roseus* L.) as an example, liposomes were prepared by film-forming, reverse-phase evaporation vesicle method, and remote loading method (pH gradient method, adjusted pH 4.0 to pH 7.4). The complex liposomal

Table 8.2 Liposomes in the pharmaceutical for drug delivery [45–47]

Application and type of liposomes	Pharmaceutical ingredients	Target site or treated disease by liposomes
General liposomes	Wogonin, usnea acid, 5-fluorouracil iohexol, hydroxycamptothecin	Cancer, tuberculosis, brain and liver, lung
Solubilization	Amphotericin b, minoxidil	Fungal infections
Site-avoidance	Doxorubicin, amphotericin b	Nephrotoxicity cardiotoxicity
Long-circulating, sustained-release	Brucine, hormones, corticosteroids, drug depot in the lungs	Stomach lung liver, cancer, biotherapeutics
Drug protection	Cytosine arabinoside, interleukins	Cancer, etc.
RES targeting	Macrophage-locate, tetanus toxoid, vaccines	Cancer, tetanus
Immunoliposomes specific targeting	Docetaxel, paclitaxel, cells bearing specific antigens	Tumor, wide therapeutic applicability
Extravasation	Leaky vasculature of tumors, inflammations, infections	Cancer, bacterial infections
Accumulation	Prostaglandins	Cardiovascular diseases
Penetration enhance	Triptolide, baicalein, topical vehicles	Lung cancer, eliminate radicals, dermatology
Drug depot	Lungs, subcutaneous, muscular, ocular	Wide therapeutic applicability
Antibiotic delivery	Mafenide acetate, streptomycin, chloramphenicol	Antibiotic therapy
Transdermal delivery	Celecoxib	Osteoarthritis, acute pain, rheumatoid arthritis
Cosmetics delivery	Tretinoin	Skin care
Delivery to parasite	Miltefosine	Parasitic diseases
Gen delivery	Magnetite cationic/DNA complex	Bioengineering

mitoxantrone and vincristine may meet the requirements of the potential use in clinical practice [49].

8.6 Conclusion

Based on liposomes' solubility in water and their ability to protect entrapped API and deliver to targeted cells, liposomes are being widely investigated and developed for a wide range of medical applications. Liposomes are expected to be a kind of drug delivery system to carry a large number of API, including those from Chinese medicines. Carrying antimicrobial, anticancer, antifungal, etc., agents, liposomes could be modified to target specific disordered cells in diseased organs. Liposomes could be taken orally, administered by injection, or applied externally. Liposomes have been approved as drug carriers to improve effects and duration of action and to decrease toxicity, dosage, and frequency of administration. With these approvals, liposomes are achieving clinical acceptance. Future research will certainly expand the breadth and extent of applications possible with these unique formulations.

References

1. Yang, F. Y., et al. (1977). Application of liposome in the research of bio-membrane and pharmacy. *Progress in Biochemistry and Biophysics*, (18), 36–40.
2. Gu, X.-q., et al. (1982). Investigation of polyphase liposome a new dosage form for antitumor agents report I—Anti-tumor activity screening of Polyphase liposome 139 and others. *Journal of Shenyang College of Pharmacy*, (15), 1–9.
3. Bangham, A. D., et al. (1962). Action of saponin on biological cell membranes. *Nature, 196* (4858), 952–955.
4. Horne, R. W., et al. (1963). Negatively stained lipoprotein membranes. *Nature, 200*(4913), 1340.
5. Bangham, A. D., et al. (1964). Negative staining of phospholipids and their structural modification by surface-active agents as observed in the electron microscope. *Journal of Molecular Biology, 8*(5), 660–668.
6. Bangham, A. D., et al. (1965). Diffusion of univalent ions across the lamellae of swollen phospholipids. *Journal of Molecular Biology, 13*(1), 238–252.
7. Bangham, A. D., et al. (1965). The action of steroids and streptolysin S on the permeability of phospholipid structures to cations. *Journal of Molecular Biology, 13*(1), 253–259.
8. Weissmann, G., et al. (1965). Abstracts. *The Journal of Clinical Investigation, 44*(6), 1109–1116.
9. Watts, G., et al. (2010). *The Lancet, 375*(9731), 2070.
10. YashRoy, R. C. (1990). Lamellar dispersion and phase separation of chloroplast membrane lipids by negative staining electron microscopy. *Journal of Biosciences, 15*(2), 93–98.
11. Forrest, L. R. (2015). Structural symmetry in membrane proteins. *Annual Review of Biophysics, 44*(1), 311–337.
12. Voet, D. (2012). *Fundamentals of biochemistry: Life at the molecular level* (4th ed.). Wiley. ISBN 978-1118129180.
13. Fahy, E., et al. (2009). Update of the LIPID MAPS comprehensive classification system for lipids. *Journal of Lipid Research, 50*(Suppl S1), S9–S14. https://doi.org/10.1194/jlr.R800095-JLR200
14. Moss, G. P., et al. (1997). IUPAC compendium of chemical terminology. In *Pure and applied chemistry* (Vol. 67, 2nd ed., pp. 1307–1375. ISBN 978-0-521-51150-6). International Union of Pure and Applied Chemistry. https://doi.org/10.1351/pac199567081307
15. Yashroy, R. C. (1987). 13C NMR studies of lipid fatty acyl chains of chloroplast membranes. *Indian Journal of Biochemistry & Biophysics, 24*(6), 177–178.
16. Devlin, T. M. (1997). *Textbook of biochemistry: With clinical correlations* (4th ed., pp. 193–195). John Wiley & Sons. ISBN 978-0-471-17053-2.
17. Lodish, H., Berk, A., Zipursky, L. S., et al. (2000). Biomembranes: Structural organization and basic functions. In *Molecular cell biology* (4th ed.). Scientific American Books. ISBN 978-0-7167-3136-8.
18. Cooper, G. M. (2000). Structure of the plasma membrane. In *The cell: A molecular approach* (2nd ed.).
19. Lentz, B. R. (2003). Exposure of platelet membrane phosphatidylserine regulates blood coagulation. *Progress in Lipid Research, 42*(5), 423–438.

20. Dougherty, R. M., et al. (1987). Lipid and phospholipid fatty acid composition of plasma, red blood cells, and platelets and how they are affected by dietary lipids: A study of normal subjects from Italy, Finland, and the USA. *The American Journal of Clinical Nutrition, 45*(2), 443–455.
21. Mitchell, B. (2019). *Cell and molecular biology* (pp. 130–131., ISBN 978-1-83947-446-0). ED-Tech Press.
22. Mashaghi, S., et al. (2013). Lipid nanotechnology. *International Journal of Molecular Sciences, 14*(2), 4242–4282.
23. Inoue, K., & Nojima, S. (1984). *Pharmacia, 20*, 869.
24. https://avantilipids.com/tech-support/liposome-preparation/lipids-for-liposome-formation
25. Marsh, D. (2012). Thermodynamics of phospholipid self-assembly. *Biophysical Journal, 102*, 1079–1087.
26. Wang, X., et al. (2018). Anti-CD133 monoclonal antibody conjugated immunomagnetic nanosensor for molecular imaging of targeted cancer stem cells. *Sensors and Actuators B: Chemical, 255*, 3447–3457.
27. Yu, F., et al. (2017). A potent germline-like human monoclonal antibody targets a pH-sensitive epitope on H7N9 influenza hemagglutinin. *Cell Host & Microbe, 22*(4), 471–483.e5.
28. Park, M. J., et al. (2013). Pulsed high-intensity focused ultrasound therapy enhances targeted delivery of cetuximab to colon cancer xenograft model in mice. *Ultrasound in Medicine & Biology, 39*(2), 292–299.
29. Lin, C., et al. (2017). Pulmonary delivery of triptolide-loaded liposomes decorated with anti-carbonic anhydrase IX antibody for lung cancer therapy. *Scientific Reports, 7*, 1097. https://doi.org/10.1038/s41598-017-00957-4
30. Riaz, M. K., et al. (2019). Pulmonary delivery of transferrin receptors targeting peptide surface-functionalized liposomes augments the chemotherapeutic effect of quercetin in lung cancer therapy. *International Journal of Nanomedicine, 14*, 2879–2902.
31. Liang, C., et al. (2015). Aptamer-functionalized lipid nanoparticles targeting osteoblasts as a novel RNA interference-based bone anabolic strategy. *Nature Medicine, 21*(3), 288–294.
32. Silindir-Gunay, M., et al. (2019). Radiolabeled, folate-conjugated liposomes as tumor imaging agents: Formulation and in vitro evaluation. *Journal of Drug Delivery Science and Technology, 50*, 321–328.
33. Verma, A., et al. (2019). Folate conjugated double liposomes bearing prednisolone and methotrexate for targeting rheumatoid arthritis. *Pharmaceutical Research, 36*(8), 123.
34. Dube, D., et al. (2010). Preparation and evaluation of galactosylated vesicular carrier for hepatic targeting of silibinin. *Drug Development and Industrial Pharmacy, 36*(5), 547–555.
35. Cevc, G., & Blume, G. (1992). Lipid vesicles penetrate into intact skin owing to the transdermal osmotic gradients and hydration force. *Biochimica et Biophysica Acta, 1104*, 226–232.
36. Gupta, A., Aggarwal, G., Singla, S., & Arora, R. (2012). Transfersomes: A novel vesicular carrier for enhanced transdermal delivery of sertraline: development, characterization, and performance evaluation. *Scientia Pharmaceutica, 80*(4), 1061–1080.
37. Dragicevic, N., Verma, D. D., & Fahr, A. (2016). Invasomes: Vesicles for enhanced skin delivery of drugs. In N. Dragicevic & H. Maibach (Eds.), *Percutaneous penetration enhancers chemical methods in penetration enhancement*. Springer. https://doi.org/10.1007/978-3-662-47862-2_5. ISBN 978-3-662-47861-5.
38. Touitou, E. (1996/1998). Compositions for applying active substances to or through the skin; Patent number: 5540934 Granted; Patent number 5716638 Granted.
39. Rybicka, K. (June 1996). Glycosomes - The organelles of glycogen metabolism. *Tissue & Cell, 28*(3), 253–265.
40. López, R. R., et al. (2020). Surface response based modeling of liposome characteristics in a periodic disturbance mixer. *Micromachines, 11*(3), 235.
41. Colas, J. C., et al. (2007). Microscopical investigations of nisin-loaded nanoliposomes prepared by Mozafari method and their bacterial targeting. *Micron, 38*(8), 841–847.
42. Mayer, L. D., et al. (1986). Vesicles of variable sizes produced by a rapid extrusion procedure. *Biochimica et Biophysica Acta, 858*, 161–168.

43. Szoka, F., Jr., et al. (1978). Procedure for preparation of liposomes with large internal aqueous space and high capture by reverse-phase evaporation. *Proceedings of the National Academy of Sciences of the United States of America, 75*(9), 4194–4198.
44. Fox, C. B., et al. (2014). Cryogenic transmission electron microscopy of recombinant tuberculosis vaccine antigen with anionic liposomes reveals formation of flattened liposomes. *International Journal of Nanomedicine, 9*, 1367–1377.
45. Karami, N., et al. (2018). Liposomes as a novel drug delivery system: Fundamental and pharmaceutical application. *Asian Journal of Pharmaceutics, 12*(1), S31–S41.
46. Li, D.-C., et al. (2009). Application of targeted drug delivery system in Chinese medicine. *Journal of Controlled Release, 138*, 103–112.
47. Lipowsky, R., et al. (1995). Chapter 10, Applications of liposomes. In *Handbook of biological physics* (Vol. 1, pp. 491–519). Elsevier Science B.V..
48. Wang, X., et al. (2013). miR-214 targets ATF4 to inhibit bone formation. *Nature Medicine, 19*(1), 93–100.
49. Chen, T., et al. (2009). Efficacy and toxicity of liposomal compound vincristine sulfate on breast cancer in nude mice. *Journal of Biomedical Engineering, 26*(1), 127–129.

Chapter 9
Microparticulate Drug Delivery Systems for Chinese Medicines

Wenping Wang

Abstract Microparticulate drug delivery system of Chinese medicine refers to particles within 1–1000 μm using microencapsulation technology to load the active ingredients, fractions, or even crude extracts from Chinese Materia Medica or natural medicines into coating materials. Microparticle is one of the hot spots in the development of novel pharmaceutical products of Chinese medicine. It can mask the undesired flavors, provide a favorable reservoir for liquid extracts and various nanocarriers, serve as a protection for unstable or sensitive ingredients against the external environment, modify the drug release pattern and target drug delivery site for improved therapeutic effect and reduced side effect, and also act as a pharmaceutical intermediate for the further fabrication of different dosage forms. Due to these advantages over conventional preparations, microparticles have found extensive applications in both pharmaceutical and bioengineering fields. This chapter reviews literature on microparticulate preparations of Chinese medicine published in the past 10 years and aims to provide a procedure for the development of microparticulate DDS for Chinese pharmaceuticals. A survey of various core/shell materials and microencapsulation techniques in the literature is presented. And we also summarize the application of microparticles of Chinese medicine in different fields. In the future, more attention should be paid to the research on the development of novel coating materials with natural origins and new microencapsulation techniques with efficient drug loading and eco-friendly processes and also on the widespread application of microparticulate DDS of Chinese medicine.

Keywords Microparticle · Microencapsulation · Microsphere · Microcapsule · Chinese medicine · Microparticulate drug delivery system · Coating material

---

W. Wang (✉)
School of Chinese Materia Medica, Yunnan University of Chinese Medicine, Kunming, China
e-mail: wangwenping@ynutcm.edu.cn

N. Feng, Z. Yang (eds.), *Novel Drug Delivery Systems for Chinese Medicines*,
https://doi.org/10.1007/978-981-16-3444-4_9

9.1 Introduction

Microparticulate drug delivery system is a very useful approach to overcome the difficulties associated with conventional dosage forms of Chinese medicine. It plays an important role aimed to protect active ingredients from the environment and reduce its side effects or provide modified-release and improved bioavailability.

Microparticles are referred to as particle systems (1–1000 μm) constituted by combinations of bioactives and biomaterials [1]. Microparticles are the resulting products of the microencapsulation process. Microencapsulation technology in the pharmaceutical industry usually aims to increase the effectiveness of active ingredients by entrapping them with polymer materials [2]. The main advantages of applying microencapsulation in Chinese medicines are listed as follows: (1) solidification of liquid or semi-solid drugs, such as volatile oils and fluid extracts from Chinese medicinal slices; (2) stabilization of active ingredients, specifically protect drugs from oxidization, reduce loss by volatilization, and avoid damage by exposure to enzymes and different pH environments in the gastrointestinal tract; (3) sustained or controlled release of drugs; (4) site-specific or even targeted delivery of active ingredients, such as gastric-retentive or liver-targeted preparations; and (5) improvement of patient compliance via taste-masking [3], less gastric-irritation, and more convenience.

On the other hand, several drawbacks are also required to be taken into consideration during the application of microencapsulation techniques [4]. First of all, the limited drug loading capacity of microparticles means higher administration dose, but improved stability and bioavailability can make up the difference. Secondly, multi-step processes are often required, which may result in potential drug loss, difficulties on scale-up production, and undesired sub-products or residues. Finally, various parameters can affect the characteristics of final microparticulate products, which may further affect their therapeutic performance.

Currently, research on microparticles for Chinese medicines is focused on developing new DDS to obtain pharmaceutical products which can reduce adverse and side effects, allow site-specific drug delivery, and provide a sustained or controlled release of drugs.

9.2 Types and Components of Microparticles of Chinese Medicine

Microparticles can be categorized as microcapsules and microspheres by their internal structure [5]. Generally, a microcapsule is a reservoir system with solid or liquid bioactive as its core material and polymers as its coating material (also called encapsulating, shell, or wall material). For microspheres, active ingredients are dispersed or even dissolved in polymers to form a matrix system.

However, microcapsules and microspheres are often used synonymously. And nowadays, the difference between microcapsule and microsphere is reduced or even disappeared with the development of microencapsulation technology [6, 7]. Novel microspheres, with a similar structure to microcapsules, are appearing one after another, including core-shell microspheres [8, 9], hollow microspheres [10, 11], and liquid-core microspheres [6].

9.2.1 Core Materials

As listed in Table 9.1, various active ingredients extracted from Chinese medicine can be adopted into microparticulate preparations. In some cases, the core material was a single active compound extracted from a specific Chinese Materia Medica. In other cases, effective fractions (or even crude extracts) from one or more Chinese medicinal slices were used as the core material and encapsulated into the particles. For the latter cases, the active component is a more complicated mixture of a variety of substances with different physio-chemical and pharmacokinetic properties, and the therapeutic mechanism is far away fully understood, in comparison with a single active compound. Therefore, more challenges might be encountered in the preparation process and qualitative assessment [44–46].

At present, a single active ingredient was more often taken as a model drug. But in the future, we can expect more research on microparticles loaded with multi-ingredient as the development of the modernization of Chinese medicine.

9.2.2 Coating Materials

The coating material and its physical structure strongly influence the fabrication process of the microparticles and play a crucial role in the drug release behavior of the final products. Therefore, the choice of coating materials is one of the key steps during the development of microparticulate products. The coating material should be non-toxic and non-irritative to the organism and is preferred to be biocompatible and biodegradable. Moreover, the physical and chemical properties of these materials should be proper for the microencapsulation and modified-release of the bioactive. Generally, polymers are applied in the microencapsulation process and can be classified into two categories as water-soluble and water-insoluble materials. The polymers should be chemically compatible and non-reactive with the encapsulating components and provide the desired coating properties such as strength, flexibility, impermeability, and stability [1, 2].

Table 9.2 presents the coating/matrix materials used in the encapsulation of Chinese medicine and their extracts. Among these materials, the most commonly used products are natural-origin and water-soluble carbohydrates and their derivatives because of their excellent biocompatibility and low cost. PLA and PLGA are

Table 9.1 Examples of microencapsulated ingredients from Chinese medicine

Categories	Active ingredients	Examples	Origin	References
Single medicinal slices	Extracts (extraction process)	Crude extract	Shanzhuyu (*Corni Fructus*)	[12]
		Volatile oil	Ezhu (*Curcumae Rhizoma*), jingjie (*Schizonepetae Herba*)	[13]
		Total alkaloids	Maqianzi (*Strychni Semen*)	[14]
		Polysaccharides	Fuling (*Poria*)	[15]
		Chuanxiong	Chuanxiong (*Chuanxiong Rhizoma*)	[16]
		Polysaccharides	Baiji (*Rhizoma Bletillae*)	[17]
		Saponins	Sanqi (*Notoginseng Radix et Rhizoma*)	[18]
	Active ingredients	Naringenin	Gusuibu (*Drynariae Rhizoma*)	[19]
		Asiaticoside	Jixuecao (*Centellae Herba*)	[20]
		Icariin	Yinyanghuo (*Epimedii Folium*)	[21, 22]
		Ligustrazine HCl	Chuanxiong (*Chuanxiong Rhizoma*)	[23]
		Ginsenoside Rg3	Renshen (*Ginseng Radix et Rhizoma*)	[24]
		Ginsenoside Rg1	Renshen (*Ginseng Radix et Rhizoma*)	[25]
		Cucurbitacin B	Guadi (*Melo Pedicellus*)	[26]
		Curcumin	Jianghuang (*Curcumae Longae Rhizoma*)	[27, 28]
		Norcantharidate	Banmao (*Mylabris*)	[29]
		Puerarin	Gegen (*Puerariae Lobatae Radix*)	[30]
		Norisoboldine	Wuyao (*Linderae Radix*)	[31]
		Sinomenine	Qingfengteng (*Sinomenii Caulis*)	[32]
		Glycyrrhetinic acid	Gancao (*Glycyrrhizae Radix et Rhizoma*)	[33, 34]
		Sophoridine	Kudouzi (*Sophora Alopecuroide Semen*)	[35]
		Breviscapine	Dengzhanhua (*Erigerontis Herba*)	[36]
Compound formula	Crude extracts	Shenmai injection	Renshen (*Ginseng Radix et Rhizoma*), Maidong (*Ophiopogonis Radix*), Wuweizi (*Schisandrae Chinensis Fructus*)	[37]
		Ethanol extracts	Compound kangai powder: Baihuasheshecao (*Hedyotis Diffusae Herba*), Shuihonghuazi (*Polygoni Orientalis Fructus*), Sanqi (*Notoginseng Radix et Rhizoma*), Chonglou (*Paridis Rhizoma*), Xiyangshen (*Panacis Quinquefolii Radix*), Chaihu (*Bupleuri Radix*)	[38]

(continued)

Table 9.1 (continued)

Categories	Active ingredients	Examples	Origin	References
		Extracts	Wuyao (*Linderae Radix*), compound Shuanghuanglian	[39]
		Extracts	Compound Shuanghuanglian	[40]
	Effective fractions	Total flavonoids	Gusuibu (*Drynariae Rhizoma*) + Yejuhua (*Chrysanthemi Indici Flos*)	[41]
		Total flavonoids	Yinyanghuo (*Epimedii Folium*) + Huangqin (*Scutellariae Radix*) + Sanqi (*Notoginseng Radix et Rhizoma*) + Yejuhua (*Chrysanthemi Indici Flos*)	[42]
		Total alkaloids	Huanglian (*Coptidis Rhizoma*) and Wuzhuyu (Euodiae Fructus) in a ratio of 6:1 (w/w)	[43]

Table 9.2 Commonly used coating materials for microencapsulation of Chinese medicine

Category	Subcategory	Materials	Ref.
Water-soluble materials	Carbohydrate and derivatives	Gums: gelatin, acacia gum	[38]
		Alginate +/− chitosan	[22, 25]
		Maltodextrin	[12]
	Protein and derivatives	BSA	[34]
		HSA	[29]
		Eudargit	[32, 40]
		HPMCP	[42]
Water-insoluble materials	Synthetic polymers	Polyesters: PLA, PLGA	[24, 33]
		EC	[13, 14, 20]
		mPEG-PMA	[18]

degradable in vivo and are approved by the FDA of the United States; therefore they are often applied to encapsulate active ingredients for prolonged-release or targeted delivery systems [47].

In some cases, extracts from Chinese medicines can be used as the matrix material for the fabrication of microparticles. Luo et al. extracted and isolated the polysaccharide fraction from *Rhizoma Bletillae* to prepare microspheres by an emulsification-cool condensation-chemical crosslinking method [48]. The obtained MSs were then applied as an embolic agent in interventional approach.

9.3 Fabrication of Microparticulate DDS of Chinese Medicine

The development of microparticles of Chinese medicine involves three stages (see Fig. 9.1): the extraction and pretreatment of active components from Chinese Materia Medica as the core materials, the dispersion of both core and shell materials in one or more liquid systems, and the microencapsulation of the active components with the coating materials.

The active components in the liquid system can be dispersed as a solution, an emulsion, or suspension, and the polymers usually as a solution. The liquid is described as an aqueous system in most cases and seldom as a non-aqueous system using organic solvents or oil as the medium. Generally, an emulsion needs to be prepared before the formation of the microparticles, especially for oil drugs or organic solutions of polymers and/or drugs. Several conventional methods can be used to form emulsion mostly with a broad size distribution, including stirring, static mixing, homogenization, and dripping [27]. But novel techniques can be adapted to produce emulsions with uniform droplets, such as membrane-emulsification technique [49] and microfluidic technique [50].

During the microencapsulation process, the active material in solid, liquid, or semi-solid state is coated with a continuous film or matrix to form particles in the micrometer to the millimeter in size. According to the formation mechanism and the consolidation method, the microencapsulation processes can be categorized into three groups [27, 49, 50]: physical methods (solvent evaporation, spray drying, supercritical fluid precipitation, and lyophilization), physicochemical methods (coacervation, ionic gelation), and chemical methods (interfacial polymerization, molecular inclusion complexation). The physical and physiochemical methods, especially solvent evaporation and coacervation, were frequently used because of their feasibility and flexibility during the preparation of microparticles of Chinese medicine.

9.3.1 Solvent Evaporation

The solvent evaporation method is widely applied for the fabrication of microparticles based on water-insoluble polymers, especially for PLA/PLGA microspheres. Typically, four steps are involved in this method [4, 51]: (1) Dissolve the polymer as a coating material in an organic solvent, and then disperse the active compound (or its aqueous solution) to form a solution, a suspension, or an emulsion. (2) Disperse the organic phase into an aqueous phase (continuous phase) to form an emulsion; sometimes an oil liquid (e.g., liquid paraffin) may be used as the continuous phase. (3) Remove the organic solvent by evaporation or liquid extraction. (4) Collect the particles by filtration or centrifugation and freeze-/vaccum-dry the microparticles.

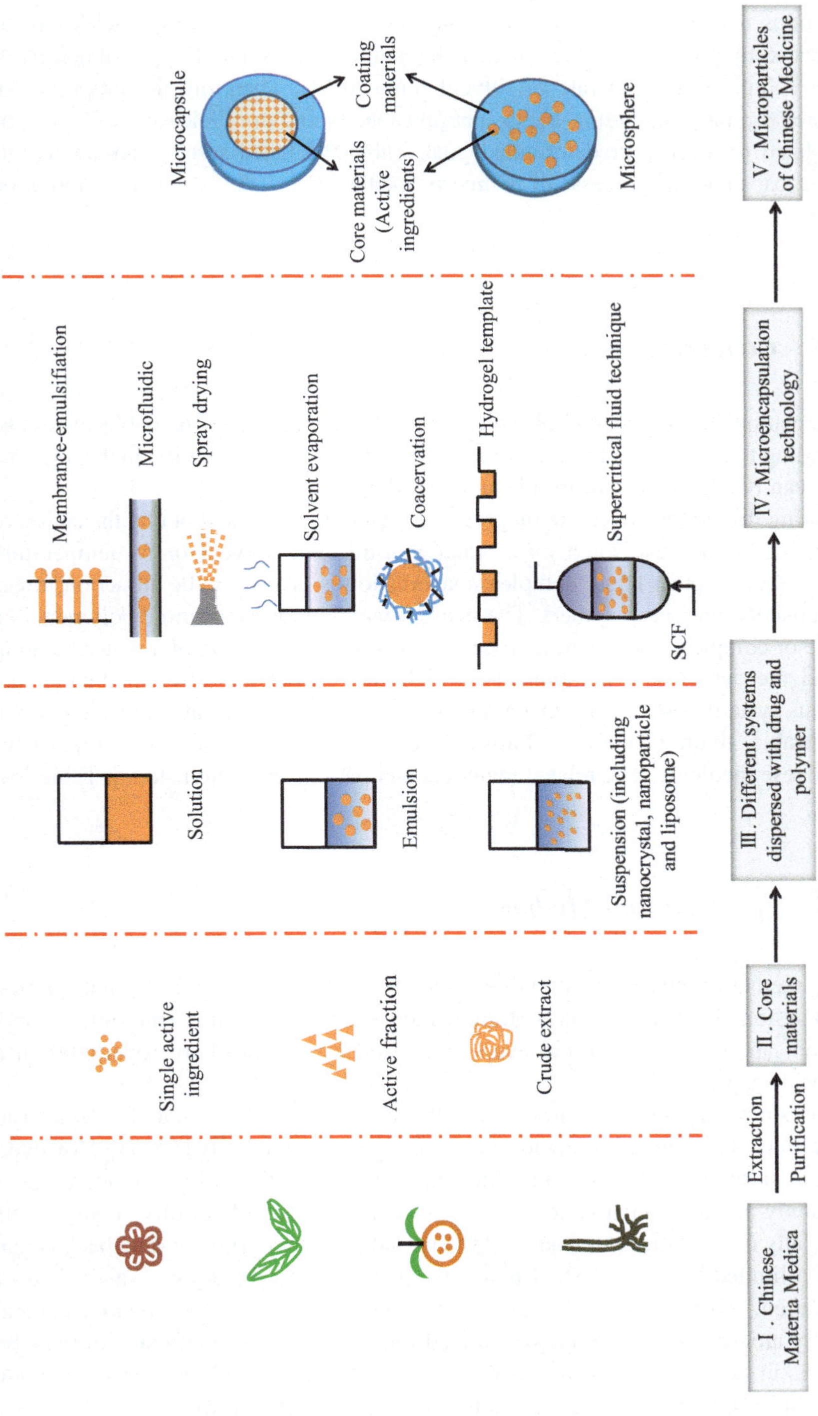

Fig. 9.1 Schematic procedures for the development of microparticulate DDS of Chinese medicine

The solvent evaporation method attracted much attention for its mild process conditions and ease of use and scale-up. The structure of microparticles can be influenced by process variables such as the nature of the solvent, types of additives, phase volume ratio, and rate of solvent removal [4]. Therefore the properties of obtained products, including encapsulation capacity and drug release profile, can be modulated to reach a predetermined goal. Table 9.3 listed some examples of the microencapsulation process of Chinese medicine by the solvent evaporation technique.

9.3.2 Coacervation

Coacervation in the aqueous phase can be used to trap water-insoluble materials. According to the involved phase separation mechanism, coacervation in the aqueous phase can be classified into simple and complex coacervation [52, 53].

During the simple coacervation process, the polymer is salted out by the action of electrolytes or is desolvated by a water non-miscible solvent or by temperature change. On the other hand, complex coacervation is driven by the attraction forces of oppositely charged polymers. The phase separation of one or more polymers in a simple or complex coacervation process results in the formation of a matrix coating around the active core components, which was suspended or emulsified in the aqueous system. The coating materials used to produce coacervates include gelatin, gum Arabic, albumin, alginate, chitosan, and EC for the fabrication of microparticles of Chinese medicine. The related materials and parameters were listed in Table 9.4.

9.3.3 Spray Drying Method

In this method, both drugs and polymers are firstly dispersed and homogenized in a liquid system. Then the liquid is atomized to form tiny drops that enter into contact with hot air, resulting in rapid evaporation and formation of microparticles in a spherical shape.

The spray drying technology is well established and suitable for industrial applications due to its relatively low cost and high reproducibility [54, 55]. However, a major disadvantage of the spray drying technique is that a high temperature is commonly applied which is not favorable for the stability of sensitive components (especially macromolecules such as proteins and peptides). Another drawback is that it has a limited number of shell materials available and therefore a small field of application. Since most spray drying processes in the Chinese pharmaceutical industry are carried out from aqueous feed formulations, the shell material must be soluble in water at an acceptable level. Typical shell materials include hydrophobically modified starch, maltodextrins, and PLGA [56].

Table 9.3 The materials and processes of the solvent evaporation method applied to microparticles of Chinese medicine

Emulsion type	Particle structure	Polymer	Active compound	Experiment conditions	Particle characteristics	References
O/W	Porous MS	EC	Asiaticoside	Emulsion method, dripping; O, drug solution in DCM; W, 1% PVA in water	44.34 ± 14.68 μm, EE = 71.8 ± 0.2%, D_{6h} > 90%	[20]
	MS	PLGA (50:50)	Naringenin	Emulsion method, dripping; O, drug solution in DCM + acetone (4:1); W, 2.5% PVA in water	44.34 ± 14.68 μm, EE = 20.1–35.9%, DL = 0.01–0.20%	[19]
	MC	EC	Strychnos alkaloids	Emulsion method, dripping; O, drug solution in EtAc; W, 2% Tween80 in water	523.7 μm, EE = 53.99%, DL = 18.25%, $D_{0.5h}$ = 10.3%, D_{12h} = 99.9%	[14]
$W_1/O/W_2$	MC	PLGA (75:25, 20 kDa)	Totoal flavonoids from Gusuibu (*Drynariae Rhizoma*) and Yejuhua (*Chrysanthemi Indici Flos*)	Emulsion method, dripping; W_1, drug solution; O, DCM + EtAc (1:2); W_2, 3% PVA + 2%NaCl	44.34 ± 14.68 μm, EE = 83.89 ± 2.30%, DL = 5.90 ± 0.07%, D_{12h} = 40%, D_{30d} = 90%	[41]
	MS	Polyethylene glycol monomethyl ether-polymandelic acid, mPEG10000-PMA (1:9)	Saponins of Sanqi (*Notoginseng Radix et Rhizoma*)	Emulsion method, dripping; W_1, drug solution in ethanol; O, DCM (1:2); W_2, 1%PVA	2.51 ± 0.21 μm, EE = 47.3 ± 1.6%, DL = 8.54 ± 0.16%, D_{12d} = 36.4%, D_{48d} = 65.9%	[18]
O_1/O_2	MS	PLGA (50:50, 20 kDa)	Sophoridine	Emulsion method, homogenization; O_1, CAN + DCM (9:1); O_2, liquid paraffin	17.2 ± 3.9 μm, EE = 65%, DL = 6.5%, D_{4h} = 14%, D_{24h} = 34%, D_{14d} = 94%	[35]
	Hollow MP	EC	Curcumin	Emulsion method, stirring; O_1, ethanol + ether (3:1); O_2, liquid paraffin (7% span)	655.6 ± 14.4 μm, DL = 3.41%, D_{24h} = 96.3%	[28]

Table 9.4 The materials and processes of the coacervation method applied to Chinese medicine

Coacervation types	Coating materials	Crosslinking agent	Core materials	References
Simple coacervation	Gelatin	Glutaraldehyde	Poria polysaccharides	[15]
	Alginate	Calcium chloride	Curcumin; *Chuanxiong* (*Chuanxiong Rhizoma*) extract	[16, 27]
	Chitosan	Glutaraldehyde	Sinomenine; norisoboldine; ligustrazine HCl;	[23, 31, 32]
	Carboxymethyl chitosan	Glutaraldehyde	Puerarin	[30]
	Human serum albumin (HAS)	Glutaraldehyde	Norcantharidate	[29]
	BSA	Zinc chloride and glutaraldehyde	Glycyrrhetinic acid	[34]
Complex coacervation	Gum Arabic, gelatin	Glutaraldehyde	Ethanol extract of compound kangai powder	[38]
	Alginate, chitosan	Calcium chloride +/glutaraldehyde	*Shenmai* injection; Ginsenoside Rg1; icariin	[22, 25, 37]

Dong et al. prepared microcapsules encapsulated with essential oil of Roudoukou (*Myristicae Semen*) by spray drying technique using either gum Arabic and maltodextrin (GA-MD) or octenyl succinic acid-modified starch and maltodextrin (OSA-MD) as the wall materials [57]. The influence of these materials on product properties is then investigated and compared. Powder property analysis indicated that GA-MD microcapsules presented larger size, higher moisture, and poorer flowability compared with OSA-MD microcapsules. Fourier-transform infrared spectroscopy and thermogravimetric analysis showed that both GA-MD and OSA-MD microcapsules improved the stability of nutmeg essential oil. However, GA-MD microcapsules exhibited higher storage stability than OSA-MD microcapsules.

9.3.4 Other Methods

A series of novel microencapsulation techniques emerged in the last decade. And some of them have been applied for the preparation of microparticles of Chinese medicine.

9.3.4.1 Supercritical Fluid Technique

The unique properties of supercritical fluid technique (SCF), in particular supercritical carbon dioxide (CO_2), provide numerous opportunities for the development of pharmaceutical processes including microencapsulation for drug delivery purposes. SCF can be used in many different ways to produce microparticles or even nanoparticles based on the properties of the core and shell materials. According to the function of SCF in the process, three types of techniques have been well established for microencapsulation of bioactive: rapid expansion of supercritical solution (RESS) method, supercritical fluid anti-solvent (SAS) method, and particles from gas-saturated solution (PGSS) method. Among them, the PGSS technique adopted SCF as the solute, not as the solvent or anti-solvent, so that it can be used for water-soluble core and shell materials [58]. Compared with conventional methods such as solvent evaporation, coacervation, and spray drying, PGSS holds several advantages on its mild process and ability to produce solvent-free and homogenous products. During the PGSS process, no elevated temperatures or organic solvents are required, which is of special benefit in preserving the stability of volatile or heat-sensitive ingredients. Despite its strength over other methods, PGSS is still not widely applied in the microencapsulation of Chinese medicine mainly due to its requirement for expensive and particular equipment.

Shanzhuyu (*Corni Fructus*), also known as cornel, was used for thousands of years as a traditional medicine in China. Its active ingredients showed high nutritional and pharmacological value. Therefore in the work of Sun et al., the active components were extracted from *Shanzhuyu* by supercritical CO_2 fluid and then entrapped into microcapsules via the PGSS process [12]. Both extraction and microencapsulation processes were optimized, the obtained extract was analyzed by GC-MS, and 17 chemical components were identified. The extract was then introduced into a self-made micro-mixing chamber via a coaxial nozzle and mixed with the coating material (gum Arabic and maltodextrin) to form the microcapsules. The process parameters, including the nozzle straight diameter and the flow rates of SCF and the shell materials, were optimized by an orthogonal design experiment. The final products showed as irregular particles with their size ranging from 2.0 to 4.5 μm.

9.3.4.2 Hydrogel-Template Technique

The template method, also known as the water-soluble polymer template method, was firstly introduced by Park's group for the fabrication of homogeneous microparticles with predefined size and shape [59]. It has shown to be useful in encapsulating different types of active compounds and using various volatile organic solvents [60], in contrast to the limited types of drugs and solvents (mostly DCM or EtAc) for the conventional oil-in-water emulsion-solvent evaporation process.

Wang et al. compared the properties of microparticles prepared by the template and solvent evaporation techniques, using glycyrrhetinic acid as a model drug and PLGA as the matrix polymer [33]. Although the obtained microparticles showed a preferable encapsulation efficiency (>70%) and mean particle size (~40 μm) for both methods, they provided two distinguished drug release profiles: drug release from MPs by the conventional method was slow before Day 50 and then accelerated, meanwhile a zero-order release profile for 3 months after an initial burst release was revealed for MPs by the template method. The researchers suggested that these two methods can be supplementary with each other in the optimization of drug formulation for achieving predetermined drug release patterns.

9.4 Characterization of Microparticulate DDS of Chinese Medicine

9.4.1 Particle Size and Size Distribution

The average or mean diameter can be determined using dynamic light scattering technique. And the homogeneity of the particle is represented with a polydispersity index (PDI) or span.

9.4.2 Morphology and Structure

Morphology of particles can be observed under optical microscopy (for larger samples), transmission electron microscopy (TEM), or atomic force microscopy (AFM). Surface or cross-sectional structure can be studied with scanning electron microscopy (SEM) after pretreated by freeze-sectioning and/or sputter-coating techniques.

The specific surface area of microparticles can be determined using the nitrogen adsorption-desorption analysis and Brunauer-Emmett-Teller (NET) absorption model. The porosity of porous samples can be analyzed via the Barrett-Joyner-Halenda (BJH) measurement [51].

9.4.3 Drug Loading Capacity and Release Pattern

Drug loading performance is usually represented with the encapsulation efficiency (EE) and drug loading (DL) of the microparticles. In vitro drug release behavior can be investigated in proper release medium using a dialysis bag or sealed tubes as the container. Samples are withdrawn at scheduled time intervals and analyzed for drug content to obtain the release pattern of microparticles.

9.4.4 Drug-Excipient Interaction

The excipients and processes of the microparticulate products may change the crystallinity and dispersion degree of the drug in the microparticle matrix and therefore influence the stability and drug release property of the microparticles. The most frequently used analytical techniques for interaction between drug and excipient include differential scanning calorimetry (DSC), differential thermal analysis (DTA), powder X-ray diffraction (PXRD), and Fourier-transform infrared spectroscopy [61].

DSC is widely used as a leading thermal analysis technique for easy detection of physical interactions, such as a change in the polymorphic form, conversion of crystalline to amorphous form. An absence, or a significant shift in the melting of the components, or appearance of a new exo-/endothermic peak and/or variation in the corresponding enthalpies of reaction on the physical mixture indicates possible interactions. DTA can also detect eutectic formation.

PXRD is a direct tool for measurement of the crystal form of a material with a typical output being a plot of intensity vs. the diffraction angle (2θ). It can detect chemical interaction by the appearance of unique diffraction peaks or physical incompatibilities like changes in amorphous/crystalline nature and polymorphic changes. The lack of crystalline API peaks when the API-loaded microparticles were analyzed could indicate that the drug is amorphous and highly dispersed in the matrix or that the loading is too low to detect using the parameters chosen [35].

FTIR is an efficient method to detect interaction on unique bands or peak shifting. But the presence of overlapping peaks in the spectra may hinder the analysis, and environmental humidity may interfere with the results.

9.5 Application of Microparticulate DDS of Chinese Medicine

9.5.1 Solidification and Powderization

Microencapsulation technology is of great value for solidification and/or powderization of liquid, semi-solid, and solid active compounds. The volatile oils [13] and crude extracts [12] of Chinese herbal medicine were usually entrapped into microcapsules for improved stability of active ingredients and better processability. The extract powder of Chinese medicine (e.g., Poria) can be microencapsulated to effectively reduce their hygroscopic effect and to improve their powder properties

[15], including bulk density, angle of repose, and specific surface area. Crude extracts from Chinese medicines generally taste bitter. Therefore in some cases, the microencapsulation technique was used for taste-masking and improved compliance by oral administration [40].

Curcumin is the primary bioactive ingredient (up to ~5%) in *Jianghuang* (*Curcumae Longae Rhizoma*). It has anti-inflammatory properties and decent evidence for indications from chronic pain to depression. But curcumin is a water-insoluble, unstable, reactive, nonbioavailable compound, necessitating special formulations to be efficiently absorbed.

Zhou et al. developed the alginate MSs for encapsulation of a liquid self-emulsifying mixture of curcumin, oil, Poloxamer 188, and PEG 400. The final products showed a drug content of 71.32 mg/g and an average size of 11.33 μm. Drug release from the MS was over 80% at 50 min in different media, which was preferable for improved oral absorption [27].

9.5.2 Prolonged-Release for Improved Bioavailability

The polymers in the microparticles, no matter water-soluble or not, provided a barrier for drug diffusion during the dissolution/release process. So one of the major advantages of microencapsulation is that it provides an easy but efficient approach for sustained or controlled release profiles to improve the bioavailability of active ingredients and to promote therapeutic effect. Therefore, many researchers adopted this strategy in their studies. Table 9.5 listed the main information on some reports.

9.5.3 Targeted or Site-Specific Drug Delivery

Targeted DDS can induce drug to be directly concentrated on the target site. It has become a hot spot in the field of pharmaceutical research on Chinese medicine due to its high therapeutic effects and low side effects [45, 62]. In the case of targeted microparticulate DDS of Chinese medicine, most researches adopted the passive or physio-chemical targeting strategy rather than an active targeting approach. Particle size and surface properties are key factors for passive targeting. Previous reports demonstrated that the particles larger than 7 μm are mostly retained by pulmonary capillaries and those smaller than 7 μm are commonly engulfed by macrophages of liver and spleen.

Zhang et al. prepared a liposome-in-microcapsule system based on chitosan for lung target delivery of ligustrazin hydrochloride as a potential lung cancer therapy [23]. The final product showed its particle size in a range of 5–8 μm and an encapsulation efficiency of 65.3%, a low loading capacity of 3%, and a slow but incomplete in vitro release pattern.

Table 9.5 In vitro and/or in vivo properties of some microparticulate DDS of Chinese medicine

Active compounds	Coating material	Type of MP	Characterization results	In vitro release properties	Pharmacokinetic/ pharmacodynamic performance	Reference
Puerarin	Carboxymethyl chitosan	MS	NA	NA	Significantly increased AUC, C_{max}, T_{max}, $T_{1/2}$, and MRT and decreased CL after oral administration. And the protective effect of MS on myocardial injury in rats was significantly greater than puerarin at the same dose	[30]
Saponins of Sanqi (*Notoginseng Radix et Rhizoma*)	mPEG10000-PMA (1:9)	MS	2.51 ± 0.21 μm, EE = 47.3%, DL = 8.5%	Drug released stably for about 12 days and degraded within 60 days	MS showed good biocompatibility, anti-inflammatory, and anti-tumor activities	[18]
Total alkaloids of Maqianzi (*Strychni Semen*)	EC	MC	523.7 μm, EE = 54.0%, DL = 18.3%	Sustained release for 12 h in artificial gastric/ intestinal juice	NA	[14]
Total flavonoids of Gusuibu (*Drynariae Rhizoma*) and Yejuhua (*Chrysanthemi Indici Flos*)	PLGA (L: G = 75:25, MW20000)	MC	44.3 ± 14.7 μm, EE = 95.3%, DL = 5.9%,	Burst of 40% in 24 h, 50% drug released at 12 days and 90% at 50 days	NA	[41]

NA not available

Wang et al. prepared a lung-targeting sophoridine-loaded PLGA MPs via a simple oil-in-oil emulsion-solvent evaporation process [35]. The obtained particles showed an average size of 17 μm with 90% of them ranging in 12–24 μm. Drug concentration in the lung tissue of rats was 220.10 μg/g for MPs and 6.77 μg/g for aqueous solution formulation after intravenous injection for 30 min, respectively. And a significantly higher drug level in lung tissue than in other major organs and blood samples was revealed for a duration of 12 days after one single injection of the MPs. Therefore, these MPs are expected to improve the treatment efficacy of sophoridine against lung cancer.

Yan et al. encapsulated norcantharidate into human serum albumin (HAS) MPs by the emulsion crosslinking method [29]. Although the obtained particles show an average size of 13.3 μm, an in vivo study revealed higher AUC inside the liver and spleen than the solution group after injection. And the AUC ratio of MPs to solution reached 3.49 for the liver but less than 1 for the heart, lung, and kidney.

Pi et al. entrapped curcumin into hollow microspheres based on EC to increase the residence time of the drug in the stomach [28]. The final products showed a DL of 3.4% and a size of around 650 μm. The floating rate at 24 h was about 90%, and the drug released over 90% at 8 h after a burst of 10% at 30 min. The oral bioavailability of MSs was 12-fold higher than that of the crude drug. Therefore, the floating MPs might be a promising strategy to achieve sustained release and increase the oral bioavailability of curcumin.

Zuojin Pills was first recorded in *Dan Xi Xin Fa* (*Danxi's Experiential Therapy*) for treating gastrointestinal disorders in the fifteenth century. Its formula involves *Huanglian* (*Coptidis Rhizoma*) and *Wuzhuyu* (*Euodiae Fructus*) in a ratio of 6:1 (w/w). For a better therapeutic effect on the gastric ulcer, Wang et al. designed a mucoadhesive microsphere based on alginate and chitosan and loaded with total alkaloids from *Zuojin* formula [43]. The obtained MPs revealed sustained release pattern and excellent gastric retention performance within both in vitro and rat stomach. Also, the MPs showed gastroprotective effects through reducing the inflammatory response on ethanol-induced acute gastric mucosal injury in rats.

They also prepared a chitosan-coated alginate microsphere for colon-targeted delivery of icariin [22]. The final MPs released 10% in simulated gastric fluid and 65.6% in stimulated colonic fluid and showed a long retention time of more than 12 h in the colon. The MPs reduced the colonic injury by decreasing the colon mucosa damage index in rats and also eliminated the inflammatory response by reducing the productions and gene expression of inflammatory mediators and cytokines in colonic mucosa.

Sinomenine is a pure alkaloid extracted from *Qingfengteng* (*Sinomenii Caulis*). It has been widely applied to treat rheumatism and other immune diseases due to its anti-inflammatory effects, inhibition of cellular and humoral immune function. Xiong et al. entrapped sinomenine into chitosan MPs followed by coating with Eudragit. The sinomenine enteric-coated microspheres were revealed as an effective and safe therapy for inflammatory bowel disease in mice via regulation of TLR/NF-κB signaling [32].

In some cases, the microparticles can be administrated directly into a specific region and retained there for a long-term effect. He et al. developed the norisoboldine-loaded chitosan microspheres for intra-articular injection to treat rheumatoid arthritis [31]. The MSs showed a burst release followed by a slow progression afterward. In vivo studies using Sprague-Dawley rats revealed that the drug-loaded chitosan microspheres were biocompatible.

9.5.4 Biomedical Engineering

Transcatheter-arterial embolization (TAE) is widely used to treat various diseases, such as tumors, vascular lesions, and hemorrhages [63]. Microparticles became one of the commonly used embolic agents due to its capability to be injected via small flow-directed and ease of manipulation.

Since 1985, Feng's group has conducted a series of studies on *Baiji* (*Bletilla Rhizoma*) on its embolic effect. According to their reports, *Bletilla striata* polysaccharide was confirmed as an extraordinary carrier and can inhibit angiogenesis and collateral circulation after TAE [48]. Then the polysaccharide was processed into MSs with their diameters around 200 μm. Embolization experiments in the renal artery of rabbit and a rabbit liver VX2 carcinoma model confirmed that MSs of *Bletilla striata* polysaccharide could be applied as a safe and efficient embolic agent in interventional approaches.

Systemic infusion of bone marrow-derived mesenchymal stem cells (BMSCs) has become a promising strategy for disease treatment and tissue regeneration. Strategies to enhance the efficiency of BMSC cell therapy are crucial to promoting its clinical application.

The compound formula of Shenmai Yin, firstly recorded in *Zheng Yin Mai Zhi* (*Symptoms*, *Causes*, *Pulses*, and *Treatment*), is consisted of two herbal medicines, *Hongshen* (*Ginseng Radix et Rhizama Rubra*) and *Maidong* (*Ophiopogonis Radix*). One of its modern pharmaceuticals, Shenmai injection, now is clinically used to treat cardiovascular diseases. Li et al. prepared Shenmai microspheres using alginate and chitosan as coating materials [37]. The obtained MS was then explored on its induction effect on the differentiation of BMSC into the neuronal cell, and the results revealed that the Wnt3a signaling pathway promoted the induction of Shenmai MS in the differentiation process. *Renshen* (*Ginseng Radix et Rhizoma*) is one of the most common medicinal plants used in China for thousands of years. Ginsenosides of ginseng have revealed decent neuroprotective effects on central nervous system disorders and neuronal diseases. And ginsenoside Rg1, one of the most abundant compounds in ginseng, also showed neuroprotective effects on neuronal cells. Guo et al. prepared Rg1-loaded alginate-chitosan microspheres and evaluated the effects of microspheres on human bone marrow (BM) stromal cells (hBMSC). The results confirmed that Rg1-loaded microspheres could promote hBMSC proliferation and differentiation and suppress hBMSC apoptosis induced by hypoxia-reoxygenation [25].

The repair and regeneration of wound and osseous tissue defects are still major medical health problems to solve in clinical. Drug-loaded microspheres have attracted much interest in the last decade for their potential applications for wound/bone repair and regeneration. Asiaticoside, a poor water-soluble ingredient with low bioavailability extracted from *Jixuecao* (*Centellae Herba*), was loaded into porous microspheres using EC as the matrix material at an EE of 71.82%. Approximately 90% of the drug was gradually released within 25 h [20]. The cellular uptake of drugs for MS formulation was 5.6–9.1 times higher than that for the solution of free drug. The drug-loaded MSs enhanced the proliferation and migration of keratinocytes and skin fibroblasts and significantly accelerated wound closure in vivo.

Chen et al. developed the organic-inorganic hybrid microspheres based on chitosan and nano-hydroxyapatite (nHAP) composite as a drug delivery carrier [64]. Icariin, the primary active ingredients of *Yinyanghuo* (*Epimedii Folium*), was loaded into the microspheres to obtain a sustained release behavior. In vitro bioactive experiments revealed that the composite microspheres provided a suitable microenvironment for osteoblast attachment and proliferation, which is favorable for bone repair.

Gusuibu (*Drynariae Rhizoma*) is a traditional herbal medicine frequently applied in the area of orthopedics and traumatology. Its extracts can induce osteoblastic proliferation and promote the differentiation of human periodontal ligament cells. Naringenin is one of active flavonoid aglycones identified in *Gusuibu*. Therefore, Liu et al. loaded naringenin into PLGA MSs and then dispersed into the agarose-gelatin solution to form a gel scaffold with uniform porous structure. The obtained scaffold could enhance the viability and biological function of chondrocytes and is a potential approach for cartilage tissue engineering [19].

9.5.5 Other Applications

Not only the microparticles can be applied as a carrier for nanocarriers (e.g., liposomes [23], nanocrystals [36], and nanoparticles [34]), but also they can be used as a pharmaceutical intermediate for further preparation of other products (e.g., aerosol).

Wang et al. developed PLGA microparticles loaded with breviscapine nanocrystals and compared them with the MSs prepared by conventional O/W emulsion-solvent evaporation method [36]. As a result, drug loading was increased from 2.4% up to 15.3% and encapsulation efficiency from 48.5% to 91.9%. Also, the obtained MP showed a relatively stable serum drug level for more than 30 days after intramuscular injection in rats. This nanocrystal-in-microparticle strategy provided a promising approach for drugs with poor solubility in organic solvents to develop long-term therapeutic products characterized with preferable in vitro and in vivo performance.

Ma et al. prepared a quantitative aerosol for lung cancer treatment by intranasal administration [38]. The extract from *kangai* powder (a compound formula) was entrapped by the coating materials of gum Arabic and gelatin to form MCs at a mean size of 6.4 μm and an EE of 84.6%. The obtained MCs were then mixed with other additives in the container followed by pressure filling of propellant to form the aerosol.

Sun et al. entrapped three flavonoid compounds extracted from Chinese medicinal plants into HPMCP to form enteric MCs as anti-veterinary preparations [42]. The influence of MCs on the immune-effect of Newcastle Disease vaccine, intestinal enzyme activities, and microbiology flora in chickens was investigated, and the results showed that the MCs could significantly increase serum antibody titers, reduce chicken morbidity and mortality after challenge, and improve the protection rate and the digestive enzyme.

Zebrafish has been recognized as an excellent animal model for the pharmacology investigation. Lin et al. developed a microparticle system for oral delivery of TCM in zebrafish so that it can be used for easy and rapid evaluation of drug effect on disease [16]. *Chuanxiong* (*Chuanxiong Rhizoma*) was encapsulated together with fish food into alginate MPs. The obtained MPs (around 1000 μm in diameter) were placed into the tank with zebrafish. It only took about 30 s for the uptake of one microparticle by a single zebrafish. The MP was moved to the end of the gastrointestinal tract after oral administration for 6 h and excreted from the body after 16 h.

9.6 Conclusion and Prospects

The favorable and tunable properties of microparticulate DDS make it a very attractive option in processing Chinese medicinal products for pharmaceutical applications, particularly regarding the microencapsulation of active ingredients for sustained release or targeted delivery. It is encouraging to recognize that more and more fractionate extracts from single Chinese Materia Medica or even compound formula (but not an only single active ingredient) were encapsulated into microparticle preparations using biocompatible and bio-renewable materials as the coating.

Despite tremendous progress having been made on both formulation and fabrication processes of microparticles, future research in this field should continue to focus on the following issues: (1) Novel carrier materials and encapsulation techniques that could improve the EE and DL of active core materials (especially water-soluble drugs), and use a green solvent in the microencapsulation process for lower cost and higher safety and provide efficient protection and tunable release pattern for various drug delivery purposes. (2) Special design and extended application of novel microparticulate DDS to make better use of the advantages of Chinese medicine. (3) Systematic evaluation of quality analysis, in vitro, and in vivo performance of the obtained microparticle products.

We believe that the in-depth knowledge of pharmacology, biopharmaceutics, and pharmacodynamics of Chinese medicine will help to realize the potential for rapid development and extensive application of microparticulate products of Chinese medicine soon.

Acknowledgments This work was financially supported by the National Natural Science Foundation of China [81360644, 81660665].

References

1. Dias, M. I., Ferreira, I. C. F. R., & Barreiro, M. F. (2015). Microencapsulation of bioactives for food applications. *Food & Function, 6*(4), 1035–1052.
2. Paulo, F., & Santos, L. (2017). Design of experiments for microencapsulation applications: A review. *Materials Science and Engineering: C, 77*, 1327–1340.
3. Al-Kasmi, B., Alsirawan, M. B., Bashimam, M., & El-Zein, H. (2017). Mechanical microencapsulation: The best technique in taste masking for the manufacturing scale - Effect of polymer encapsulation on drug targeting. *Journal of Controlled Release, 260*, 134–141.
4. Ozkan, G., Francob, P., De Marco, I., Xiao, J., & Capanoglu, E. (2019). A review of microencapsulation methods for food antioxidants: Principles, advantages, drawbacks and applications. *Food Chemistry, 272*, 494–506.
5. Herrero-Vanrell, R., Bravo-Osuna, I., Andrés-Guerrero, V., et al. (2014). The potential of using biodegradable microspheres in retinal diseases and other intraocular pathologies. *Progress in Retinal and Eye Research, 42*, 27–43.
6. Manabu, T. (2018). Microfluidic devices for drug delivery systems. *Advanced Drug Delivery Reviews, 128*, 1–2.
7. Sanjay, S. T., Zhou, W., Dou, M., Tavakolia, H., Ma, L., et al. (2018). Recent advances of controlled drug delivery using microfluidic platforms. *Advanced Drug Delivery Reviews, 128*, 3–28.
8. Perez, R. A., & Kim, H. W. (2015). Core–shell designed scaffolds for drug delivery and tissue engineering. *Acta Biomaterialia, 21*, 2–19.
9. Hiraoka, S., Uchida, S., & Namiki, N. (2014). Preparation and characterization of high-content aripiprazole-loaded core–shell structure microsphere for long-release injectable formulation. *Chemical & Pharmaceutical Bulletin, 62*(7), 654–660.
10. Yang, H., Gao, H., & Wang, Y. (2016). Hollow hydroxyapatite microsphere: A promising carrier for bone tissue engineering. *Journal of Microencapsulation, 33*(5), 421–426.
11. Gao, X., Hai, X., Baigude, H., Guan, W., & Liu, Z. (2016). Fabrication of functional hollow microspheres constructed from MOF shells: Promising drug delivery systems with high loading capacity and targeted transport. *Scientific Reports, 6*, 37705.
12. Sun, F. (2018). *Cornus officinalis effective components extracted and micro-encapsulated by supercritical CO_2*. Dissertation. Zhengzhou University.
13. Wang, F. (2011). *Study on preparation and evaluation of zedoary, schizonepetae volatile oil microcapsules*. Dissertation. East China University of Science and Technology.
14. Pan, J. (2014). *The preparation and evaluation of strychnos alkaloids microcapsules and compound volatile oile microcapsules*. Dissertation. East China University of Science and Technology.
15. Yi, P. (2013). *The microencapsulation reduce Medicine extract powder hygroscopic and evaluation*. Dissertation. Chengdu University of Traditional Chinese Medicine.
16. Lin, L. J., Chiang, C. J., Chao, Y. P., Wang, S. D., Chiou, Y. T., et al. (2016). Development of alginate microspheres containing chuanxiong for oral administration to adult zebrafish. *BioMed Research International, 2016*, 4013071.

17. Luo, S. H., Song, S. L., Zheng, C. S., Li, W. Y., Wang, Y., et al. (2017). Embolic effects of Bletilla striata microspheres in renal artery and transplanted VX2 liver tumor model in rabbits. *Chinese Journal of Integrative Medicine, 25*(6), 1–8.
18. He, Y., Li, H. L., Zheng, X. Y., Yuan, M. W., Yang, R. Y., et al. (2019). Preparation, in vivo and in vitro release of polyethylene glycol monomethyl ether-polymandelic acid microspheres loaded panax notoginseng saponins. *Molecules, 24*(10), E2024.
19. Liu, Y. (2014). *Preparation of agarose-geltain scaffold integrated with PLGA/Naringenin microspheres on repairing of articular cartilage injury*. Disseration. Nanjing University of Chinese Medicine.
20. Xie, S. (2019). *Construction of asiaticoside loaded porous microspheres for wound repair and regeneration*. Dissertation. Zhejiang University.
21. Pan, P. (2016). *Preparation and characterization of two hybrid sestems-magnetic drug-loaded microsphere and self-healing hydrogel for bone repair*. Dissertation. Fuzhou University.
22. Wang, Q. S., Wang, G. F., Zhou, J., Gao, L. N., & Cui, Y. L. (2016). Colon targeted oral drug delivery system based on alginate-chitosan microspheres loaded with icariin in the treatment of ulcerative colitis. *International Journal of Pharmaceutics, 515*(1–2), 176–185.
23. Zhang, Y. (2014). *Preparation and cytotoxicity investigation of ligustrazine hydrochloride particles*. Dissertation. Chongqing Medical University.
24. Liu, C. (2009). *Study on effective composition extracting and microencapsulation of traditional Chinese medicine*. Dissertation. Jilin University.
25. Guo, Y. H., Zhao, S., Du, Y. X., Xing, Q. J., Chen, B. L., et al. (2017). Effects of ginsenoside Rg1-loaded alginate-chitosan microspheres on human bone marrow stromal cells. *Bioscience Reports, 37*(3), BSR20160566.
26. Zhou, L. Y., Guan, J., Nie, S. F., & Pan, W. S. (2009). Preparation and optimization of formulation of PLGA microspheres containing chinese herbal extract cucurbitacin B. *China Pharmacy, 20*(33), 2588–2592.
27. Zhou, L., Liu, Y. H., & Jia, J. (2015). Preparation and in vitro release characteristics of curcumin in self-emulsifying microsphere. *Chinese Journal of Clinical Rational Drug Use, 8*(15), 31–33.
28. Pi, C., Yuan, J. W., Liu, H., Zuo, Y., Feng, T., et al. (2018). In vitro and in vivo evaluation of curcumin loaded hollow microspheres prepared with ethyl cellulose and citric acid. *International Journal of Biological Macromolecules, 115*, 1046–1054.
29. Yan, F., Li, B., Shen, F. P., Fu, Q., et al. (2014). Formulation and characterization of albumin microspheres containing norcantharidate for liver tumor targeting. *Drug Delivery, 22*(6), 862–868.
30. Song, X., Bai, X., Liu, S., Dong, L., Deng, H., et al. (2016). A novel microspheres formulation of puerarin: pharmacokinetics study and in vivo pharmacodynamics evaluations. *Evidence-based Complementary and Alternative Medicine, 2016*, 4016963.
31. He, M., Wang, H., Dou, W., Chou, G., Wei, X., et al. (2016). Preparation and drug release properties of norisoboldine-loaded chitosan microspheres. *International Journal of Biological Macromolecules, 91*, 1101–1109.
32. Xiong, H., Tian, L., Zhao, Z., Chen, S., Zhao, Q., et al. (2017). The sinomenine enteric-coated microspheres suppressed the TLR/NF-kappa B signaling in DSS-induced experimental colitis. *International Immunopharmacology, 50*, 251–262.
33. Wang, H., Zhang, G. X., Sui, H., Liu, Y. H., Parkd, K., & Wang, W. P. (2015). Comparative studies on the properties of glycyrrhetinic acid-loaded PLGA microparticles prepared by emulsion and template methods. *International Journal of Pharmaceutics, 496*(2), 723–731.
34. Wang, W. P., Lei, Y. Y., Sui, H., Zhang, W. P., Zhu, R. Y., et al. (2016). Fabrication and evaluation of nanoparticle-assembled BSA microparticles for enhanced liver delivery of glycyrrhetinic acid. *Artificial Cells, Nanomedicine, and Biotechnology, 45*(4), 740–747.
35. Wang, W. P., Cai, Y. Q., Zhang, G. X., Liu, Y. H., Sui, H., et al. (2016). Sophoridine-loaded PLGA microspheres for lung targeting: Preparation, in vitro, and in vivo evaluation. *Drug Delivery, 23*(9), 3674–3680.

36. Wang, H., Zhang, G. X., Ma, X. Q., Liu, Y. H., Feng, J., et al. (2017). Enhanced encapsulation and bioavailability of breviscapine in PLGA microparticles by nanocrystal and water-soluble polymer template techniques. *European Journal of Pharmaceutics and Biopharmaceutics, 115*, 177–185.
37. Li, Z. B., Guo, Y. H., Xing, Q. J., & Liu, Q. F. (2019). Shenmai microspheres and its induction effects on differentiation of bone marrow mesenchymal stem cell under Wnt signaling pathway. *Guangxi Medicial Journal, 41*(08), 999–1003.
38. Ma, L. (2015). *The preparation and quality standard of microcapsules aerosol for treating lung cancer*. Wuhan University of Technology.
39. Ruofei Du, Y. F., Liu, Y., & Desheng, X. (2008). Data analysis and characterization of hygroscopicity of Chinese herbal extracts. *Chinese Traditional Patent Medicine, 30*(12), 1767–1771.
40. Wang, Y., Feng, Y., & Xu, D. S. (2007). Studies on taste-masking technology of traditional Chinese medicine compounds. *China Journal of Chinese Materia Medica, 32*(13), 35–38.
41. Chen, N. N., Ma, N., Che, H. Z., Jiao, P., Chen, F., et al. (2017). Preparation of compound TF-PLGA microcapsule and its drug release characteristics in vitro. *Journal of Jilin University (Medicine Edition), 43*(3), 593–599.
42. Sun, Z. (2013). *Pharmcological effects of Traditional Chinese Medicine flavonoids compound and enteric microcapsules*. Dissertation. Nanjing Agricultural College.
43. Wang, Q. S., Zhu, X. N., Jiang, H. L., Wang, G. F., & Cui, Y. L. (2015). Protective effects of alginate–chitosan microspheres loaded with alkaloids from Coptis chinensis Franch. and Evodia rutaecarpa (Juss.) Benth. (Zuojin Pill) against ethanol-induced acute gastric mucosal injury in rats. *Drug Design, Development and Therapy, 9*, 6151–6165.
44. Gao, C. F., Liu, L. J., Zhou, Y. Y., Bian, Z. X., Wang, S. P., et al. (2019). Novel drug delivery systems of Chinese medicine for the treatment of inflammatory bowel disease. *Chinese Medicine, 14*, 23.
45. Xu, W., Xing, F. J., Dong, K., You, C., Yan, Y., et al. (2015). Application of traditional Chinese medicine preparation in targeting drug delivery system. *Drug Delivery, 22*(3), 258–265.
46. Ma, Z., Zhang, B., Fan, Y. Q., Wang, M., Kebebe, D., et al. (2019). Traditional Chinese medicine combined with hepatic targeted drug delivery systems: A new strategy for the treatment of liver diseases. *Biomedicine & Pharmacotherapy, 117*, 109128.
47. Han, F. Y., Thurecht, K. J., Whittaker, A. K., & Smith, M. T. (2016). Bioerodable PLGA-based microparticles for producing sustained-release drug formulations and strategies for improving drug loading. *Frontiers in Pharmacology, 7*, 185.
48. Luo, S. H., Song, S. L., Zheng, C. S., Li, W. Y., Wang, Y., et al. (2019). Embolic effects of bletilla striata microspheres in renal artery and transplanted VX2 liver tumor model in rabbits. *Chinese Journal of Integrative Medicine, 25*(06), 431–438.
49. Giorno, L., Dragosavac, M., & Piacentini, E. (2017). Pharmaceutical particles design by membrane emulsification: preparation methods and applications in drug delivery. *Current Pharmaceutical Desgin, 23*(2), 302–318.
50. Li, W., Zhang, L. Y., Ge, X. H., & Xu, B. Y. (2018). Microfluidic fabrication of microparticles for biomedical applications. *Chemical Society Reviews, 47*(15), 5646–5683.
51. Ghosh, D. D., Sourabh, S., & Moumita, C. (2018). Porous microspheres: Synthesis, characterisation and applications in pharmaceutical & medical fields. *International Journal of Pharmaceutics, 548*(1), 34–48.
52. Timilsena, Y. P., Akanbi, T. O., Khalid, N., Adhikari, B., & Barrow, C. J. (2018). Complex coacervation: Principles, mechanisms and applications in microencapsulation. *International Journal of Biological Macromolecules, 121*, 1276–1286.
53. Xiao, Z. B., Liu, W. L., Zhu, G., Zhou, R., & Niu, Y. W. (2014). A review of the preparation and application of flavour and essential oils microcapsules based on complex coacervation technology. *Journal of the Science of Food and Agriculture, 94*(8), 1482–1494.
54. Davis, M., & Walker, G. (2017). Recent strategies in spray drying for the enhanced bioavailability of poorly water-soluble drugs. *Journal of Controlled Release, 269*, 110–127.

55. Sosnik, A., & Seremeta, K. P. (2015). Advantages and challenges of the spray-drying technology for the production of pure drug particles and drug-loaded polymeric carriers. *Advances in Colloid and Interface Science, 223*, 40–54.
56. Wan, F., & Yang, M. (2016). Design of PLGA-based depot delivery systems for biopharmaceuticals prepared by spray drying. *International Journal of Pharmaceutics, 498*(1–2), 82–95.
57. Dong, X. Y., Wu, B. F., Deng, Q. C., Wei, F., Chen, H., et al. (2018). Microencapsulation of nutmeg essential oil by spray-drying with different wall materials. *Oil Crop Science, 3*(04), 258–269.
58. Soh, S. H., & Lee, L. Y. (2019). Microencapsulation and Nanoencapsulation Using Supercritical Fluid (SCF) Techniques. *Pharmaceutics, 11*(1), 21.
59. Acharya, G., Shin, C. S., Mcdermott, M., Mishra, H., Park, H., et al. (2010). The hydrogel template method for fabrication of homogeneous nano/microparticles. *Journal of Controlled Release, 141*(3), 314–319.
60. Lu, Y. S., Sturek, M., & Park, K. (2014). Microparticles produced by the hydrogel template method for sustained drug delivery. *International Journal of Pharmaceutics, 461*(1–2), 258–269.
61. Chadha, R., & Bhandari, S. (2014). Drug–excipient compatibility screening—Role of thermoanalytical and spectroscopic techniques. *Journal of Pharmaceutical and Biomedical Analysis, 87*, 82–97.
62. Patel, M. M. (2017). Formulation and development of di-dependent microparticulate system for colon-specific drug delivery. *Drug Delivery and Translational Research, 7*(2), 312–324.
63. Teichgräber, U., Aschenbach, R., Diamantis, I., von Rundstedt, F. C., Grimm, M. O., et al. (2018). Prostate artery embolization: Indication. *Technique and Clinical Results. Röfo, 190*(09), 847–855.
64. Chen, J. D., Pan, P. P., Zhang, Y. J., Zhong, S. N., & Zhang, Q. Q. (2015). Preparation of chitosan/nano hydroxyapatite organic-inorganic hybrid microspheres for bone repair. *Colloids and Surfaces. B, Biointerfaces, 134*, 401–407.

Chapter 10
Hydrogels for Delivery of Chinese Medicines

Tianyuan Ci, Jing Zang, and Nianping Feng

Abstract Hydrogels are three-dimensional water-swollen networks and have widespread biomedical applications. This chapter focuses on the hydrogel systems for delivering Chinese medicines. The hydrogels could improve in vivo performance of drugs by modifying their releasing profile, enhancing the local drug contents, and achieving multi-drug synergy. The general classification, gelling mechanisms, and commonly adopted characterization modalities of hydrogels are also addressed. Further, we highlight the latest strategies and applications of hydrogels classified by their delivery routes and indications. Challenges in clinical translation of hydrogel systems and future research opportunities are discussed.

Keywords Hydrogel · Chinese medicines · Delivery systems · Delivery routes · Pharmaceutical efficacy

10.1 Introduction

Hydrogels are three-dimensional polymer networks that could hold large amounts of water due to the water absorbance of the hydrophilic groups and their resistance to dissolution arising from cross-linking structures [1, 2]. Its water-containing state resembles human extracellular matrix that renders the hydrogels one of the earliest material used in human body [2]. The history of biomedical hydrogel could date back to 1960, when Wichterle and Lim first reported their synthesized glycol methacrylate-based gel as the filling material after enucleation of the eye [3]. However, both fundamental and clinical research of hydrogels developed slowly at that time, and the total publications of hydrogel were under 100/year before 1970s

Tianyuan Ci and Jing Zang contributed equally to this work.

T. Ci · J. Zang · N. Feng (✉)
Department of Pharmaceutical Sciences, Shanghai University of Traditional Chinese Medicine, Shanghai, China
e-mail: npfeng@shutcm.edu.cn

N. Feng, Z. Yang (eds.), *Novel Drug Delivery Systems for Chinese Medicines*,
https://doi.org/10.1007/978-981-16-3444-4_10

[4]. Until 2000, hydrogels gradually received attentions and experienced rapid developments in bio-related fields, such as tissue engineering, drug delivery, and biosensors [5, 6].

In drug delivery, the porous structure enables the hydrogel to hold a variety of drugs with high loading capacities, including small-molecule drugs, macromolecular drugs, other nano- or micro-based particles, and even cells, providing spatial and temporal controlled release of these encapsulated contents [7]. In general, the hydrogel systems enable the active ingredients higher content and longer time at the lesion sites [8] and sometimes could also protect the drugs from degradation [9], realize multi-drug synergy, and help enhance the fraction of the active forms [10].

Both natural materials and synthetic polymers could be the components to build up a hydrogel, but the compositions of the hydrogels dramatically influence their functions and properties. Natural polymers, such as sodium alginate, collagen, gelatin, or fibrous proteins, are components of plants or animal tissues, which have good biocompatibility and low toxicity but usually with limited mechanical strength and large porous size [6]. And synthetic polymer-based hydrogels can be further modified to obtain specific strength, degradability, and functionality, to satisfy various biomedical demands, such as longer releasing time (even weeks to months) and stimuli-responsive release of the loaded drugs [6]. These hydrogels could achieve smart delivery of drugs at special tissue microenvironment, accomplishing on-demand administration and better efficacy in vivo.

In this chapter, we will focus on the applications of hydrogels in delivering Chinese medicines and summarize the clinical-used gel formulations of Chinese medicines (Table 10.1). In addition, regarding various novel hydrogels that have been developed, this chapter will highlight the latest strategies and applications of Chinese medicine-delivering hydrogels. Further, the hydrogels that are simply assembled by small molecules of Chinese medicines will also be addressed.

10.2 Effects of Hydrogels in Improving In Vivo Efficacies of Drugs

The active ingredients directly extracted from natural herbs and plants usually suffer from undesirable physicochemical properties and poor pharmacokinetic profiles, such as fast in vivo clearance, low bioavailability, and weak stability, which hinders their clinical applications. Proper leverage of the hydrogel systems could improve the druggability of Chinese medicines, in specific, to realize the sustained and local release, achieve multi-drug synergistic combination, and increase the stability of drugs.

Table 10.1 Clinical gels of Chinese medicines in China

Product	Active ingredients	Administration route	Indications
Chunru gel	Cortex ailanthic, sophora, moutan bark, etc.	Cavitary (vaginal)	Chronic cervicitis
Kushen gel	Alkaloids, sophora	Cavitary (vaginal)	Vaginitis
Baofukang gel	Zedoary turmeric oil, borneol, etc.	Cavitary (vaginal)	Vaginitis
Shukang gel	Hawthorn kernel essence, etc.	Cavitary (vaginal)	Pudendum pruritus
Kangfu gel	Elecampane, angelica dahurica, etc.	Cavitary (vaginal)	Vaginal congestion
Huangtengsu gel	Palmatine	Cavitary (vaginal)	Vaginitis
Tujingpi gel	Cortex pseudolaricis, benzoic acid, etc.	Topical	Tinea
Liushen gel	Artificial musk, realgar, borneol, etc.	Topical	Furunculosis
Chansuzhentong gel	Venenum bufonis, nux vomica, radix aconiti kusenzoffii, etc.	Topical	Muscle pain
Lajiaojian gel	Capsaicin	Topical	Arthritis, joint pain
Lajiaofengshi gel	Pepper, menthol, borneol, etc.	Topical	Joint pain
Fengshidieda gel	Radix aconiti, radix angelicae sinensis, etc.	Topical	Traumatic injuries
Chanwu gel	Radix aconiti, zanthoxylum, etc.	Topical	Pain
Heidouliuyou gel	Black soybean tar, eucalyptus oil, etc.	Topical	Dermatitis
Zhongtong gel	Scandent schefflera root, panax notoginseng, etc.	Topical	Traumatic injuries
Qiyezaoganna gel	Sodium aescinate, diethylamine salicylate	Topical	Soft tissue injury, tenosynovitis
Deproteinized calf blood extract eye gel	Deproteinized calf blood extract	Ophthalmic	Keratohelcosis, corneal injury
Pilocarpine nitrate eye gel	Pilocarpine nitrate	Ophthalmic	Miotic
Yiyajianpi gel	Chinese yam, coix seed, etc.	Oral	Infantile anorexia

Drugs@ State Food and Drug Administration of China: Approved Drug Products; website: https://www.nmpa.gov.cn/yaopin/index.html

10.2.1 Sustained Release

One of the merits of the hydrogel-based systems is the sustained release of drugs, enabling the drug concentration maintained in a relatively stable range for long time, which reduces the frequency of drug administration and further improves the drugs' in vivo pharmacokinetics [11, 12].

The mechanism of this "controlled" fate of drugs in hydrogels lies in the "mesh size" of the innate hydrogel structure, which is largely influenced by the material types, polymer concentrations, and gelling mechanisms (chemical crosslinking or physical packing). The typical mesh sizes reported for hydrogels range from 5 to 100 nm [7], thus could be utilized to sustain release most hydrophobic drug crystals or macromolecular drugs, such as IgG (size ~10 nm) [13]. As for small molecular hydrophilic drugs (size <1 nm), direct loading into hydrogels will not achieve desired sustained releasing profiles, and composite systems combining liposomes [14], nanoparticles [15], or microspheres [16] with hydrogels could be a choice. For example, in order to achieve sustained release and avoid the burst release of doxorubicin (DOX), a small hydrophilic drug, Cao et al. developed a liposome/hydrogel composite system, in which DOX was first encapsulated in liposomes (particle size ~75 nm) and then further loaded into the hydrogel [17]. For merely DOX/hydrogel system, 66% of DOX was released within 12 h, while in DOX liposome/hydrogel system, only 20% of DOX was released during 12 h. Then, the drug was gradually released up to 11 days.

The releasing mechanisms could also be speculated based on the ratio of hydrogel mesh size/drug size, which could be divided as fast diffusion (ratio >1), slow diffusion (ratio ~1), and swelling/degradation controlling (ratio <1) (Fig. 10.1) [7]. However, in the experimental level, the releasing mechanisms could be deduced by the experimental releasing profiles' fitting with Peppas equation of $Q_t = K \cdot t^n$, in which Q_t is the drug release amount at time t; K is the rate constant; and n is the diffusion index [18]: $n = 0.5$, diffusion-controlled; $n = 1$, degradation-controlled; and $n = 0.5$–1, diffusion and degradation controlled.

10.2.2 Enhancing Local Drug Content

With the exception of porous structures, the hydrogels are usually with high viscosity which is prospected by the Mark-Houwink empirical equation of $[\eta] = K\overline{M}_v^a$ that the intrinsic viscosity is directly proportional to the molecular weights of the polymers. For hydrogel, its crosslinking structure makes the overall molecular weight of the polymers close to "infinity," which means a high intrinsic viscosity. This behavior enabled the gel un-flowable without external force and stay at the lesion site for a long time [19]. In special, besides "un-flowable," the bioadhesive hydrogels could further strictly stick to mucosa based on the complex interactions between the materials and tissue proteins [20]. For example, poly(acrylic acid) or polyacrylate-based hydrogels are widely used in transdermal or cavitary delivery systems [21, 22]. The obvious advantage of this "un-flowable" or "bioadhesive" property is to significantly enhance the local drug content [23], leading to obvious improvement of drug efficacy.

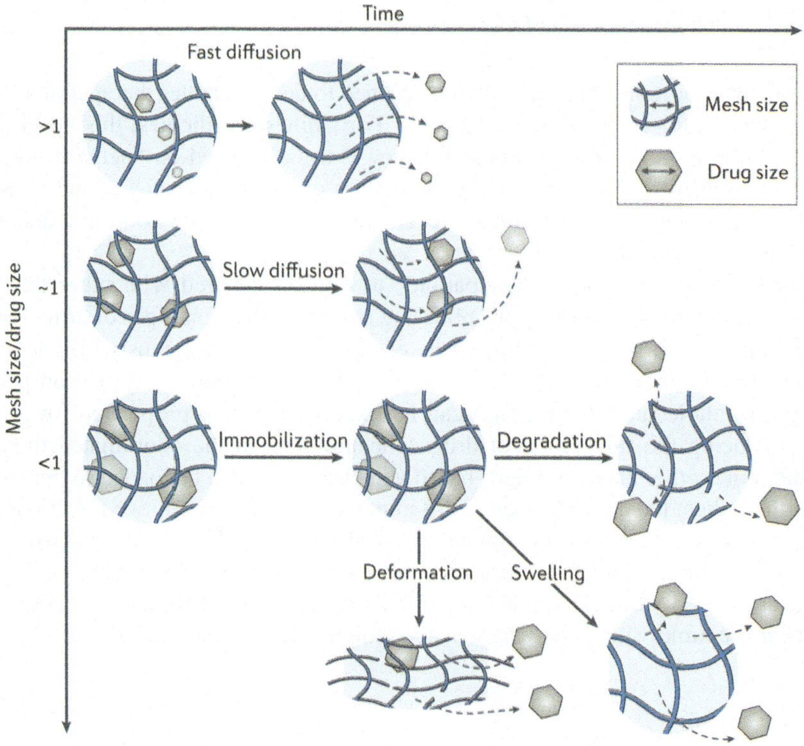

Fig. 10.1 Releasing mechanisms of drugs out of hydrogels, as determined by the ratio of mesh size/drug size. (Reprinted with permission from Ref [7]. Copyright 2016 Nature Publishing Group)

In addition, hydrogels also have unique advantages for the disease treatments of particular tissues, such as brain and joint cavity [24]. Blood-brain barrier (BBB) in the brain prevents many drugs from entering the brain through the blood [25], and articular cartilage has limited blood supply. These obstacles make the drugs in the blood difficult to reach these sites [26]. Injectable hydrogels can be injected into the lesion sites directly and significantly increase the local drug content [27]. For example, the therapeutic efficacy of cyclosporin A (CsA), an effective drug for stroke, is limited by intravenously injection, but with severe adverse effects such as nephrotoxicity and hepatotoxicity. Caicco et al. loaded CsA in the microspheres/hydrogel composite system and found CsA could be maintained at a constant effective concentration in the subventricular zone for at least 24 days post-implant [28].

10.2.3 Multi-drug Synergy

In clinic, two or more drugs are often combined to achieve better therapeutic effects and reduce multi-drug resistance [29–31]. For Chinese medicines, this synergistic combination is more crucial, whose efficacy is usually relied on "network targets, multi-components." Moreover, the combination of Western medicine and Chinese medicine is gaining more attention in recent years, especially for antitumor and anti-infection treatments [32].

For hydrogel, it is more "compatible" to drugs compared with other delivery vehicles and could be served as the releasing matrix of different types of drugs. More importantly, multiple drugs can be easily encapsulated simultaneously [33], and due to the structural characteristics of hydrogels, drugs with similar physical properties (solubility, molecular weight, etc.) can be fixed in a certain proportion for a long time, reducing the fluctuation of drug concentrations in the coordinated therapy. Furthermore, other nano- or micro-based vehicles could also be loaded in hydrogels to further adjust the drug releases of different components, to achieve the maximum drug synergetic efficacy. For example, Nihal Medatwal et al. co-loaded celastrol and doxorubicin in the lithocholic acid dipeptide conjugate-based hydrogel at a desired drug ratio. The hydrogel mediated a combination release of celastrol and doxorubicin near the tumor site, achieving a synergistic therapeutic effect [34].

10.2.4 Increasing the Stability of Drugs

Lots of drugs suffer instability during storage in their free state, and utilizing proper delivery vehicles has been proved to be an effective strategy. For example, curcumin is an active ingredient extracted from turmeric and is reported to have various pharmaceutical functions including antioxidant and anti-inflammation. However, it has poor chemical stability in water and low oral bioavailability. Zheng et al. encapsulated curcumin in chitosan gel beads and proved this gel system could significantly decrease the degradation rate of the drug [35]. The authors stated the underlying mechanism could be attributed to the encapsulation of the hydrophobic curcumin within hydrogels, which protected them from interacting with reactive substances in aqueous phase [35].

A question might arise: how hydrogels protect drugs from the reactive substances in water in the case that the hydrogel itself is full of water? The reason lies in the fact that there are still hydrophobic microstructures in hydrogel. For example, the gelling mechanism of the polyester-polyether hydrogel, such as poly(D,L-lactide-*co*-glycolide)-*b*-poly(ethylene glycol)-*b*-poly(D,L-lactide-*co*-glycolide) (PLGA-PEG-PLGA) thermosensitive hydrogel, is the hydrophobic interactions between inner micelles [36]. These hydrophobic micro-domains could adsorb hydrophobic drugs and decrease the degradation in water.

10.2.5 Stimuli-Triggered Drug Release

The stimuli-responsive hydrogels could realize triggered drug release in certain tissue microenvironments, achieving on-demand administration, maintaining a constant concentration of drugs in the lesion, and improving the drug bioavailability [37]. The stimuli could be temperature, pH, enzyme, external force, and light. For example, Raza et al. prepared a paclitaxel (PTX) drug delivery system that utilized a pH-responsive peptide hydrogel as the delivery vehicle [38]. At pH 7.4, the peptide self-assembled to form a stable and drug-loaded hydrogel, while under acidic pH conditions, degradation of peptide hydrogel and drug release could be observed. At pH 5.5, the drug-loaded hydrogel continuously released PTX for nearly 1 week. Similarly, enzyme-responsive hydrogel is also one of the research hotspots. Liu et al. prepared a matrix metalloproteinase 9 (MMP9)-responsive curcumin microsphere and then loaded the microsphere into a thermosensitive hydrogel to form MMP 9-responsive and thermosensitive composite system [39]. There have been reports that the diabetic skin wound is difficult to heal [40] and MMP9 is usually overexpressed in the diabetic unhealed wounds. The microspheres in the hydrogel reacted with MMP9 and released curcumin to promote wound healing. The results showed that the wound healing rate of curcumin hydrogel was over 90% on Day 12 post-therapy.

10.2.6 Increasing the Fraction of the Drugs' Active Form

In some occasions, the hydrogels could increase the fraction of the drugs' active forms, such as camptothecin and its analogues. Camptothecin is a potent antitumor ingredient extracted from the Chinese herb *Xishu* (*Camptotheca acuminata* Decne.). Camptothecin has two chemical forms, active lactone and inactive carboxylate [41, 42]. However, at physiological conditions, the active lactone fraction is only around 10% [43], which largely hinders its clinical use. Ci et al. discovered that after loading the camptothecin analogues into a polyester-based hydrogel, its lactone fraction could be sharply increased to nearly 50% (irinotecan) and 70% (10-hydroxycamptothecin), further increasing the drugs' antitumor efficacy and alleviating their side effects [44, 45]. The mechanisms are attributed to the hydrophobic interactions between drug molecules and the hydrophobic core in the microstructure of the hydrogel, which increased the equilibrium constant between lactone and carboxylate [46].

10.3 Classification and Gelation Mechanisms of Hydrogels

Since the hydrogels are 3D crosslinking networks, the gel systems could be generally divided into two categories, chemical and physical crosslinking hydrogels, whose driving forces of the gelling process are covalent bonds and non-covalent interactions, respectively [47]. The steps of the hydrogel preparation are first dissolving the material that could form a hydrogel in water, followed by the treatments with crosslinkers, irradiations, or microenvironment change (pH, temperature, ion strength, etc.), to trigger the chemical or physical crosslinking between monomers or polymer chains.

10.3.1 Chemical Crosslinking Hydrogels

For chemical crosslinking hydrogels, the synthesis process could be the crosslinking of monomers or polymers by radiation and crosslinking of polymers via reactions between functional groups (Fig. 10.2) [47]. More specific crosslinking methods as well as the possible chemical reactions, suitable compositions, etc. have been thoroughly reviewed by Hennink et al. [48]. In any case, the linkage between monomers or polymers is set up through chemical ways, and a global internal network (gel) is formed.

The obvious advantage of the chemical crosslinking hydrogels is the feasible regulation of hydrogel properties in a wide range, such as strength, hydrophilicity, and biodegradability, via the adjustment of composite monomers and polymers, or controlling the crosslinking density. For example, Hubbell et al. synthesized a hydrogel made from poly(ethylene glycol)-*b*-poly(a-hydroxy acid) diacrylate. The introduction of oligo(aliphatic ester) realized the formed gels to be biodegradable and could be used as implantable drug carrier [49].

However, obvious disadvantages of the chemical crosslinking hydrogels lie in the potential safety problems when being utilized in biomedical fields. The crosslinking agents are sometimes toxic to human bodies and need to be removed out clearly from the synthesized hydrogel systems [50]. Meanwhile, the encapsulated cargos could also suffer from degradation by irradiation or generated heat during the crosslinking process. Thus, the chemical crosslinking hydrogels are generally fading in bio-related applications, replaced by the physical crosslinking hydrogels correspondingly.

10.3.2 Physical Crosslinking Hydrogels

In contrast to chemical hydrogels, the crosslinking in physical hydrogels is driven by physical associations, such as ionic interactions, hydrogen bonds, hydrophobic

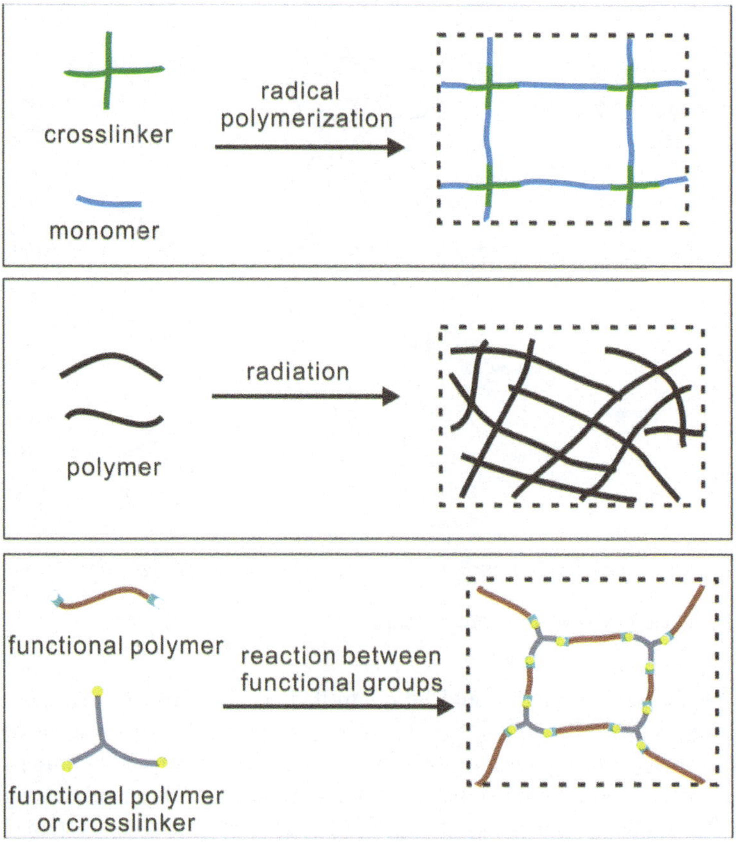

Fig. 10.2 Scheme of the synthesis of chemical crosslinking hydrogels

interactions, inclusion complexation, or formation of crystallites. The mild gelation process enables a variety of drugs or even cells to be incorporated into the matrix with the retention of full biological activities of the payloads, thus leading to better biocompatibility and wider biomedical applications (Fig. 10.3).

10.3.2.1 Ionic Interactions

Alginate hydrogel is a representative of physical gels formed by ionic interactions. Alginate is a linear anionic polysaccharide with the repeating units of β-1,4-linked D-mannuronic acid (M) and L-guluronic acid (G) [51]. Coordination interactions occur between G-blocks and divalent cations, such as Ca^{2+}, resulting in an "egg-box" structure; thus a physical crosslinking network could be formed if mixing calcium ions and alginate solutions under neutral or basic conditions.

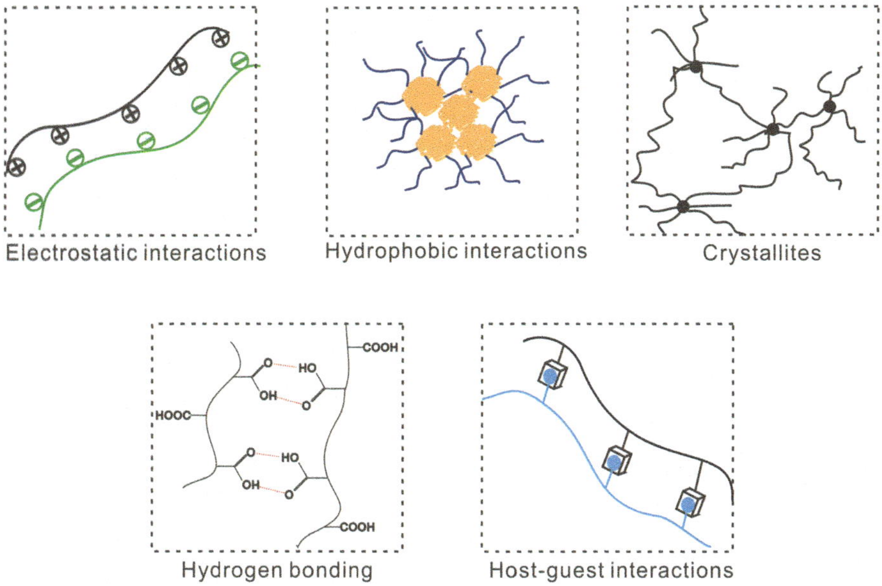

Fig. 10.3 Gelling mechanisms of physical gels

The mechanical strength could be controlled by the types of divalent cations, concentrations, specific preparation steps, etc. For example, Kuo et al. prepared alginate beads via dripping alginate solution into the medium containing calcium ions [52]. The authors found slower gelation systems ($CaCO_3$ suspension) generate more uniform and mechanically stronger gels than faster gelation systems ($CaSO_4$ solution). The compressive modulus and strength increased with alginate concentration, total calcium content, molecular weight, and guluronic acid (G) content of the alginate.

However, the ionically crosslinked hydrogels are easy to swell and will quickly dissolve in an aqueous environment (such as less divalent cations), thus are unable to achieve long-term retention at the lesion sites.

10.3.2.2 Hydrophobic Interactions

Hydrophobic interactions are usually the driving force of the gelation of hydrophobic-hydrophilic copolymers, such as Pluronic® (poly(ethylene glycol)-poly(propylene glycol)-poly(ethylene glycol), PEO-PPO-PEO) and ReGel® (poly (D,L-lactide-*co*-glycolide)-*b*-poly(ethylene glycol)-*b*-poly(D,L-lactide-*co*-glycolide), PLGA-PEG-PLGA) [36, 53]. In these systems, the copolymer would first self-assemble into micelles above the critical micelle concentration (CMC) with a hydrophobic core and a hydrophilic corona. Along with the increase of temperature, the hydrophilic chains of PEO become desolvated as a result of the breakage of the hydrogen bonds, leading to the system favoring hydrophobic interactions among the hydrophobic cores in a style of "micelle packing" or "percolated micelle network" [54], which indicates the gel formation.

Compared with the ionic interactions mentioned above, the gels formed by hydrophobic interactions usually "last" for long time against dilution of body fluid and could be used as the vehicles for long-term drug release. For example, Yang et al. utilized Pluronic® F127 hydrogel to load docetaxel, and the drug could be sustainedly released for over 6 days [55]. OncoGel, a depot of ReGel which is clinically in phase II stage for neck tumor treatment, could continuously release paclitaxel directly to the tumor and surrounding tissues for 6 weeks [56].

10.3.2.3 Hydrogen Bonds

Hydrogen bond is another important driving force of physical gels made of polypeptides [57], polynucleotide [58], or polymers full of hydroxy or carboxyl groups [59]. Due to the easy dissociation in physiological medium, hydrogen bonds usually cooperate with other molecular physical interactions to trigger the gelation of polymers. For example, Naskar et al. synthesized a water-soluble oligopeptide of H_2N-Gly-Phe-Ile-Leu-COOH and demonstrated this peptide could form hydrogels at physiological pH (pH 6–8.5) with a minimum gelation concentration of only 2.65% (w/v). The authors proposed the gelling mechanism of this peptide hydrogel is the combination of hydrogen bonds between C=O and N-H groups in different molecules and π-π interactions between the aromatic rings on the backbone of peptides.

10.3.2.4 Formation of Crystallites

Poly(vinyl alcohol) (PVA) is a water-soluble biocompatible synthetic polymer, and its aqueous solution could form a hydrogel after repeated "freeze-thaw" process [60]. The gel mechanical property could be adjusted by the polymer concentration, PVA molecular weight, as well as the repeating circles. The authors proposed PVA gel formation is ascribed to the formation of crystallites that act as physical crosslinking points in the system [60]. Due to its superior biocompatibility and easy preparation process, PVA hydrogel has been widely used in biomedical areas, such as wound dressing or drug delivery [61, 62]. The mechanical property of PVA hydrogel is sometimes limited, and its pore size is usually too large to enable sustained drug release of most small molecular drugs. Thus, various blended systems combining other hydrogel materials were also developed for specific applications. For example, Takamura et al. added sodium alginate or Pluronic L62 in PVA solution and prepared the hybrid hydrogel via freeze-thaw process [63]. The mechanical strength of the hydrogel was positively related with the amount of alginate or Pluronic L62 added, and drug release rate was negatively related [63].

10.3.2.5 Inclusion Complexation

Suitable leveraging host-guest interactions could also prepare physical hydrogels. The most commonly used host molecule in drug delivery is cyclodextrin (CD), and it can couple with linear polymers, such as polyethylene glycol (PEG), or small guest molecules (azobenzene, ferrocene, etc.) [64]. Thus, when mixing CD with PEG or other small guest molecule-modified polymers, a physical gel will be formed. Different with other physical interactions, the host-guest interaction is of high stability, and the formed hydrogel usually is capable of well mechanical strength. Manakker et al. prepared a series of supramolecular hydrogels with β-cyclodextrin and 8-arm or linear cholesterol-derivatized PEG with storage moduli in the range of 10–500 kPa [65]. The gel mechanical properties depend on temperature, concentration of polymers, molecular weight, and architecture of PEG [65]. In addition, due to the mild preparation conditions, the complexation hydrogel could be loaded with various small molecular and biomacromolecular drugs. Through adjusting the specific guest polymer or cyclodextrin derivate, the encapsulated drugs could be released in a sustained, rapid, or environmental responsive manner [66]. For example, the PEGylated drugs could be incorporated in CD-based hydrogel system in a high drug loading capacity via the inclusion complexation, achieving different drug in vivo biodistribution and therapeutic significance [67].

10.4 Characterization of Hydrogels

The physiochemical properties of hydrogel will influence the function and applications of the systems; thus proper characterization of materials is a necessity before use. Generally, it could be divided into morphology-, mechanical- and biomedical-related characterizations for the hydrogels in drug delivery. Morphology reflects the actually "gel" state of hydrogels; besides directly visualized by taking images by camera, its internal structures could be evaluated by scanning electron microscope (SEM), transmission electron microscope (TEM), and atomic force microscopy (AFM). Mechanical properties of hydrogels are mainly characterized by rheometer, which is the most important equipment in studying hydrogels. Besides that, other tests, such as phase diagram and degradation behavior, are also adopted to study the physiochemical properties of hydrogels. Moreover, for the hydrogels with biomedical applications, their biosafety is upmost. According to the delivery routes and their duration of exposure, the specific requirements are different. For oral, topical, or cavitary hydrogels, cell cytotoxicity test, irritation test (skin, mucosa), and sensitization test are necessities for the application of FDA approval. For implanted hydrogels, besides the above tests, the hemocompatibility, histocompatibility, short-term and long-term toxicity, etc. are sometimes required as well.

In this section, we will concentrate on the general tests for hydrogels when conducting a fundamental research, which include rheology, phase diagram, and morphology-related characterizations.

10.4.1 Rheology

Rheology studies the deformation and flow laws of materials in terms of stress, strain, temperature, and time [68] and is the most important evaluation modality for hydrogels. Hydrogel has a variety of rheological parameters, such as elastic modulus (G'), viscous modulus (G''), and viscosity (η), which could directly or indirectly reflect the hydrogels' strength, gelling point, and internal structure [69]. G' represents the ability of materials to store elastic deformation energy and represents the rebound index of materials after deformation, which is usually used to characterize the "solid" behavior of materials. G'' refers to the heat dissipation caused by deformation when the applied force is removed, which indicates the "liquid" behavior of the material [70]. η is a physical quantity to reflect the viscosity of a fluid [71].

In specific, the two parameters "gel strength" and "gelling transition point" are usually paid more attention in biomedical applications. Gel strength could be reflected by the value of modulus, especially G', which shows reference for the application of hydrogels. For example, in tissue engineering, if the hydrogels are leveraged as the sealant to seal wounds, it has to be subjected to the pressure of blood or tissue fluids, and its mechanical property (modulus) needs to be high [72, 73]. For example, the strength of interpenetrating polymer network (IPN) or double network (DN) hydrogels is significantly enhanced by double crosslinking [74]. Liu et al. designed a cell-encapsulating hydrogel based on the IPN of gelatin and dextran functionalized with methacrylate (MA) and aldehyde (AD), whose modulus could be high up to 10^4 Pa and could be used in vascular tissue engineering [75]. In some occasions, the modulus of hydrogel could be adjusted to 10^6 Pa via special chemical and physical modifications to satisfy higher demand of the hydrogels' mechanical strength [76]. In contrast, in drug delivery, the high modulus of hydrogel is usually unnecessary; a value around 10^3 Pa is enough.

The gelling point is another important indicator, especially for stimuli-responsive hydrogels, which could also be determined by rheology. In general, sol state, $G' < G''$; gel state, $G' > G''$; gelling point, $G' = G''$. Taking reverse thermosensitive hydrogel as an example, the material will undergo sol-to-gel transition along the increase of temperature. At low temperature, it is a "sol" with low modulus; when temperature increases, the modulus is sharply elevated; it becomes a "gel" when $G' > G''$. The crossover point in the rheology figure is the gelling point (Fig. 10.4) [77].

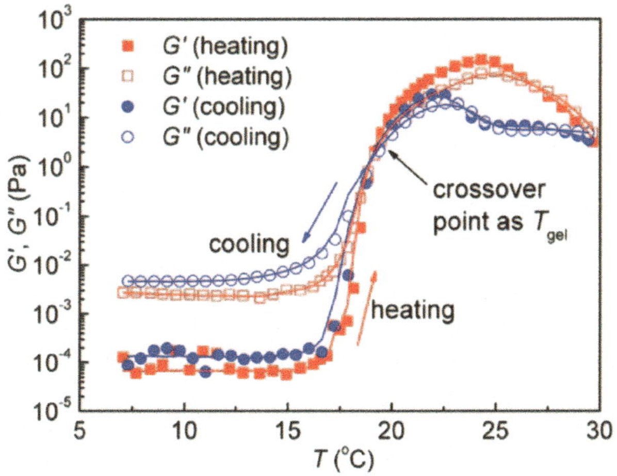

Fig. 10.4 G' and G'' of two typical reverse thermosensitive hydrogels along temperature. (Reprinted with permission from Ref [77]. Copyright 2008 American Chemical Society)

10.4.2 Phase Diagram

In comparison to rheology, phase diagram provides a clear outline of the state of hydrogels in different conditions and sometimes is more feasible in practical use. Usually, the phase diagram of hydrogels is depicted via the results of inverting tube test. That is, a gel state is defined as no flow within 30 s after the vials are inverted 180°.

For example, in the thermosensitive hydrogel PLGA-PEG-PLGA, its hydrogel state is related to temperature, polymer concentration, and the drug-encapsulating or not (Fig. 10.5) [44]. Direct phase diagram could help clarify the effects of these factors on the gelling process of material. Critical gelation concentration (CGC, the lowest polymer concentration the system needs to form a gel) and critical gelation temperature (CGT, the lowest temperature the system needs to form a gel) could be easily deduced from the phase diagram. As shown in Fig. 10.5, the CGC for polymer itself was 5 wt% while increased to 10 wt% after loading drugs. CGT remained almost unchanged for hydrogel or drug-loaded hydrogel, both around 35 °C, which guaranteed the gel state in the body and a sol state at room temperature.

10.4.3 Morphology

The structure of hydrogel is also a critical parameter in hydrogel characterization and is crucial in adjusting drug release. Scanning electron microscope (SEM), transmission electron microscope (TEM), and atomic force microscopy (AFM) are commonly used instruments to observe the microstructure of hydrogel.

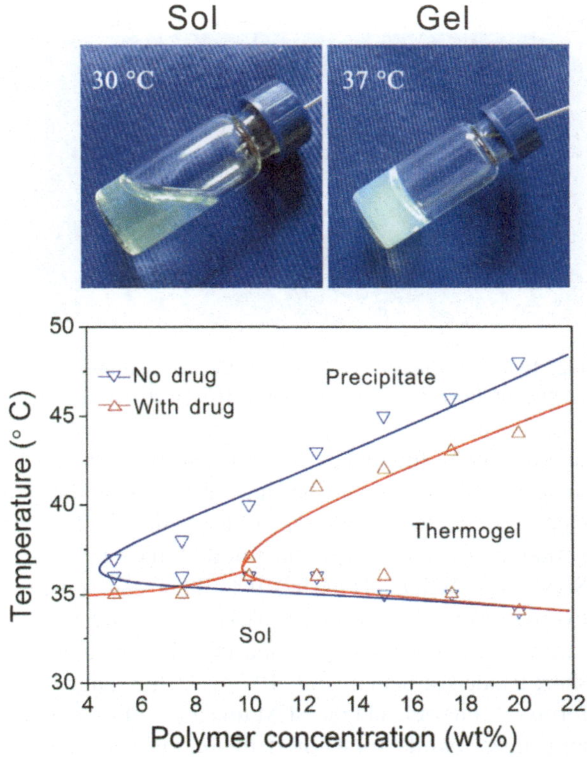

Fig. 10.5 The phase diagram of thermosensitive hydrogels via inverting tube method. (Reprinted with permission from Ref [44]. Copyright 2014 Nature Publishing Group)

10.4.3.1 Transmission Electron Microscope

TEM utilizes electron beam of extremely short wavelength as the illumination source and electromagnetic lens to focus the image [78]. Since TEM uses transmitted electrons to image, TEM can provide internal structure of the samples, such as crystal structure, morphology, and stress state information. For example, Chen et al. designed an amphiphilic peptide which could first self-assemble into nanoribbons in aqueous solution (Fig. 10.6a) and underwent sol-to-gel transition with the existence of glutamine transaminase (TGase), to realize quick hemostasis [79]. The authors stated this enzyme-triggered gelation was due to the physical crosslinking between already-existed nanoribbons with the newly created thin nanofibers (Fig. 10.6b). Utilizing TEM, the images of the microstructure of the system before and after gelation could be clearly observed.

10.4.3.2 Scanning Electron Microscope

SEM utilizes an incident electron beam with a certain energy to scan the sample and excites secondary electrons derived from the interactions between the incident electron and the sample. SEM allows a large area, a few nanometers to tens of

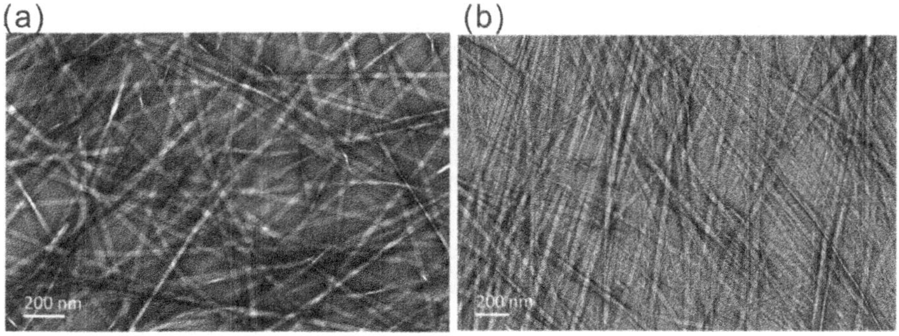

Fig. 10.6 TEM images of I3QGK before (**a**) and after (**b**) addition of TGase. (Reprinted with permission from Ref [79]. Copyright 2016 American Chemical Society)

microns, to be focused at one time and produces high-resolution three-dimensional images [80], thus could be utilized to assess the gelling process besides merely characterizing the morphology of the hydrogel at certain state. For example, the self-gelling process of the gel composed by the small molecular rhein was evaluated by SEM [81]. When pH is 8.0–9.4, rhein can self-assemble to form a transparent hydrogel (Fig. 10.7a). Once pH is higher than 9.4, the hydrogel disintegrates and forms a blood red solution, and the SEM images show that the solution contains short banded structure (Fig. 10.7b). In the range of pH 6.8 to pH 8.0, the sample forms viscous gel, and the SEM images confirm that the hydrogel structure is mainly long fibers, while some short fibers are observed on the surface (Fig. 10.7c). In addition, when pH value is lower than 8.0, there are short rod-like precipitates in the gel (Fig. 10.7d). In summary, the formation of rhein hydrogel is highly dependent on the pH value of the medium and could be observed by SEM.

10.4.3.3 Atomic Force Microscopy

AFM adopts the micro cantilever to sense and amplify the force between the tip of the cantilever and the atom of the sample with atomic resolution [82]. AFM is capable of high resolution, wide application range, and easy preparation of testing samples. However, the tip of AFM will cause the soft nanostructure to be significantly flattened, and its image will be wider and shallower than its actual state [80]. AFM can be used to obtain a three-dimensional image of the sample "surface," which can distinguish atomic-level surface changes and measure the height difference between two positions accurately to calculate the surface roughness of the sample. In SEM it is difficult to detect the subtle height changes of the sample surface; thus in the nm-level scanning range, the image of AFM is significantly better than SEM. For example, AFM is used to observe hydrogel scaffolds consisting of silk fibroin peptide (SF16) in the treatment of peripheral nerve injury. From the AFM images, long self-assembled nanofiber fragments formed by SF16 peptide can be observed (Fig. 10.8) [83].

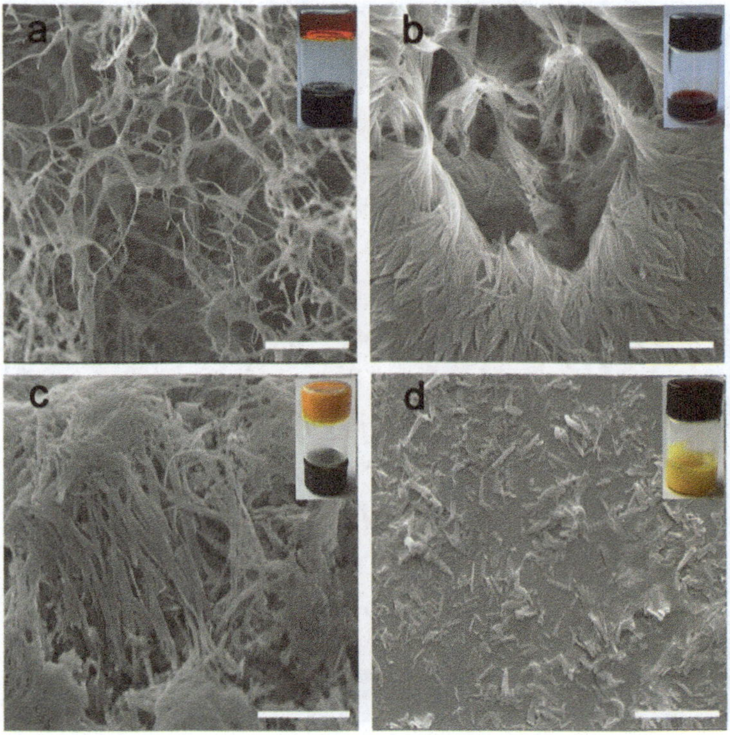

Fig. 10.7 SEM images of rhein hydrogel at different pH. (**a**) pH = 8.3, (**b**) pH = 10.2, (**c**) pH = 7.4, (**d**) pH = 6.5. Scale bar, 5μm. (Reprinted with permission from Ref [81]. Copyright 2019 Nature Publishing Group)

10.5 Hydrogel Systems for Delivering Active Ingredients of Chinese Medicines

Given the merits of hydrogels, various Chinese medicines are encapsulated in the gel to pursue better in vivo performance (Table 10.2). In the section, we will classify these hydrogel systems according to their delivery routes: injectable hydrogels, transdermal (topical) hydrogels, cavitary hydrogels and ophthalmic hydrogels, and oral hydrogels.

10.5.1 Injectable Hydrogels

Injectable hydrogel refers to a system that is a fluid liquid before injection and changes from a sol state to a solid gel under physiological conditions after administration via injection [116]. The factors that promote the transformation are specific

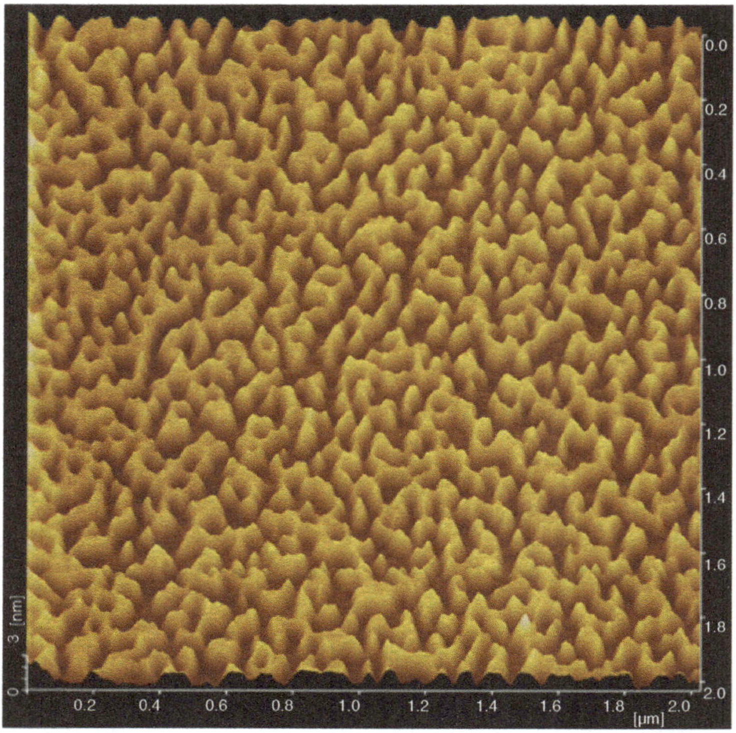

Fig. 10.8 Atomic force microscope image of the silk fibroin peptide (SF16) hydrogel scaffold. (Reprinted with permission from Ref [83]. Copyright 2013 Dove Press)

chemical reactions or external stimuli, such as temperature, pH, light irradiation, etc. [117]. Currently, injectable hydrogels have been widely used in cancer treatments [118], cartilage regeneration [84], tissue engineering [119], etc. Compared with non-injectable hydrogels, injectable hydrogels can be injected into the lesion site after simple mixing with drugs in the sol state and thus has shown a promising prospect for long-term drug delivery [120].

10.5.1.1 Cartilage Regeneration

Osteoarthritis (OA) is a joint disease of cartilage wear and meniscus damage and is accompanied by severe pain that seriously dampens people's life quality [121]. Articular cartilage is an avascular tissue with complex structure, which is mainly composed of cartilage cells wrapped in proteoglycan and collagen matrix [122]. As there are no blood vessels, lymph vessels, and progenitor cells in articular cartilage, its self-repair ability after damage is extremely limited [123]. Due to the well biocompatibility and high water content, hydrogels are suitable materials to simulate the extracellular matrix (ECM) of natural cartilage [124]. The hydrogels can be injected

Table 10.2 Typical hydrogel systems for delivery of Chinese medicines

Delivery route	Therapeutic drugs	Gel material	Gel property	Indications	Results	Ref
Intra-articular injection	Magnoflorine	Hyaluronic acid	/	Osteoarthritis	Increasing the number of chondrocytes and forming ECM of chondrocytes on 3 weeks	[84]
Intra-articular injection	Hedysarum heteropoly polysaccharides	Hyaluronic acid	/	Osteoarthritis	Expand the extension angle of the knee joint and reduce the thickness of joint synovium	[85]
Intratumoral injection	Embelin	PECT	Thermosensitive	Cancer	The therapeutic effect for the hydrogel group (0.5 mg/mouse) was equivalent to that of embelin solution (6 mg/mouse)	[86]
Intratumoral injection	Dihydroartemisinin	Agarose	Photothermal sensitive	Cancer	In vivo temperature of hydrogel group was raised by about 15 °C within 5 min; the tumor growth was significantly lowered	[87]
Subcutaneous injection	Irinotecan	PLGA-PEG-PLGA	Thermosensitive	Cancer	Tumor inhibition ratios of IRN/thermogel groups were 86.2–98.2%, while that of the free IRN groups were 52.3–80.5% at the same drug doses	[44]
Myocardial injection	Polydopamine	Thiolate-modified hyaluronic acid	ROS sensitive	Postinfarcted cardiac	Significant improvement of cardiac functions was achieved, accompanied by inhibition of the expression of inflammation factors	[88]
Intrauterine injection	β-Estradiol	Aloe and poloxamer	Thermosensitive	Intrauterine adhesion	Promote the proliferation of endometrial stromal cells and	[89]

(continued)

Table 10.2 (continued)

Delivery route	Therapeutic drugs	Gel material	Gel property	Indications	Results	Ref
					endometrial regeneration, and prevent re-adhesion	
Subcutaneous injection	Radix ophiopogonis polysaccharide	PLGA	/	Myocardial ischemia	Low but lasting ROP plasma concentrations, long-term pre-caution and cure of myocardial ischemia	[90]
Subcutaneous injection	Radix ophiopogonis polysaccharide	Poloxamer	Thermosensitive	Myocardial ischemia	Full ROP exposure, short-term acute therapies of myocardial ischemia	[90]
Subcutaneous injection	Ibuprofen	Liquidambaric acid	/	Inflammation	Inhibit the release of TNF-α and PGE2	[91]
Transdermal administration	Cortex moutan	Poloxamer 407 and sodium carboxymethyl cellulose	/	Atopic dermatitis	High drug permeability percent-age with the highest percentage around 8%	[92]
Transdermal administration	Gallic acid	Pluronic F-127	Dual responsive (pH/temperature)	Atopic dermatitis	Enhanced percutaneous perme-ability and high bioavailability	[93]
Transdermal administration	Danggui buxue extract	Poloxamer 407	Thermosensitive	Wound	The wound healing rate was 93% after gel treatment on the 14th day	[94]
Transdermal administration	Aloe vera	carbopol 934	/	Wound	The wound healing rate was 80% after gel treatment on the 14th day	[95]
Transdermal administration	Curcumin	PF127-CHO	pH sensitive	Wound	The wound contraction area could reach 72% after using it in wound for 5 days	[96]
Transdermal administration	Brucine	Carbopol	/	Pain	The prohibition of the nocicep-tive response by hydrogel at the dosage of 30 mg/kg could reach 38.0%	[97]

Transdermal administration	Evodiamine and rutaecarpine	Hyaluronic acid	/	Pain	Downregulate serum levels of prostaglandin E2, interleukin 6, and tumor necrosis factor	[98]
Transdermal administration	Haifengteng, luoshiteng, chuanshanlong, etc.	Carbopol	/	Cancer pain	Decreased the levels of ICTP and BAP, inhibits bone metastasis	[99]
Transdermal administration	Anemonin	HPMC and Carbomer 934	/	Rheumatoid arthritis	49% inhibitory effect on ear swelling	[100]
Transdermal administration	*Urtica dioica*	Carbopol 934	/	Rheumatoid arthritis	The positive rate of analgesia reached 58%	[101]
Transdermal administration	Baicalin	Glycerol monooleic acid	/	/	Stronger skin permeability, sustained drug release	[102]
Transdermal administration	Marigold, chrysanthemum, and *Salvia miltiorrhiza*	Carbomer 940, glycerin, propylene glycol	/	Hand-foot syndrome	Positive rate of 71%, significant improvement compared to the placebo	[103]
Nasal	Paeonol	Poloxamer 407	Thermosensitive	Allergic rhinitis	Improve the pathological changes, IgE, LTE 4, nasal mucosa eosinophil ↓	[104]
Nasal	Cicada slough, bezoar, borneol, etc.	Glycerin	/	Allergic rhinitis	LTE4, IgE, nasal mucosa eosinophil ↓	[105]
Nasal	Radix Bupleuri	Gellan gum	/	Fever	Hydrogel could control the temperature of the experimental animals for 20–30 h	[106]
Vaginal	Copper-curcumin	Carbopol 974p	/	Contraception	Inhibiting sperm motility within 30 s	[107]
Vaginal	Gentianae radix et rhizoma, Stemonae radix, etc.	Carbopol 941 and xanthan gum	/	Cervicitis	Reduce pathological damage of cervix and vagina IL-2, IL-17, and MCP-1 ↓	[108]

(continued)

Table 10.2 (continued)

Delivery route	Therapeutic drugs	Gel material	Gel property	Indications	Results	Ref
Ocular administration	Puerarin	Carbopol/HPMC	pH sensitivity	/	The constant of absorption rate of hydrogel exhibited 1.82-fold greater than that of aqueous solution, enhancing ocular bio-availability and patient compliance	[109]
Ocular administration	Quercetin	F127 and CMCS	Temperature and pH sensitivity	/	Slow release of quercetin	[110]
Ocular administration	Curcumin	Pluronic P123	Ion-sensitive	/	The cumulative curcumin per-meation amount of hydrogel 1.32-fold higher than curcumin solution	[111]
Intratumoral injection	Doxorubicin	Triterpenoids	/	Cancer	Prolong the survival of tumor-bearing mice by 63%, the tumor inhibition of the hydrogel group could reach 97.6% on the 14th day after treatment	[112]
Intratumoral injection	Doxorubicin	Poricoic acid A	/	Cancer	The tumors appeared 35.1% atrophy after treatment; the inhi-bition rate of hydrogel group was 116.58%	[113]
Injectable	Rhein	Rhein	/	Neural inflammation	Downregulating the levels of TNF-α, IL-6, IL-12, and iNOS	[81]
Oral	Bovine serum albumin	Chinese quince seed gum, poly (*N*,*N*-diethylacryl amide-co-methacrylic acid)	pH sensitivity	/	Protecting protein drugs from degrading in the stomach	[114]
Oral	Berberine hydrochloride	Bacterial cellulose	/	Gastrointestinal infections	Exhibiting sustained drug release under different pH conditions (cumulative release rate >68% within 72 h)	[115]

into the closed joint cavity to provide a bionic microenvironment for the adhesion, growth, and reconstitution of cartilage cells [121] and can also encapsulate anti-osteoarthritis drugs and growth factors to promote cartilage regeneration [125].

Saponins have proved to exhibit cartilage protective effects by reducing the degradation of extracellular matrix and chondrocyte damage. Jeon et al. designed saponins (Sa)-loaded gellan gum (GG) hydrogel for cartilage regeneration [84]. The results revealed the chondrocytes could proliferate faster if seeding on the Sa/GG hydrogels and the expression of type I and type II collagen also increased. The hydrogel was proved to maintain the chondrocyte phenotype and enhance the biological activity of cartilage ECM. Zhang et al. prepared hedysarum heteropoly polysaccharide-loaded hyaluronic acid hydrogel and observed its therapeutic effects for osteoarthritis in rats [85]. The results showed that the hydrogel group could significantly expand the extension angle of the knee joint of OA rats (control group $150.9 \pm 9.0°$ vs. hydrogel group $169.1 \pm 6.9°$) and reduce the thickness of joint synovium (control group 368.9μm vs. hydrogel group 249.9μm). Moreover, the hydrogel group reduced the administration frequency (once a week), and the compliance of patients was improved.

10.5.1.2 Cancer Treatments

Cancer therapy is an important application for injectable Chinese medicine-encapsulated hydrogels. Peng et al. constructed an embelin-loaded thermosensitive hydrogel with the amphiphilic triblock copolymer of poly (ε-caprolactone-co-1,4,8-trioxa[4.6]spiro-9-undecanone)-poly (ethylene glycol)-poly (ε-caprolactone-co-1,4,8-trioxa[4.6]spiro-9-undecanone) (PECT) [86]. Embelin was reported to be an effective therapeutic drug in treating cancer; however, its high hydrophobicity and low oral bioavailability limited its direct use in clinic [46]. The application of PECT gel increased the local drug content in tumor tissue, prolonged the drug's effective time, and reduced systemic toxicity. After administrating into the body, embelin/PECT solution transformed into the gel state within a few seconds due to its thermosensitivity and then continuously released the drug. In vivo antitumor test showed that the therapeutic effect for the hydrogel group at a low dose of 0.5 mg per mouse was equivalent to that of embelin solution at the dose of 6 mg per mouse.

Similarly, Ci et al. loaded a camptothecin analogue of irinotecan into the thermogel composed of poly(D,L-lactide-co-glycolide)-*b*-poly(ethylene glycol)-*b*-poly(D,L-lacitide-glycolid) (PLGA-PEG-PLGA) [44]. Besides sustainably releasing the drug for 2 weeks, the hydrogel significantly increased the equilibrium lactone fraction of irinotecan to approximate 50% through hydrophobic interactions. After the tumor-bearing mice being treated with the irinotecan-loaded hydrogel, the tumor was significantly regressed with very mild side effects.

Besides traditional chemotherapy, Chinese medicine-based hydrogels can also be used in photothermal therapy. Chen et al. used agarose hydrogel to load Hu Kaiwen ink and ferric trichloride [87]. In this system, Hu Kaiwen ink acted as a photosensitizer to convert light into heat under near-infrared radiation, further inducing

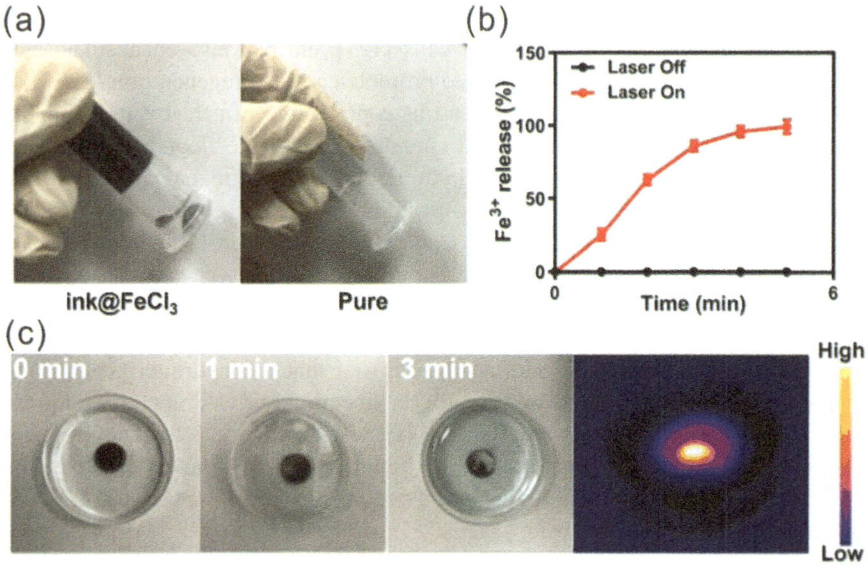

Fig. 10.9 (**a**) Typical images of the ink and ferric trichloride-loaded hydrogel. (**b**) Release profile of Fe^{3+} from the ink@hydrogel with (red) and without (black) laser irradiation. (**c**) Disassembly of the hydrogel by the 1064-nm laser irradiation (1 W/cm^2). (Reprinted with permission from Ref [87]. Copyright 2020 Frontiers Media S.A)

hydrogel disintegration to release the loaded ferric ions (Fig. 10.9). The photothermal conversion efficiency (η) of the ink was high up to 35%, which is significantly higher than conventional photothermal materials, such as Au nanorods (21%) and graphene quantum dots (29%). Meanwhile, the released Fe^{3+} would soon be reduced to Fe^{2+} in the tumor microenvironment and produce reactive ROS with the existence of pre-injecting trichloride and dihydroartemisinin (DHA) to promote tumor cell apoptosis. This hydrogel system was proved to realize the synergistic effect of DHA-Fe^{2+} in chemodynamic therapy and photothermal therapy, achieving higher tumor-suppressing efficacy.

10.5.2 Topical Hydrogels

Hydrogel is a popular delivery strategy for topical and transdermal formulations to increase the drug retention on the skin and extended drug release, realizing enhancement in drug effectiveness compared to the liquid forms. The topical hydrogels have been widely used in wound healing [94], topic dermatitis [92], and analgesia [99].

10.5.2.1 Atopic Dermatitis

Atopic dermatitis (AD) is a chronic inflammatory skin disease, manifested by itching, inflammation, swelling, redness, and exudation [126]. The drug-loaded hydrogel provides long-lasting relief for AD patients and is the most important indication for topical-used hydrogels. In clinic, corticosteroids are typical Western medicines to improve the condition of AD patients; however, long-term use may cause serious side effects such as high blood pressure and atrophy [127]. Traditional Chinese medicine (TCM) believes that AD is mainly caused by improper diet, excessive internal heat, and spleen failure. The treatment could focus on clearing the internal heat and dampness, strengthening the function of the spleen and liver [128]. Many Chinese medicines such as *Gancao* (*Glycyrrhizae Radix et Rhizoma*) [129], *Jinyinhua* (*Lonicerae Japonicae Flos*) [130], and *Bajiaohuixiang* (*Anisi Stellati Fructus*) [131] have obvious effect on the treatment of AD. Thus, encapsulating these drugs in hydrogel is a preferable delivery strategy for mild AD treatments.

Wang et al. used poloxamer 407 and sodium carboxymethyl cellulose as the gel matrix to prepare the gallic acid (GA)-loaded hydrogel for the treatment of AD [92]. Carboxymethyl cellulose sodium was added into the system to adjust the porous size of the gel, rheological properties, and gelation temperature and further modify the release profile of GA. The cumulative drug released was about 80% in 48 h. Similarly, Szekalska et al. prepared cymaroside-encapsulated hydrogel using alginate as hydrogel matrix for AD treatment (Fig. 10.10) [132]. In vivo experiments indicated that drug-loaded hydrogel could significantly reduce the number of

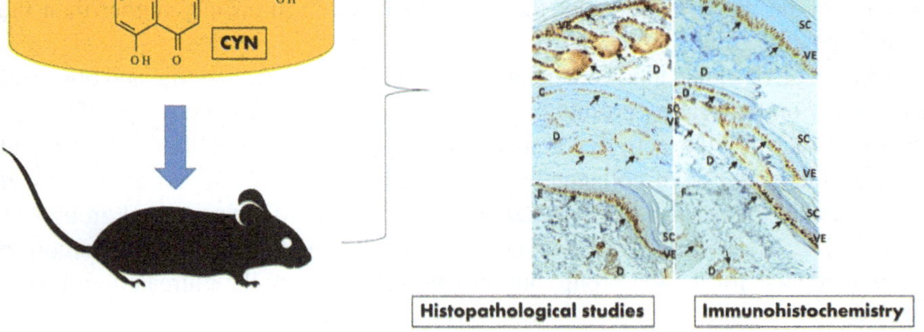

Fig. 10.10 Preparation of and anti-inflammatory efficacy of cymaroside-loaded hydrogels. (Reprinted with permission from Ref [132]. Copyright 2020 Elsevier)

granulocytes in the skin, reflecting obvious anti-inflammatory effects in AD model mice.

10.5.2.2 Wound Healing

Skin wounds refer to the destruction of the integrity of skin tissues and are often accompanied by the loss of body materials [133]. Wound healing is a complex process, generally including hemostasis (vascular constriction and thrombosis), local inflammation (infiltration of immune cells), proliferation of tissue cells (re-epithelialization, angiogenesis, collagen synthesis, extracellular matrix formation), and tissue remodeling (collagen remodeling, vascular maturation, and regression) [134]. These processes are easily affected by various factors, such as bacteria, oxygen, and nutrients. For example, hypoxia will block the fibroblast proliferation and remodeling [135]; insufficient supply of nutrition will lead to high possibility of wound infection and decrease wound tensile strength [136]; bacteria in the wound can easily cause inflammation and make the wound difficult to heal [137]. Hydrogels can absorb tissue exudates and allow fresh oxygen to penetrate [138] and adhere to the surface of the wound to isolate bacteria and reduce the occurrence of infection [138], thus promoting wound healing.

Cui et al. loaded *Danggui Buxue* extract in liposomes and further dispersed the drug/liposome in a thermosensitive gel [94]. Liposomes have good skin permeability and can be used as a drug carrier for skin wound healing [139]. However, the low viscosity of liposomal solution leads to the fast shedding from skin surface. Dispersing liposomes into hydrogels can improve their stability and increase the retention time of drugs in skin wounds. *Danggui Buxue* extract can activate the VEGF/PI3K/Akt and TGF-β/Smads signaling pathways, accelerating wound healing. On the seventh day post-administration of the drug-loaded hydrogel, tissue edema in rats almost disappeared with microvessels and fibroblasts arranging orderly. In contrast, tissue edema and inflammatory infiltration could be observed in the control group (blank liposomes in hydrogel), and wound healing still retained in an early stage. The percentage of wound contraction of the hydrogel group was about 93% on the 14th day after therapy, which was significantly higher than the vehicle control group (70%).

Khan et al. designed aloe vera gel with carbomer 934 as gel material and observed its efficacy on the healing promotion of skin wounds in rats after surgery [95]. Aloe vera can increase the activity of macrophages, stimulate fibroblast activity, and increase the synthesis of collagen to promote wound contraction. After 14 days of gel treatment, the healing rate reached 80.1%, while that of the untreated group was only 52.7%. Meanwhile, there was no obvious inflammation and pus formation in the wound sites for the gel group, but they were obvious in the untreated group.

10.5.2.3 Analgesia

The pain sensation is people's inherent response to noxious stimuli that acts on the body [140], and the application of Chinese medicines for analgesia has a long history. The ancient medical record of *Compendium of Materia Medica* denoted a large number of pain-relieving and analgesic medicines, such as datura flower, poppy shell, etc. [141]. The analgesic mechanism of Chinese medicines can be roughly attributed to their effects on the central and peripheral nervous systems [142]. The effect of Chinese medicines on the central nervous system is mainly through increasing the content of opioid peptides, inhibiting the release of neurotransmitter NO, and reducing the content of prostaglandin E2 (PGE 2) in the brain. And the analgesic mechanisms of the peripheral nervous system mainly include reducing the secretion of peripheral pain-causing substances and increasing the release of peripheral endogenous analgesic substances [143]. Drug-loaded hydrogels are convenient to use and can directly act on the painful area and thus are widely used for analgesia.

Wang et al. prepared a composite system of liposome/hydrogel to load brucine for enhancing its antalgic effectiveness [97]. Due to the low solubility and poor skin permeability, free brucine has difficulty to penetrate the skin layer. Liposomes can help drugs penetrate deeper in the skin due to its high affinity with the stratum corneum. Moreover, after encapsulating in hydrogel, the system can further realize long-term drug retention, promoting the skin accumulation of drugs. The results indicated the pain alleviating rate was high up to 38%, which was greater than that of the positive control *Yunnan Baiyao* Tincture (31.3%).

Similar as the composite system of liposome/hydrogel, other nano- or micro-based particles can also be capsulated in hydrogel to further improve the drugs' efficacy. Wang et al. prepared a microemulsion/hydrogel (ME-Gel) to load evodiamine and rutaecarpine to realize sustained release and long effective time of the drug [98]. Three days post-treatment with ME-Gel, no erythema or edema was observed, and the analgesic effects of ME-Gel containing evodiamine and rutaecarpine were strongest compared with all other control groups. In addition, the administration of ME-Gel effectively downregulated the serum levels of PGE 2, IL-6, and TNF-α, indicating well analgesic effects.

10.5.3 Cavitary Hydrogels

Compared with injectable and topical administration, delivering drugs via cavity could sometimes achieve a balance between patients' compliance and effective drug contents for the easy penetration of the drugs into the cavitary mucosa than skin. Besides leveraging as local delivery systems to treat rhinitis [104], vaginitis [144], or colitis [145], cavitary delivery could also exert systematic effects to tackle fever [106], contraception [107], and candidiasis [146].

The advantages of cavity administration are obvious due to the abundant blood vessels and lymphatics under the cavity mucosa [147], such as quick absorbance of drugs and the avoidance of first-pass effects. Thus, various cavitary-administrated hydrogels have been developed to enhance the in vivo effectiveness of Chinese medicines.

10.5.3.1 Nasal Hydrogel

Nasal hydrogel was a representative in this field. Chu et al. used poloxamer 407 as the gel material to prepare paeonol thermosensitive hydrogel to treat allergic rhinitis (AR) [104]. Through adjusting poloxamer content, this hydrogel underwent sol-gel transition at around 34 °C, realizing the easy administration into the nasal cavity in a sol state and the quick gelation after delivery. Paeonol was gradually released for 12 h, which significantly decreased the inflammatory factors of IgE, LTE4, and the number of eosinophils in the guinea pig model of AR.

Nasal hydrogel could exhibit systematic therapeutic efficacy as well. Cao et al. loaded Radix Bupleuri with gellan gum 0.5% (m/v) to control fever [106]. Compared with the traditional bupleurum nasal solution, bupleurum nasal hydrogel could control the temperature of the experimental animals for 20–30 h, while the effective time of oral bupleurum was only 6 h.

10.5.3.2 Vaginal Hydrogel

Chinese medicine-encapsulating vaginal hydrogels also attract widespread attention in both research and clinical use. Chauhan Gaurav et al. prepared a composite system to load curcumin and copper, in which curcumin and copper were first incorporated into β-cyclodextrin and further loaded in carbopol gel for contraception by vaginal delivery [107]. Both copper ions and curcumin were sustainedly released and prevent pregnancy by damaging the function of sperm membrane and decreasing sperm activity. The results revealed the vaginal gel can completely inhibit sperm movement within 30 s after administration.

Cervicitis treatment is another example as the indications of vaginal hydrogels. In clinical practice, the drug resistance is a major obstacle in tackling cervicitis by antibiotics. Therefore, the efficacy of vaginal gel containing Chinese medicines was gradually focused by researchers. Mao et al. studied the effects of Feilin vaginal gel (FVG) in cervicitis therapy, which contained various Chinese medicine components of *Baixianpi* (*Dictamni Cortex*), *Baibu* (*Stemonae Radix*), *Qinpi* (*Fraxini Cortex*), *Chishao* (*Paeoniae Radix Rubra*), etc. [108]. The clinical manifestations of cervicitis are cervical epithelial hyperplasia and inflammatory cell infiltration. After FVG (1.1 g/kg) treatment, cervical lesions and infiltration immune cells were improved, and the reticulate bodies were significantly reduced.

10.5.4 Ophthalmic Hydrogel

In clinic, ophthalmic diseases are often treated by drug-containing eye drops [148]. However, many external forces, such as eye blinking and tearing, easily extrude the liquid droplets from the eye, leading to low bioavailability of the drug [149]. Ophthalmic-used hydrogels, especially the bioadhesive types, have strong adhesion to the cornea, which can promote the retention and corneal absorption of the active drugs [150].

Yu et al. used F127 and carboxymethyl chitosan (CMCS) as the gel matrix to develop a quercetin-loaded hydrogel [151]. Leveraging the pH sensitivity of CMCS and the thermosensitivity of F127, this hydrogel was capable of dual responsiveness of temperature and pH. The results confirmed this hydrogel has a maximum swelling rate at 35 °C and pH 7.4 and can achieve slow release of quercetin for 72 h.

Wu et al. prepared a pH-triggered puerarin ophthalmic gel with carbopol 980 as the gelling agent and hydroxypropyl methyl cellulose (HPMC) as the bioadhesion-enhancing agent [109]. Puerarin is an osajin isoflavone extracted from *Gegen* (*Puerariae Lobatae Radix*), which can reduce intraocular pressure, improve eye blood flow, and ameliorate retinal function and microcirculation. However, due to tear secretion and nasolacrimal duct drainage, puerarin eye drops have a short pre-corneal retention time. In addition, puerarin may cause respiratory and gastro-intestinal side effects if drained into the gastrointestinal tract through the nasolacrimal duct. Puerarin gel can significantly extend the drug's residence in the cornea and improve its bioavailability. Compared with puerarin solution, the area under the curve ($AUC_{0\text{–}24h}$) of the in situ gel within 24 h was 2.17 times higher than that of the puerarin solution.

10.5.5 Oral Hydrogel

Oral delivery of drugs has obvious advantages in improving patients' compliance and is convenient in both carrying and administering, which is the most widely adopted administration route in clinic [152]. However, due to the microenvironment of gastrointestinal tract as well as the innate properties of some drugs, oral delivery could not be suitable for all drug candidates. For example, gastric acid and digestive enzymes will degrade proteins or pH-nonstable drugs [153]; the drugs with poor solubility and low-permeability drugs are usually with undesired bioavailability due to its bad absorption in the gastrointestinal tract [115]. The application of hydrogels can sometimes effectively solve these problems. For example, Xie et al. constructed a pH-sensitive polymer as hydrogel skeleton with Chinese quince seed gum and poly (*N*,*N*-diethylacryl amide-co-methacrylic acid). Bovine serum albumin (BSA) was used as model drug to investigate the release behavior of hydrogels in vitro [114]. The swelling degree of hydrogel in different pH environments is different, which can effectively control the release behavior of drugs in the gastrointestinal tract. Experiments showed that the release of BSA in simulated gastric juice (pH 1.2) was less than 40% within 12 h, while under the condition of pH 7.4, the release rate of BSA in hydrogel increased sharply with the cumulative release of 77.3% within 12 h. The hydrogel can effectively protect the protein drugs from being destroyed in the acid environment and promote its release in the intestinal tract in the meantime.

Similarly, Lin et al. developed a berberine hydrochloride (BBH)-encapsulated hydrogel [115]. BBH is used to treat diarrhea and other gastrointestinal diseases, but its insolubility dramatically affected its curative effect. In this system, the authors first prepared the inclusion complex of BBH with cyclodextrin (CDS) to improve the solubility of BBH. Subsequently, the drug/cyclodextrin complex was loaded in the nanocellulose-reinforced chitosan hydrogel to achieve sustained release and improved bioavailability. Due to the hyperfine network of hydrogel matrix, BBH/hydrogel exhibited sustained release under gastrointestinal pH conditions (pH 1.2 and pH 6.8), and in vitro antibacterial experiments showed that BC/IC hydrogel had better antibacterial effects and was expected to become a candidate for oral treatment of gastrointestinal infections.

10.6 Chinese Medicine-Skeleton Hydrogels

Besides loading in the hydrogels to be the active ingredients, Chinese medicines could also composite hydrogels themselves and act as the gel "matrix" to construct Chinese medicine-skeleton hydrogel.

Zheng et al. prepared a rhein hydrogel, in which the only gel matrix is the small molecular compound of rhein with the structure shown in Fig. 10.11a. They confirmed the gel was formed due to π-π stacking, hydrogen bonds, and other non-covalent interactions among rhein molecules [81]. The microscopic morphology of the rhein hydrogel was fibers (Fig. 10.11b, c), and the gelation exhibits mechanical force and temperature responsiveness (Fig. 10.11d). The gel could sustain release rhein for 24 h, prolonging the retention time of the drug. Moreover, the rhein nanofiber in the system of rhein hydrogel more easily entered into the cells and inhibited TLR4/NFκB pathway to exert anti-inflammatory effects. Compared with equivalent dose of free rhein, rhein hydrogels significantly downregulated the levels of various pro-inflammatory cytokines and neurotoxic factors, such as TNF-α, IL-6, IL-12, and iNOS, and thus was proved to be a better neuroinflammation alleviation system.

The formed Chinese medicine-skeleton hydrogels could also encapsulate other drugs to behave as delivery vehicles and exert synergetic therapeutic efficacies. Zhi et al. extracted triterpenoid of liquidambaric acid from liquidambar to prepare injectable natural product gels (NPG) [112]. The gel preparation process is simple and feasible, that is, after dissolving the extracted compound into certain mixed solvent of ethanol/water, the triterpenoid solution could form a gel even at a low drug concentration (0.25% w/v). Based on the weak non-covalent force, the molecules of liquidambaric acid self-assembled into one-dimensional fibers and then changed to

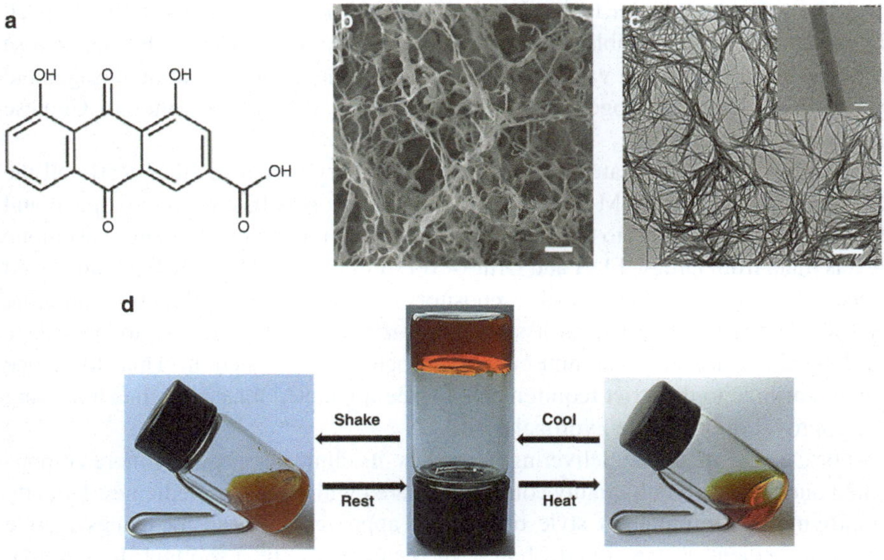

Fig. 10.11 Chemical structure of rhein (**a**) and the microstructure of the formed rhein-skeleton hydrogel (**b**, **c**). (**d**) Mechanical and temperature responsiveness of rhein-skeleton hydrogel. (Reprinted with permission from Ref [81]. Copyright 2019 Nature Publishing Group)

the gel state with a three-dimensional fiber network with the participation of solvents. DOX was encapsulated into the gel to construct DOX-3/NPG, and the release of DOX in DOX-3/NPG could last for 10 days. On the contrary, for DOX-EW (DOX solution in mixed solvent of ethanol and water), DOX would be quickly cleared out of the blood, as revealed by the in vivo fluorescence signal. The results indicated it is difficult to detect the free drug signal in DOX-EW group, but for DOX-3/NPG group the fluorescence was still visible at Day 7. The tumor suppression rate of DOX-3/NPG group was 22.1% higher than that of DOX-loaded glycerol gelatin (DOX-GG) group.

10.7 Discussion and Perspectives

Hydrogels have experienced fast development in the past decades, and various polymers or small molecular compounds are leveraged to construct the network of hydrogel via chemical or physical crosslinking [154]. Through controlling the compositions, the hydrogels' mechanical properties, environmental responsiveness, bioadhesive functions, as well as biodegradation could be finely adjusted, which boosts their applications in tissue engineering, drug delivery, and medical devices. In drug delivery, small hydrophilic and hydrophobic drugs as well as macromolecular drugs all could be sustained release in hydrogel or hydrogel-based composite systems. Furthermore, the loading capacity and encapsulating efficacy of hydrogels are relatively much larger than other nano- or micro-based systems. In this aspect, hydrogels are more suitable as the delivery vehicle of Chinese medicines, whose efficacy usually relied on various components and large administration dosage, and proper leverage of hydrogels could enhance the in vivo performance of Chinese medicines.

The current clinical status of the hydrogel delivery systems is that nearly all the approved Western or TCM drug-encapsulating hydrogels belong to the topical and vaginal delivery systems to treat local skin or vaginal infections and control hormone levels (data from Drug@FDA and Drug@SFDA in China). The only FDA-approved injectable hydrogel is Acthar Gel, a repository corticotropin formulation for infantile spasms, which is supplied as a sterile preparation in 16% gelatin to provide a prolonged release after intramuscular or subcutaneous injection. This difference might attribute to the strict requirements for the implanted materials, thus hindering the approval of injectable hydrogels.

For Chinese medicine-delivering hydrogels, its clinical approval is more complicated due to the difficult quality control compared with Western medicines. Directly improving the formulation style of existing approved Chinese medicines (single active ingredient or compound Chinese medicines) may be a shortcut. In addition, the hydrogels simply composed of the active drugs (Chinese medicine-skeleton hydrogels) can also be a promising delivery strategy.

Overall, hydrogel is a promising delivery strategy in enhancing Chinese medicines' efficacies. Together with the developments of materials science, pharmaceutics, pharmacology, and the processing techniques of Chinese medicines, more useful Chinese medicine/hydrogel formulations could be designed and move to clinic use, to cure diseases and improve people's life.

References

1. Ahmed, E. M. (2015). Hydrogel: Preparation, characterization, and applications: A review. *Journal of Advanced Research, 6*(2), 105–121.
2. Kopecek, J. (2007). Hydrogel biomaterials: A smart future? *Biomaterials, 28*(34), 5185–5192.
3. Wichterle, O., & LíM, D. (1960). Hydrophilic gels for biological use. *Nature, 185*(4706), 117–118.
4. Lee, S. C., Kwon, I. K., & Park, K. (2013). Hydrogels for delivery of bioactive agents: A historical perspective. *Advanced Drug Delivery Reviews, 65*(1), 17–20.
5. Yuk, H., Lu, B., & Zhao, X. (2019). Hydrogel bioelectronics. *Chemical Society Reviews, 48*(6), 1642–1667.
6. Zhu, J., & Marchant, R. E. (2011). Design properties of hydrogel tissue-engineering scaffolds. *Expert Review of Medical Devices, 8*(5), 607–626.
7. Li, J., & Mooney, D. J. (2016). Designing hydrogels for controlled drug delivery. *Nature Reviews Materials, 1*(12), 16071.
8. Tiller, J. C. (2003). Increasing the local concentration of drugs by hydrogel formation. *Angewandte Chemie, International Edition, 42*(27), 3072–3075.
9. McClements, D. J. (2017). Recent progress in hydrogel delivery systems for improving nutraceutical bioavailability. *Food Hydrocolloids, 68*, 238–245.

10. Chang, G., Ci, T., Yu, L., & Ding, J. (2011). Enhancement of the fraction of the active form of an antitumor drug topotecan via an injectable hydrogel. *Journal of Controlled Release, 156*(1), 21–27.
11. Crommelin, D. J. A., & Florence, A. T. (2013). Towards more effective advanced drug delivery systems. *International Journal of Phytoremediation, 454*(1), 496–511.
12. El-Sherbiny, I. M., & Yacoub, M. H. (2013). Hydrogel scaffolds for tissue engineering: Progress and challenges. *Global Cardiology Science & Practice, 2013*(3), 316–342.
13. Lai, W. F., & Rogach, A. L. (2017). Hydrogel-based materials for delivery of herbal medicines. *ACS Applied Materials & Interfaces, 9*(13), 11309–11320.
14. Gao, W., Vecchio, D., Li, J., Zhu, J., Zhang, Q., Fu, V., Li, J., Thamphiwatana, S., Lu, D., & Zhang, L. (2014). Hydrogel containing nanoparticle-stabilized liposomes for topical antimicrobial delivery. *ACS Nano, 8*(3), 2900–2907.
15. Numata, K., Yamazaki, S., & Naga, N. (2012). Biocompatible and biodegradable dual-drug release system based on silk hydrogel containing silk nanoparticles. *Biomacromolecules, 13*(5), 1383–1389.
16. Soppirnath, K. S., & Aminabhavi, T. M. (2002). Water transport and drug release study from cross-linked polyacrylamide grafted guar gum hydrogel microspheres for the controlled release application. *European Journal of Pharmaceutics and Biopharmaceutics, 53*(1), 87–98.
17. Cao, D., Zhang, X., Akabar, M., Luo, Y., Wu, H., Ke, X., & Ci, T. (2019). Liposomal doxorubicin loaded PLGA-PEG-PLGA based thermogel for sustained local drug delivery for the treatment of breast cancer. *Artificial Cells Nanomedicine and Biotechnology, 47*(1), 181–191.
18. Siepmann, J., & Peppas, N. A. (2011). Higuchi equation: Derivation, applications, use and misuse. *International Journal of Phytoremediation, 418*(1), 6–12.
19. Wang, W., Zhao, Y., Yi, H., Chen, T., Kang, S., Zhang, T., Rao, F., & Song, S. (2019). Pb (II) removal from water using porous hydrogel of chitosan-2D montmorillonite. *International Journal of Cast Metals Research, 128*, 85–93.
20. Peppas, N. A., & Sahlin, J. J. (1996). Hydrogels as mucoadhesive and bioadhesive materials: A review. *Biomaterials, 17*(16), 1553–1561.
21. Chansai, P., Sirivat, A., Niamlang, S., Chotpattananont, D., & Viravaidya-Pasuwat, K. (2009). Controlled transdermal iontophoresis of sulfosalicylic acid from polypyrrole/poly(acrylic acid) hydrogel. *International Journal of Phytoremediation, 381*(1), 25–33.
22. Lee, T. W., Kim, J. C., & Hwang, S. J. (2003). Hydrogel patches containing Triclosan for acne treatment. *European Journal of Pharmaceutics and Biopharmaceutics, 56*(3), 407–412.
23. Huang, D., Sun, M., Bu, Y., Luo, F., Lin, C., Lin, Z., Weng, Z., Yang, F., & Wu, D. (2019). Microcapsule-embedded hydrogel patches for ultrasound responsive and enhanced transdermal delivery of diclofenac sodium. *Journal of Materials Chemistry B, 7*(14), 2330–2337.
24. Li, S., Zhang, Q., & Dai, W. (2020). Research progress in hydrogels for local drug delivery in postoperative treatment of tumor. *Progress in Pharmaceurical Sciences, 44*(5), 351–360.
25. Abbott, N. J., Ronnback, L., & Hansson, E. (2006). Astrocyte-endothelial interactions at the blood-brain barrier. *Nature Reviews. Neuroscience, 7*(1), 41–53.
26. Makris, E. A., Gomoll, A. H., Malizos, K. N., Hu, J. C., & Athanasiou, K. A. (2015). Repair and tissue engineering techniques for articular cartilage. *Nature Reviews Rheumatology, 11*(1), 21–34.
27. Naahidi, S., Jafari, M., Logan, M., Wang, Y., Yuan, Y., Bae, H., Dixon, B., & Chen, P. (2017). Biocompatibility of hydrogel-based scaffolds for tissue engineering applications. *Biotechnology Advances, 35*(5), 530–544.
28. Caicco, M. J., Cooke, M. J., Wang, Y., Tuladhar, A., Morshead, C. M., & Shoichet, M. S. (2013). A hydrogel composite system for sustained epi-cortical delivery of Cyclosporin A to the brain for treatment of stroke. *Journal of Controlled Release, 166*(3), 197–202.
29. Wu, D.-C., Hsu, P.-I., Wu, J.-Y., Opekun, A. R., Kuo, C.-H., Wu, I. C., Wang, S. S. W., Chen, A., Hung, W.-C., & Graham, D. Y. (2010). Sequential and concomitant therapy with four

drugs is equally effective for eradication of H pylori infection. *Clinical Gastroenterology and Hepatology, 8*(1), 36–41.
30. Reiichiro, S., Yasunori, S., Ken, O., Hideharu, O., & Kazutaka, Y. (2019). Evaluation of marsupialization combined with long-term administration of antibacterial agents in calves with omphalophlebitis and secondary liver abscess. *Large Animal Review, 25*(3), 107–110.
31. Katsumata, K., Musiake, N., Shibuya, K., Nakajima, T., Watanabe, M., Sasaki, M., & Sugiyama, Y. (2011). A review of the anti-tumor effect of the combined administration of a cyclooxygenase-2 selective inhibitor and a non-specific immunostimulant protein-bound polysaccharide on an advanced colon cancer model using colon cancer cell lines. *Oncology Letters, 2*(3), 509–514.
32. Huang, Q., Lu, G., Sben, H. M., Cbung, M. C. M., & Ong, C. N. (2007). Anti-cancer properties of anthraquinones from rhubarb. *Medicinal Research Reviews, 27*(5), 609–630.
33. Perale, G., Rossi, F., Santoro, M., Peviani, M., Papa, S., Llupi, D., Torriani, P., Micotti, E., Previdi, S., Cervo, L., Sundstrom, E., Boccaccini, A. R., Masi, M., Forloni, G., & Veglianese, P. (2012). Multiple drug delivery hydrogel system for spinal cord injury repair strategies. *Journal of Controlled Release, 159*(2), 271–280.
34. Medatwal, N., Ansari, M. N., Kumar, S., Pal, S., Jha, S. K., Verma, P., Rana, K., Dasgupta, U., & Bajaj, A. (2020). Hydrogel-mediated delivery of celastrol and doxorubicin induces a synergistic effect on tumor regression via upregulation of ceramides. *Nanoscale, 12*(35), 18463–18475.
35. Zheng, B., Zhang, Z., Chen, F., Luo, X., & McClements, D. J. (2017). Impact of delivery system type on curcumin stability: Comparison of curcumin degradation in aqueous solutions, emulsions, and hydrogel beads. *Food Hydrocolloids, 71*, 187–197.
36. Cui, S., Yu, L., & Ding, J. (2019). Thermogelling of amphiphilic block copolymers in water: ABA type versus AB or BAB type. *Macromolecules, 52*(10), 3697–3715.
37. Xia, L.-W., Xie, R., Ju, X.-J., Wang, W., Chen, Q., & Chu, L.-Y. (2013). Nano-structured smart hydrogels with rapid response and high elasticity. *Nature Communications, 4*, 2226.
38. Raza, F., Zhu, Y., Chen, L., You, X., Zhang, J., Khan, A., Khan, M. W., Hasnat, M., Zafar, H., Wu, J., & Ge, L. (2019). Paclitaxel-loaded pH responsive hydrogel based on self-assembled peptides for tumor targeting. *Biomaterials Science, 7*(5), 2023–2036.
39. Liu, J., Chen, Z., Wang, J., Li, R., Li, T., Chang, M., Yan, F., & Wang, Y. (2018). Encapsulation of curcumin nanoparticles with MMP9-responsive and thermos-sensitive hydrogel improves diabetic wound healing. *ACS Applied Materials & Interfaces, 10*(19), 16315–16326.
40. Patel, S., Srivastava, S., Singh, M. R., & Singh, D. (2019). Mechanistic insight into diabetic wounds: Pathogenesis, molecular targets and treatment strategies to pace wound healing. *Biomedicine & Pharmacotherapy, 112*, 108615.
41. Potmesil, M. (1994). Camptothecins - From bench research to hospital wards. *Cancer Research, 54*(6), 1431–1439.
42. Beretta, G. L., & Zunino, F. (2007). Relevance of extracellular and intracellular interactions of camptothecins as determinants of antitumor activity. *Biochemical Pharmacology, 74*(10), 1437–1444.
43. Fassberg, J., & Stella, V. J. (1992). A kinetic and mechanistic study of the hydrolysis of camptothecin and some analogues. *Journal of Pharmaceutical Sciences, 81*(7), 676–684.
44. Ci, T., Chen, L., Yu, L., & Ding, J. (2014). Tumor regression achieved by encapsulating a moderately soluble drug into a polymeric thermogel. *Scientific Reports, 4*, 5473.
45. Ci, T., Shen, Y., Cui, S., Liu, R., Yu, L., & Ding, J. (2017). Achieving high drug loading and sustained release of hydrophobic drugs in hydrogels through in situ crystallization. *Macromolecular Bioscience, 17*(3).
46. Agostino, D., & Cliffton, E. E. (1962). Anticoagulants and the development of pulmonary metastases. Anticoagulant effect on the Walker 256 carcinosarcoma in rats. *Archives of Surgery, 84*, 449–453.

47. Buwalda, S. J., Boere, K. W. M., Dijkstra, P. J., Feijen, J., Vermonden, T., & Hennink, W. E. (2014). Hydrogels in a historical perspective: From simple networks to smart materials. *Journal of Controlled Release, 190*, 254–273.
48. Hennink, W. E., & van Nostrum, C. F. (2012). Novel crosslinking methods to design hydrogels. *Advanced Drug Delivery Reviews, 64*, 223–236.
49. Sawhney, A. S., Pathak, C. P., & Hubbell, J. A. (1993). Bioerodible hydrogels based on photopolymerized poly(ethylene glycol)-co-poly(.alpha.-hydroxy acid) diacrylate macromers. *Macromolecules, 26*(4), 581–587.
50. Cadée, J. A., van Steenbergen, M. J., Versluis, C., Heck, A. J. R., Underberg, W. J. M., den Otter, W., Jiskoot, W., & Hennink, W. E. (2001). Oxidation of recombinant human interleukin-2 by potassium peroxodisulfate. *Pharmaceutical Research, 18*(10), 1461–1467.
51. Zhang, M., & Zhao, X. (2020). Alginate hydrogel dressings for advanced wound management. *International Journal of Biological Macromolecules, 162*, 1414–1428.
52. Kuo, C. K., & Ma, P. X. (2001). Ionically crosslinked alginate hydrogels as scaffolds for tissue engineering: Part 1. Structure, gelation rate and mechanical properties. *Biomaterials, 22*(6), 511–521.
53. Escobar-Chavez, J. J., Lopez-Cervantes, M., Naik, A., Kalia, Y. N., Quintanar-Guerrero, D., & Ganem-Quintanar, A. (2006). Applications of thermoreversible pluronic F-127 gels in pharmaceutical formulations. *Journal of Pharmacy & Pharmaceutical Sciences, 9*(3), 339–358.
54. Li, T., Ci, T., Chen, L., Yu, L., & Ding, J. (2014). Salt-induced reentrant hydrogel of poly (ethylene glycol)-poly(lactide-co-glycolide) block copolymers. *Polymer Chemistry, 5*(3), 979–991.
55. Yang, Y., Wang, J., Zhang, X., Lu, W., & Zhang, Q. (2009). A novel mixed micelle gel with thermo-sensitive property for the local delivery of docetaxel. *Journal of Controlled Release, 135*(2), 175–182.
56. Elstad, N. L., & Fowers, K. D. (2009). OncoGel (ReGel/paclitaxel) - Clinical applications for a novel paclitaxel delivery system. *Advanced Drug Delivery Reviews, 61*(10), 785–794.
57. Fichman, G., & Gazit, E. (2014). Self-assembly of short peptides to form hydrogels: Design of building blocks, physical properties and technological applications. *Acta Biomaterialia, 10*(4), 1671–1682.
58. Mo, F., Jiang, K., Zhao, D., Wang, Y., Song, J., & Tan, W. (2021). DNA hydrogel-based gene editing and drug delivery systems. *Advanced Drug Delivery Reviews, 168*, 79.
59. Alves, M.-H., Jensen, B. E. B., Smith, A. A. A., & Zelikin, A. N. (2011). Poly(vinyl alcohol) physical hydrogels: New vista on a long serving biomaterial. *Macromolecular Bioscience, 11*(10), 1293–1313.
60. Yokoyama, F., Masada, I., Shimamura, K., Ikawa, T., & Monobe, K. (1986). Morphology and structure of highly elastic poly(vinyl alcohol) hydrogel prepared by repeated freezing-and-melting. *Colloid & Polymer Science, 264*(7), 595–601.
61. Fan, L., Yang, H., Yang, J., Peng, M., & Hu, J. (2016). Preparation and characterization of chitosan/gelatin/PVA hydrogel for wound dressings. *Carbohydrate Polymers, 146*, 427–434.
62. Jiang, S., Liu, S., & Feng, W. (2011). PVA hydrogel properties for biomedical application. *Journal of the Mechanical Behavior of Biomedical Materials, 4*(7), 1228–1233.
63. Takamura, A., Ishii, F., & Hidaka, H. (1992). Drug release from poly(vinyl alcohol) gel prepared by freeze-thaw procedure. *Journal of Controlled Release, 20*(1), 21–27.
64. Chen, G., & Jiang, M. (2011). Cyclodextrin-based inclusion complexation bridging supramolecular chemistry and macromolecular self-assembly. *Chemical Society Reviews, 40*(5), 2254–2266.
65. van de Manakker, F., Kroon-Batenburg, L. M. J., Vermonden, T., van Nostrum, C. F., & Hennink, W. E. (2010). Supramolecular hydrogels formed by β-cyclodextrin self-association and host–guest inclusion complexes. *Soft Matter, 6*(1), 187–194.
66. Zhang, J. X., & Ma, P. X. (2013). Cyclodextrin-based supramolecular systems for drug delivery: Recent progress and future perspective. *Advanced Drug Delivery Reviews, 65*(9), 1215–1233.

67. Harris, J. M., & Chess, R. B. (2003). Effect of pegylation on pharmaceuticals. *Nature Reviews. Drug Discovery, 2*(3), 214–221.
68. Chen, D. T. N., Wen, Q., Janmey, P. A., Crocker, J. C., & Yodh, A. G. (2010). Rheology of soft materials. In J. S. Langer (Ed.), *Annual Review of Condensed Matter Physics* (Vol. 1, pp. 301–322).
69. Bonino, C. A., Samorezov, J. E., Jeon, O., Alsberg, E., & Khan, S. A. (2011). Real-time in situ rheology of alginate hydrogel photocrosslinking. *Soft Matter, 7*(24), 11510–11517.
70. Liu, Z., Bhandari, B., Prakash, S., Mantihal, S., & Zhang, M. (2019). Linking rheology and printability of a multicomponent gel system of carrageenan-xanthan-starch in extrusion based additive manufacturing. *Food Hydrocolloids, 87*, 413–424.
71. Mahbubul, I. M., Saidur, R., & Amalina, M. A. (2012). Latest developments on the viscosity of nanofluids. *International Journal of Heat and Mass Transfer, 55*(4), 874–885.
72. Lu, D., Wang, H., Te, L., Li, Y., Wang, X., Niu, P., Guo, H., Sun, S., Wang, X., Guan, X., Ma, H., & Lei, Z. (2017). Versatile surgical adhesive and hemostatic materials: Synthesis, properties, and application of thermoresponsive polypeptides. *Chemistry of Materials, 29*(13), 5493–5503.
73. Lin, P., Ma, S., Wang, X., & Zhou, F. (2015). Molecularly engineered dual-crosslinked hydrogel with ultrahigh mechanical strength, toughness, and good self-recovery. *Advanced Materials, 27*(12), 2054–2059.
74. Gong, Z., Zhang, G., Zeng, X., Li, J., Li, G., Huang, W., Sun, R., & Wong, C. (2016). High-strength, tough, fatigue resistant, and self-healing hydrogel based on dual physically cross-linked network. *ACS Applied Materials & Interfaces, 8*(36), 24030–24037.
75. Liu, Y., & Chan-Park, M. B. (2009). Hydrogel based on interpenetrating polymer networks of dextran and gelatin for vascular tissue engineering. *Biomaterials, 30*(2), 196–207.
76. Tuncaboylu, D. C., Argun, A., Algi, M. P., & Okay, O. (2013). Autonomic self-healing in covalently crosslinked hydrogels containing hydrophobic domains. *Polymer (Guildf), 54*(23), 6381–6388.
77. Zhang, H., Yu, L., & Ding, J. (2008). Roles of hydrophilic homopolymers on the hydrophobic-association-induced physical gelling of amphiphilic block copolymers in water. *Macromolecules, 41*(17), 6493–6499.
78. Haider, M., Rose, H., Uhlemann, S., Schwan, E., Kabius, B., & Urban, K. (1998). A spherical-aberration-corrected 200 kV transmission electron microscope. *Ultramicroscopy, 75*(1), 53–60.
79. Chen, C., Zhang, Y., Fei, R., Cao, C., Wang, M., Wang, J., Bai, J., Cox, H., Waigh, T., Lu, J. R., & Xu, H. (2016). Hydrogelation of the short self-assembling peptide I(3)QGK regulated by transglutaminase and use for rapid hemostasis. *ACS Applied Materials & Interfaces, 8*(28), 17833–17841.
80. Yu, G., Yan, X., Han, C., & Huang, F. (2013). Characterization of supramolecular gels. *Chemical Society Reviews, 42*(16), 6697–6722.
81. Zheng, J., Fan, R., Wu, H., Yao, H., Yan, Y., Liu, J., Ran, L., Sun, Z., Yi, L., Dang, L., Gan, P., Zheng, P., Yang, T., Zhang, Y., Tang, T., & Wang, Y. (2019). Directed self-assembly of herbal small molecules into sustained release hydrogels for treating neural inflammation. *Nature Communications, 10*, 1604.
82. Garcia, R., & Perez, R. (2002). Dynamic atomic force microscopy methods. *Surface Science Reports, 47*(6–8), 197–301.
83. Wei, G.-J., Yao, M., Wang, Y.-S., Zhou, C.-W., Wan, D.-Y., Lei, P.-Z., Wen, J., Lei, H.-W., & Dong, D.-M. (2013). Promotion of peripheral nerve regeneration of a peptide compound hydrogel scaffold. *International Journal of Nanomedicine, 8*, 3217–3225.
84. Jeon, H. Y., Shin, E. Y., Choi, J. H., Song, J. E., Reis, R. L., & Khang, G. (2018). Evaluation of saponin loaded gellan gum hydrogel scaffold for cartilage regeneration. *Macromolecular Research, 26*(8), 724–729.

85. Zhang, Y., Zhou, S., Yan, Y., Guo, M., & Wang, Z. (2019). Therapeutic effects of hedysarum heteropoly polysaccharides and hyaluronic acid hydrogel on osteoarthritis in rats. *Immunlogical Journal, 35*(1), 65–70.
86. Peng, M., Xu, S., Zhang, Y., Zhang, L., Huang, B., Fu, S., Xue, Z., Da, Y., Dai, Y., Qiao, L., Dong, A., Zhang, R., & Meng, W. (2014). Thermosensitive injectable hydrogel enhances the antitumor effect of embelin in mouse hepatocellular carcinoma. *Journal of Pharmaceutical Sciences, 103*(3), 965–973.
87. Chen, D., Chen, C., Huang, C., Chen, T., & Liu, Z. (2020). Injectable hydrogel for NIR-II photo-thermal tumor therapy and dihydroartemisinin-mediated chemodynamic therapy. *Frontiers in Chemistry, 8*, 251.
88. Wang, W., Chen, J., Li, M., Jia, H., Han, X., Zhang, J., Zou, Y., Tan, B., Liang, W., Shang, Y., Xu, Q., Sigen, A., Wang, W., Mao, J., Gao, X., Fan, G., & Liu, W. (2019). Rebuilding postinfarcted cardiac functions by injecting TIIA@PDA nanoparticle-cross-linked ROS-sensitive hydrogels. *ACS Applied Materials & Interfaces, 11*(3), 2880–2890.
89. Yao, Q., Zheng, Y.-W., Lan, Q.-H., Wang, L.-F., Huang, Z.-W., Chen, R., Yang, Y., Xu, H.-L., Kou, L., & Zhao, Y.-Z. (2020). Aloe/poloxamer hydrogel as an injectable beta-estradiol delivery scaffold with multi-therapeutic effects to promote endometrial regeneration for intrauterine adhesion treatment. *European Journal of Pharmaceutical Sciences, 148*, 105316.
90. Shi, X., Lin, X., Yao, C., Shen, L., & Feng, Y. (2015). Injectable long-acting in situ forming systems for Radix Ophiopogonis polysaccharide. *International Journal of Cast Metals Research, 72*, 553–559.
91. Zhi, K., & Wang, J. (2020). A self-assembled supramolecular natural product gel from liquidambaric acid in traditional Chinese medicine with inherent anti-inflammatory activity for drug delivery. *Journal of Materials Chemistry B, 8*(4), 715–726.
92. Wang, W., Hui, P. C. L., Wat, E., Ng, F. S. F., Kan, C.-W., Wang, X., Wong, E. C. W., Hu, H., Chan, B., Lau, C. B. S., & Leung, P.-C. (2016). In vitro drug release and percutaneous behavior of poloxamer-based hydrogel formulation containing traditional Chinese medicine. *Colloids and Surfaces, B: Biointerfaces, 148*, 526–532.
93. Chatterjee, S., Hui, P C.-l., Wat, E., Kan, C.-w., Leung, P.-C., & Wang, W. (2020). Drug delivery system of dual-responsive PF127 hydrogel with polysaccharide-based nano-conjugate for textile-based transdermal therapy. *Carbohydrate Polymers, 236*, 116074.
94. Cui, M.-D., Pan, Z.-H., & Pan, L.-Q. (2017). Danggui buxue extract-loaded liposomes in thermosensitive gel enhance in vivo dermal wound healing via activation of the VEGF/PI3K/Akt and TGF-beta/Smads signaling pathway. *Evidence-based Complementary and Alternative Medicine, 2017*, 8407249.
95. Khan, A. W., Kotta, S., Ansari, S. H., Sharma, R. K., Kumar, A., & Ali, J. (2013). Formulation development, optimization and evaluation of aloe vera gel for wound healing. *Pharmacognosy Magazine, 9*(36), 6–10.
96. Qu, J., Zhao, X., Liang, Y., Zhang, T., Ma, P. X., & Guo, B. (2018). Antibacterial adhesive injectable hydrogels with rapid self-healing, extensibility and compressibility as wound dressing for joints skin wound healing. *Biomaterials, 183*, 185–199.
97. Wang, J., Yuan, Y., Liu, C., Zhu, D., Shen, X., & Yang, B. (2009). Preparation and pharmaceutical/pharmacodynamic evaluation of topical brucine-loaded liposomal hydrogel. *Journal of Materials Science. Materials in Medicine, 20*(10), 2075–2084.
98. Zhang, Y.-T., Li, Z., Zhang, K., Zhang, H.-Y., He, Z.-H., Xia, Q., Zhao, J.-H., & Feng, N.-P. (2017). Co-delivery of evodiamine and rutaecarpine in a microemulsion-based hyaluronic acid hydrogel for enhanced analgesic effects on mouse pain models. *International Journal of Phytoremediation, 528*(1–2), 100–106.
99. Wang, J., Zhang, R., Dong, C., Jiao, L., Xu, L., Liu, J., Wang, Z., Ying, Q. L. M., Fong, H., & Lao, L. (2012). Topical treatment with Tong-Luo-San-Jie gel alleviates bone cancer pain in rats. *Journal of Ethnopharmacology, 143*(3), 905–913.
100. Ning, Y., Rao, Y., Yu, Z., Liang, W., & Li, F. (2016). Skin permeation profile and anti-inflammatory effect of anemonin extracted from weilingxian. *Die Pharmazie, 71*(3), 134–138.

101. Liao, J.-C., Wei, Z.-X., Ma, Z.-P., Zhao, C., & Cai, D.-Z. (2016). Evaluation of a root extract gel from Urtica dioica (Urticaceae) as analgesic and anti-inflammatory therapy in rheumatoid arthritis in mice. *Tropical Journal of Pharmaceutical Research, 15*(4), 781–785.
102. Zhang, Y., Zhang, K., Guo, T., Li, Y., Zhu, C., & Feng, N. (2015). Transdermal baicalin delivery using diethylene glycol monoethyl ether-mediated cubic phase gel. *International Journal of Phytoremediation, 479*, 219–226.
103. Karimi, E., Gharib, B., Rostami, N., Navidpour, L., & Afshar, M. (2019). Clinical efficacy of a topical polyherbal formulation in the management of fluorouracil-associated hand-foot syndrome. *Journal of Herbal Medicine, 17–18*, 100270.
104. Chu, K., Chen, L., Xu, W., Li, H., Zhang, Y., Xie, W., & Zheng, J. (2013). Preparation of a paeonol-containing temperature-sensitive in situ gel and its preliminary efficacy on allergic rhinitis. *International Journal of Molecular Sciences, 14*(3), 6499–6515.
105. Ai, S., Zheng, J., Chu, K.-d., & Zhang, H.-s. (2015). Effects of Xingbi gel on leukotriene E4 and immunoglobulin E production and nasal eosinophilia in a guinea pig model for allergic rhinitis. *Asian Pacific Journal of Allergy and Immunology, 33*(2), 99–106.
106. Cao, S.-L., Chen, E., Zhang, Q.-Z., & Jiang, X.-G. (2007). A novel nasal delivery system of a Chinese traditional medicine, Radix Bupleuri, based on the concept of ion-activated in situ gel. *Archives of Pharmacal Research, 30*(8), 1014–1019.
107. Gaurav, C., Goutam, R., Rohan, K. N., Sweta, K. T., Abhay, C. S., & Amit, G. K. (2014). (Copper-curcumin) beta-cyclodextrin vaginal gel: Delivering a novel metal-herbal approach for the development of topical contraception prophylaxis. *European Journal of Pharmaceutical Sciences, 65*, 183–191.
108. Mao, X., Zhao, R., Yao, R., Guo, S., Bao, L., Gao, Y., Sun, J., Bao, Y., Shi, Y., & Cui, X. (2019). Chinese herbal formula feilin vaginal gel prevents the cervicitis in mouse model. *Evidence-based Complementary and Alternative Medicine, 2019*, 4168126.
109. Wu, C., Qi, H., Chen, W., Huang, C., Su, C., Li, W., & Hou, S. (2007). Preparation and evaluation of a Carbopol (R)/HPMC-based in situ gelling ophthalmic system for puerarin. *Yakugaku Zasshi-Journal of the Pharmaceutical Society of Japan, 127*(1), 183–191.
110. Yu, Y., Feng, R., Yu, S., Li, J., Wang, Y., Song, Y., Yang, X., Pan, W., & Li, S. (2018). Nanostructured lipid carrier-based pH and temperature dual-responsive hydrogel composed of carboxymethyl chitosan and poloxamer for drug delivery. *International Journal of Biological Macromolecules, 114*, 462–469.
111. Duan, Y., Cai, X., Du, H., & Zhai, G. (2015). Novel in situ gel systems based on P123/TPGS mixed micelles and gellan gum for ophthalmic delivery of curcumin. *Colloids and Surfaces, B: Biointerfaces, 128*, 322–330.
112. Zhi, K., Wang, J., Zhao, H., & Yang, X. (2020). Self-assembled small molecule natural product gel for drug delivery: A breakthrough in new application of small molecule natural products. *Acta Pharmaceutica Sinica B, 10*(5), 913–927.
113. Zhi, K., Sun, Y., Zhao, H., Zhang, C., Peng, H., & Yang, X. (2020). Self-assembled supramolecular material derived from traditional Chinese medicine: Injectable self-assembled natural product gel for drug delivery with biological activity. *Materials Today Communications, 23*, 101149.
114. Xie, A.-J., Yin, H.-S., Liu, H.-M., Zhu, C.-Y., & Yang, Y.-J. (2018). Chinese quince seed gum and poly (N,N-diethylacryl amide-co-methacrylic acid) based pH-sensitive hydrogel for use in drug delivery. *Carbohydrate Polymers, 185*, 96–104.
115. Xiao, L., Poudel, A. J., Huang, L., Wang, Y., Abdalla, A. M. E., & Yang, G. (2020). Nanocellulose hyperfine network achieves sustained release of berberine hydrochloride solubilized with beta-cyclodextrin for potential anti-infection oral administration. *International Journal of Cast Metals Research, 153*, 633–640.
116. Yu, L., & Ding, J. (2008). Injectable hydrogels as unique biomedical materials. *Chemical Society Reviews, 37*(8), 1473–1481.
117. Minh Khanh, N., & Lee, D. S. (2010). Injectable biodegradable hydrogels. *Macromolecular Bioscience, 10*(6), 563–579.

118. Yin, Y., Wu, C., Wang, J., Song, F., Yue, W., & Zhong, W. (2017). A simply triggered peptide-based hydrogel as an injectable nanocarrier of tanshinone IIA and tanshinones. *Chemical Communications, 53*(3), 529–532.
119. Liu, J., Fang, Q., Lin, H., Yu, X., Zheng, H., & Wan, Y. (2020). Alginate-poloxamer/silk fibroin hydrogels with covalently and physically cross-linked networks for cartilage tissue engineering. *Carbohydrate Polymers, 247*, 116593.
120. Norouzi, M., Nazari, B., & Miller, D. W. (2016). Injectable hydrogel-based drug delivery systems for local cancer therapy. *Drug Discovery Today, 21*(11), 1835–1849.
121. Bijlsma, J. W. J., Berenbaum, F., & Lafeber, F. P. J. G. (2011). Osteoarthritis: An update with relevance for clinical practice. *Lancet, 377*(9783), 2115–2126.
122. Madeira, C., Santhagunam, A., Salgueiro, J. B., & Cabrall, J. M. S. (2015). Advanced cell therapies for articular cartilage regeneration. *Trends in Biotechnology, 33*(1), 35–42.
123. Chuah, Y. J., Peck, Y., Lau, J. E. J., Heec, H. T., & Wang, D.-A. (2017). Hydrogel based cartilaginous tissue regeneration: Recent insights and technologies. *Biomaterials Science, 5*(4), 613–631.
124. Qi, C., Liu, J., Jin, Y., Xu, L., Wang, G., Wang, Z., & Wang, L. (2018). Photo-crosslinkable, injectable sericin hydrogel as 3D biomimetic extracellular matrix for minimally invasive repairing cartilage. *Biomaterials, 163*, 89–104.
125. Li, D., Yuan, T., Zhang, X., Xiao, Y., Wang, R., Fan, Y., & Zhang, X. (2012). Icariin: A potential promoting compound for cartilage tissue engineering. *Osteoarthritis and Cartilage, 20*(12), 1647–1656.
126. Leung, D. Y. M., & Bieber, T. (2003). Atopic dermatitis. *Lancet, 361*(9352), 151–160.
127. Charman, C. R., Morris, A. D., & Williams, H. C. (2000). Topical corticosteroid phobia in patients with atopic eczema. *The British Journal of Dermatology, 142*(5), 931–936.
128. Lin, H., Li, Z., Peng, J., & Tu, S. (2019). New progress in the treatment of atopic dermatitis with traditional Chinese medicine. *Journal of Liaoning University of TCM, 21*(11), 29–32.
129. Saeedi, M., Morteza-Semnani, K., & Ghoreishi, M. R. (2003). The treatment of atopic dermatitis with licorice gel. *The Journal of Dermatological Treatment, 14*(3), 153–157.
130. Hon, K. L. E., Leung, T. F., Ng, P. C., Lam, M. C. A., Kam, W. Y. C., Wong, K. Y., Lee, K. C. K., Sung, Y. T., Cheng, K. F., Fok, T. F., Fung, K. P., & Leung, P. C. (2007). Efficacy and tolerability of a Chinese herbal medicine concoction for treatment of atopic dermatitis: A randomized, double-blind, placebo-controlled study. *The British Journal of Dermatology, 157*(2), 357–363.
131. Schempp, C. A., Windeck, T., Hezel, S., & Simon, J. C. (2003). Topical treatment of atopic dermatitis with St. John's wort cream - A randomized, placebo controlled, double blind half-side comparison. *Phytomedicine, 10*, 31–37.
132. Szekalska, M., Sosnowska, K., Tomczykowa, M., Winnicka, K., Kasacka, I., & Tomczyk, M. (2020). In vivo anti-inflammatory and anti-allergic activities of cynaroside evaluated by using hydrogel formulations. *Biomedicine & Pharmacotherapy, 121*, 109681.
133. Rodrigues, M., Kosaric, N., Bonham, C. A., & Gurtner, G. C. (2019). Wound healing: A cellular perspective. *Physiological Reviews, 99*(1), 665–706.
134. Guo, S., & DiPietro, L. A. (2010). Factors affecting wound healing. *Journal of Dental Research, 89*(3), 219–229.
135. Desmet, C. M., Preat, V., & Gallez, B. (2018). Nanomedicines and gene therapy for the delivery of growth factors to improve perfusion and oxygenation in wound healing. *Advanced Drug Delivery Reviews, 129*, 262–284.
136. Stechmiller, J. K. (2010). Understanding the role of nutrition and wound healing. *Nutrition in Clinical Practice, 25*(1), 61–68.
137. Wong, T. W., & Ramli, N. A. (2014). Carboxymethylcellulose film for bacterial wound infection control and healing. *Carbohydrate Polymers, 112*, 367–375.
138. Murakami, K., Aoki, H., Nakamura, S., Nakamura, S.-i., Takikawa, M., Hanzawa, M., Kishimoto, S., Hattori, H., Tanaka, Y., Kiyosawa, T., Sato, Y., & Ishihara, M. (2010).

Hydrogel blends of chitin/chitosan, fucoidan and alginate as healing-impaired wound dressings. *Biomaterials, 31*(1), 83–90.
139. Zhang, Y., Shen, L., Zhang, K., Guo, T., Zhao, J., Li, N., & Feng, N. (2015). Enhanced antioxidation via encapsulation of isooctyl p-methoxycinnamate with sodium deoxycholate-mediated liposome endocytosis. *International Journal of Phytoremediation, 496*(2), 392–400.
140. Cohen, M., Quintner, J., & van Rysewyk, S. (2018). Reconsidering the international association for the study of pain definition of pain. *PAIN Reports, 3*(2), e634–e634.
141. Wang, S., Zhang, D., Hu, J., Jia, Q., Xu, W., Su, D., Song, H., Xu, Z., Cui, J., Zhou, M., Yang, J., & Xiao, J. (2017). A clinical and mechanistic study of topical borneol-induced analgesia. *EMBO Molecular Medicine, 9*(6), 802–815.
142. Wang, R., Han, L., Gao, Q., Chen, D., Wang, Y., Zhang, X., Yu, X., Zhang, Y., Li, Z., & Bai, C. (2018). Progress on active analgesic components and mechanisms of commonly used traditional Chinese medicines: A comprehensive review. *Journal of Pharmacy & Pharmaceutical Sciences, 21*, 437–480.
143. Lu, Y., Zhu, Y., Zhu, G., & Pan, Y. (2015). Research on analgesia mechanism of traditional Chinese medicine. *World Chinese Medicine, 10*(4), 629–636.
144. Najafi, M. N., Rezaee, R., Najafi, N. N., Mirzaee, F., Burykina, T. I., Lupuliasa, D., Arsene, A. L., & Ghazanfarpour, M. (2019). Herbal medicines against bacterial vaginosis in women of reproductive age: A systematic review. *Farmácia, 67*(6), 931–940.
145. Xu, J., Tam, M., Samaei, S., Lerouge, S., Barralet, J., Stevenson, M. M., & Cerruti, M. (2017). Mucoadhesive chitosan hydrogels as rectal drug delivery vessels to treat ulcerative colitis. *Acta Biomaterialia, 48*, 247–257.
146. Vigani, B., Faccendini, A., Rossi, S., Sandri, G., Bonferoni, M. C., Grisoli, P., & Ferrari, F. (2019). Development of a mucoadhesive in situ gelling formulation for the delivery of lactobacillus gasseri into vaginal cavity. *Pharmaceutics, 11*(10), 511.
147. Wang, Y., He, Y., Zhao, X., Ji, X., Hong, Y., Wang, Y., Zhu, Q., Xu, B., & Sun, Y. (2015). Crinone gel for luteal phase support in frozen-thawed embryo transfer cycles: A prospective randomized clinical trial in the Chinese population. *PLoS One, 10*(7), e0133027.
148. Geerling, G., MacLennan, S., & Hartwig, D. (2004). Autologous serum eye drops for ocular surface disorders. *The British Journal of Ophthalmology, 88*(11), 1467–1474.
149. Huang, W., Zhang, N., Hua, H., Liu, T., Tang, Y., Fu, L., Yang, Y., Ma, X., & Zhao, Y. (2016). Preparation, pharmacokinetics and pharmacodynamics of ophthalmic thermosensitive in situ hydrogel of betaxolol hydrochloride. *Biomedicine & Pharmacotherapy, 83*, 107–113.
150. Yu, S., Zhang, X., Tan, G., Tian, L., Liu, D., Liu, Y., Yang, X., & Pan, W. (2017). A novel pH-induced thermosensitive hydrogel composed of carboxymethyl chitosan and poloxamer cross-linked by glutaraldehyde for ophthalmic drug delivery. *Carbohydrate Polymers, 155*, 208–217.
151. Yu, Y., Feng, R., Yu, S., Li, J., Wang, Y., Song, Y., Yang, X., Pan, W., & Li, S. (2018). Nanostructured lipid carrier-based pH and temperature dual-responsive hydrogel composed of carboxymethyl chitosan and poloxamer for drug delivery. *International Journal of Cast Metals Research, 114*, 462–469.
152. Lin, Y. H., Liang, H. F., Chung, C. K., Chen, M. C., & Sung, H. W. (2005). Physically crosslinked alginate/N,O-carboxymethyl chitosan hydrogels with calcium for oral delivery of protein drugs. *Biomaterials, 26*(14), 2105–2113.
153. Chaturvedi, K., Ganguly, K., Nadagouda, M. N., & Aminabhavi, T. M. (2013). Polymeric hydrogels for oral insulin delivery. *Journal of Controlled Release, 165*(2), 129–138.
154. Billiet, T., Vandenhaute, M., Schelfhout, J., Van Vlierberghe, S., & Dubruel, P. (2012). A review of trends and limitations in hydrogel-rapid prototyping for tissue engineering. *Biomaterials, 33*(26), 6020–6041.

Chapter 11
Cocrystallization and Coamorphization for Druggability Enhancement of Chinese Medicines

Hao Cheng, Weili Heng, Jiawei Han, Yuanfeng Wei, Linghe Zhang, Shuai Qian, Jianjun Zhang, and Yuan Gao

Abstract Cocrystallization and coamorphization techniques incorporating active ingredient of Chinese medicine and an or more appropriate coformer(s) into a homogeneous single-phase system have been employed as promising formulation strategies to improve the druggability (e.g., solubility, dissolution, stability, hygroscopicity, and tabletability, etc.) of Chinese medicines. Over the past decade, increasing reports have been published on investigations of cocrystal and coamorphous drug delivery systems of Chinese medicines. This chapter summarizes recent findings of cocrystallization and coamorphization for druggability improvement of Chinese medicines and provides their updates as a comprehensive overview in terms of definition and classification, preparation methods, druggability-related pharmaceutical properties, in vivo performances, and physicochemical characterizations.

Keywords Cocrystallization · Coamorphization · Chinese medicine · Druggability

11.1 Introduction

Traditional Chinese medicine (TCM) has recently attracted growing interest for its advantages in health care (multi-ingredients, multi-links, and multi-targets) [1, 2] as well as drug innovation and discovery [3]. However, many active ingredients

---

Hao Cheng and Weili Heng contributed equally to this work.

H. Cheng · W. Heng · J. Han · Y. Wei · S. Qian · Y. Gao (✉)
School of Traditional Chinese Pharmacy, China Pharmaceutical University, Nanjing, China
e-mail: gaoyuan@cpu.edu.cn

L. Zhang
Department of Chemistry, Smith College, Northampton, MA, USA

J. Zhang
School of Pharmacy, China Pharmaceutical University, Nanjing, China

N. Feng, Z. Yang (eds.), *Novel Drug Delivery Systems for Chinese Medicines*,
https://doi.org/10.1007/978-981-16-3444-4_11

isolated from Chinese herbs are poorly soluble [4], which has always been considered as one of the most challenging properties associated with various formulation-related performance issues. Other physicochemical defects like stability issues and hygroscopicity issues, together with poorly aqueous solubility and related low bioavailability, reduce the druggability of these TCM drug candidates. To overcome these limitations, various strategies have been applied in recent decades, including salt formation [5], cyclodextrin inclusion complexes [6], liposomes [7], amorphous solid dispersions (ASDs) [8], self-emulsifying drug delivery systems [9], nanoparticles [10], polymeric micelles [11], cocrystals [12], etc. Among these strategies, cocrystallization has emerged as a promising approach to improve solubility, dissolution, and other physicochemical properties of poorly soluble active ingredients [13–15], such as baicalein-nicotinamide [16], quercetin-caffeine [17], and hesperidin-hesperidin [18] cocrystals. Cocrystals can be prepared for neutral drugs that are not able to form salts. Also, for ionizable drugs, the number of suitable ligands for cocrystallization always exceeds that of suitable counterions for saltation [14], which could significantly expand the number and diversity of solid drug forms available as well as intellectual properties.

On the other hand, amorphization by disrupting crystal lattice is one of the most effective techniques to improve the aqueous solubility/dissolution of these drug candidates and hence their bioavailabilities [19–21]. However, inherent poor physical stability due to higher energy state and the subsequent risk of devitrification during manufacturing, storage, and dissolution have greatly restricted the applications of most amorphous drugs in formulation development [22]. To improve their physical stability, polymers with a high glass transition temperature (T_g) were usually employed to form ASDs with these drugs [20, 23]. The increased T_g strengthened intermolecular force, and reduced molecular mobility would increase the physical stability of amorphous drugs. However, when drugs are poorly miscible with polymeric carriers, to incorporate a therapeutic drug dose into the ASDs, usage of large quantities of polymers would be inevitable, which would lead to a high polymer-drug ratio and subsequently large bulk volume/mass of final dosage forms [20, 24]. Furthermore, a large number of water-soluble polymers used in ASDs often absorb moisture easily, which would accelerate the recrystallization of the incorporated amorphous drugs [20, 23]. Therefore, alternative or additional strategies are urgently needed to overcome the above issues.

Over the past decade, the coamorphous drug delivery system has aroused wide interest to overcome the limitations of ASDs. Different from polymer-based ASDs, the coamorphous system possesses a lower volume/mass of dosage with superior physical stability. For example, the clinical dose of insoluble drug curcumin in adults is about 1–2 g/day. Curcumin ASD, composed of curcumin and the polymer HPMCAS in a weight ratio of 1:9, caused a high volume/mass of dosage (10–20 g/day), which is not compliant for patients [25]. However, the coamorphization of curcumin with a low molecular coformer piperine in 1:1 molar ratio showed a significant decrease in the volume of dosage form, as well as obvious enhancement in the dissolution, bioavailability, and physical stability compared with crystalline/amorphous curcumin [19]. Furthermore, combining two pharmacologically relevant drugs in the coamorphous system also has potential benefits to generate combination therapy such as synergic effects and fewer side effects [26].

This review summarizes recent findings of cocrystal and coamorphous systems in druggability improvement for Chinese medicines and provides their updates as a comprehensive overview in terms of definition and classification, preparation methods, druggability-related pharmaceutical properties (e.g., solubility, dissolution, taste masking, tabletability, etc.), in vivo performances, and physicochemical characterizations.

11.2 Definition and Classification

A pharmaceutical cocrystal, composed of an active pharmaceutical ingredient (API) and an or more appropriate cocrystal coformer(s) (usually small molecules in the Generally Recognized as Safe (GRAS) list or, for example, flavonoids and nutraceuticals such as quercetin, pterostilbene, and *p*-coumaric acid), is considered to be a stoichiometric multi-component system, where its components are connected by noncovalent interactions (e.g., hydrogen bonds, π-π stacking) in the same crystal lattice [27, 28]. Generally, it is distinguished from solvates in that cocrystal components are solids at room temperature and salts in which cocrystal components are connected via noncovalent interactions instead of ionic bonds between acids and bases. However, for cocrystals, solvates, and salts, these classifications cannot be mutually exclusive given the practical reality that there are some overlaps among these three categories in the scientific and patent literature. For example, lithium salts are widely used as APIs, and amino acid cocrystals of lithium salts were recently reported [29]. Velaga et al. reported a new pharmaceutical cocrystal with an organic counter ion, i.e., norfloxacin saccharinate-saccharin dihydrate cocrystal [30]. Therefore, the nature of multi-component solid forms is such that there is a significant overlap between salts, cocrystals, and hydrates (Fig. 11.1).

The pharmaceutical coamorphous system is prepared by coamorphization of a drug with a or more coformer(s) (e.g., low molecular weight excipient or another drug), to form a single amorphous phase in a certain stoichiometric ratio, in which components are associated by weak and discrete intermolecular interactions [32, 33]. Differentiated from the pure amorphous phase, coamorphous systems are composed of binary or multi-components, which is similar to cocrystal systems. However, this system differs from cocrystal primarily by its amorphous nature which lacks periodicity in the lattice. More comparisons between cocrystals and coamorphous systems are shown in Table 11.1.

Based on the selection of coformers, cocrystals/coamorphous systems can be categorized into drug-excipient and drug-drug cocrystals/coamorphous systems (Table 11.2). In drug-excipient binary systems, some low molecular weight excipients, such as amino acids, organic acids, low molecular saccharides, saccharin, nicotinamide, and isonicotinamide, have been employed as potential coformers.

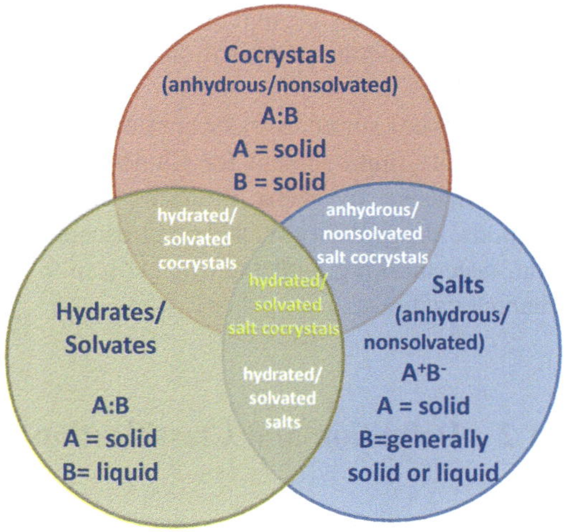

Fig. 11.1 Multi-component solid forms inherently overlap with one another. (Adapted and modified from ref. [31])

Table 11.1 Comparisons between cocrystals and coamorphous systems

Items	Cocrystals	Coamorphous systems
Solid form	Crystalline solid	Amorphous solid
Molecular packing	Periodic molecular arrangement	Long-range disorder molecular packing
Components	Binary or multi-components	
Coformer	Small molecules (excipients or drugs)	
Intermolecular interactions	Noncovalent interactions	Noncovalent interactions/no interaction
Stoichiometric ratio	A certain stoichiometric ratio	No limitation in principle
Melting temperature (T_m)	A single T_m	N/A
Glass transition temperature (T_g)	N/A	A single T_g
Thermodynamics	Low-energy state	High-energy state
Hygroscopicity	Lower hygroscopicity	Higher hygroscopicity
Solubility	Improved (depending on the nature of coformer)	
Dissolution	Improved (depending on the nature of coformer)	

N/A not available

Besides, drug combinations are also designed to form cocrystals and coamorphous systems to not only enhance solubility/dissolution of poorly soluble drugs but also achieve the synergistic effect of combined therapy, which is more in line with the characteristics of TCM.

Table 11.2 Cocrystals and coamorphous systems containing active ingredients of Chinese medicines

API	Coformer	Molar ratio	Preparation method	Formation mechanism	Outcome	Refs.
Cocrystals						
Artesunate	Nicotinamide	N/A	Solvent evaporation	Hydrogen bonds	N/A	[34]
			Slurry method			
Baicalein	Nicotinamide	1:1	Slow evaporation	Hydrogen bonds	In vitro	[16]
			Rotary evaporation		Solubility: 1.5–2-fold ↑	
			Grinding		Dissolution rate: 2.5-fold ↑	
					In vivo (rats)	
					C_{max}: 2.49-fold ↑	
					AUC: 2.8-fold ↑	
Curcumin	Catechol	1:1	Grinding	Hydrogen bonds	N/A	[35]
	Isoniazid	1:2	Solution evaporation	Hydrogen bonds	N/A	[36]
	Pyrogallol	1:1	Solvent-drop grinding	Hydrogen bonds	Dissolution rate: ~12-fold ↑	[37, 38]
	Resorcinol	1:1	Solvent-drop grinding	Hydrogen bonds	Dissolution rate: ~5-fold ↑	[38]
Emodin	Berberine chloride	1:1	Slurry method	Hydrogen bonds	Solubility: ↑	[39]
				π-π stacking	Bioavailability: ~1.7-fold ↑	
Fisetin	Nicotinamide	1:2	Solvent-drop grinding	O–H···Narom heterosynthon	N/A	[40]
	Isonicotinamide	1:1	Solution evaporation			
Genistein	Isonicotinamide	1:2	Slow evaporation	Hydrogen bonds	N/A	[41]
	4,4′-Bipyridine	1:1	Solution evaporation	Hydrogen bonds	Solubility: 1.5-fold ↑	[42]
					Antibacterial activity: ↑	
Hesperidin	Adenine	2:1	Solvent-drop grinding	Hydrogen bonds	Solubility: 1.5-fold ↑	[18]
					Dissolution: 2–4-fold ↑	
					Antihemolytic activity: 1.5-fold ↑	
	Caffeine	N/A	Solvent-drop grinding	Hydrogen bonds	In vitro	[43]

(continued)

Table 11.2 (continued)

API	Coformer	Molar ratio	Preparation method	Formation mechanism	Outcome	Refs.
					Solubility: 4-fold ↑	
					In vivo	
					Antioxidant activity: 50% ↑	
					Bioavailability: 1.6-fold ↑	
	Gallic acid	1.5:1	Solvent-drop grinding	Hydrogen bonds	In vitro	[18]
					Solubility: 3.5-fold ↑	
					Dissolution rate: 2–4-fold ↑	
					In vivo	
					Antioxidant activity: 50% ↑	
					Antihemolytic activity: 2.5-fold ↑	
	Nicotinamide	N/A	Solvent-drop grinding	Hydrogen bonds	In vitro	[43]
					Solubility: 4.5-fold ↑	
					In vivo	
					Antioxidant activity: 30% ↑	
					Bioavailability: 1.6-fold ↑	
	Picolinic acid	N/A	Solvent-drop grinding	Hydrogen bonds	In vitro	
					Solubility: 4-fold ↑	
					In vivo	
					Antioxidant activity: 20% ↑	
					Bioavailability: 1.4-fold ↑	
	Theobromine	2:1	Solvent-drop grinding	Hydrogen bonds	In vitro	[18]
					Solubility: 2.5-fold ↑	
					Dissolution rate: 2–4-fold ↑	
					In vivo	

					Antioxidant activity: 30% ↑	
					Antihemolytic activity: 2-fold ↑	
	Theophylline	1:1.5	Solvent-drop grinding	Hydrogen bonds	In vitro	
					Solubility: 3-fold ↑	
					Dissolution rate: 2–4-fold ↑	
					In vivo	
					Antioxidant activity: 30% ↑	
					Antihemolytic activity: 2-fold ↑	
Luteolin	Isonicotinamide	1:1	Solvent-drop grinding	O–H···N_{arom} heterosynthon	N/A	[40]
			Solution evaporation			
	4,4′-Bipyridine	1:3	Solution evaporation	Hydrogen bonds	Solubility: 8-fold ↑	[44]
				π-π stacking	Antibacterial activity: ↑	
Myricetin	4,4′-Bipyridine	1:1, 1:2	Solution evaporation	Hydrogen bonds	Solubility: 60-fold ↑	[45]
				π-π stacking		
	Caffeine	1:1	Slurry method	Hydrogen bonds	Dissolution rate: 17-fold ↑	[46, 47]
	Piracetam	1:1	Solvent-drop grinding	Hydrogen bonds	N/A	[48]
Naringenin	Isonicotinamide	1:2	Slow evaporation	Hydrogen bonds	Solubility: 1.3-fold ↑	[49]
					Dissolution rate: 1.6-fold ↑	
	Picolinic acid	1:1	Slurry method	Hydrogen bonds	Solubility: 1.3-fold ↑	
					Dissolution rate: 3.1-fold ↑	
Naringin	Betaine	1:1	Slurry method	Hydrogen bonds	Solubility: 1.3-fold ↑	[49]
				π-π stacking	Dissolution rate: 1.8–2-fold ↑	
Pterostilbene	Caffeine	1:1	Solvent-drop grinding	Hydrogen bonds	Dissolution rate: ~27-fold ↑	[50]
					Stability: ↑	
	Carbamazepine	1:1	Solvent evaporation	Hydrogen bonds	Solubility:	
					Carbamazepine 7-fold ↓	
					Pterostilbene 2.5-fold ↓	

(continued)

Table 11.2 (continued)

API	Coformer	Molar ratio	Preparation method	Formation mechanism	Outcome	Refs.
	Piperazine	2:1	Slow cooling	Hydrogen bonds	Dissolution rate: ~6-fold ↑	[51]
					Stability: ↑	
	Glutaric acid	1:1		Hydrogen bonds	Solubility: ↑	
					Stability: ↑	
Quercetin	4,4′-Bipyridine	1:1.5	Solution evaporation	Hydrogen bonds	Antibacterial activity: ↑	[45]
				π-π stacking		
	Caffeine	1:1	Slurry method	Hydrogen bonds	Solubility: 14-fold ↑	[17]
					Bioavailability: ~10-fold ↑	
Taxifolin	4,4′-Bipyridine	2:3	Solution evaporation	Hydrogen bonds	Antibacterial activity: ↑	[44]
				π-π stacking		
Coamorphous systems						
Curcumin	Artemisinin	1:1	Rotation evaporation	Hydrogen bonds	Dissolution rate: 2.6-fold ↑	[52]
					Bioavailability: ↑	
	Folic acid dihydrate	N/A	Liquid-assisted grinding	Hydrogen bonds	Solubility: ↑	[53]
					Dissolution rate: ↑	
					Stability: ↑	
	Piperazine	1:2	Liquid-assisted grinding	Hydrogen bonds	Solubility: 4-fold ↑	[54]
					Dissolution rate: ↑	
	Piperine	1:1	Quench cooling	Hydrogen bonds	Dissolution rate: ↑	[19]
					AUC: ~2-fold ↑	
					Stability: ↑	
Myricetin	Docetaxel	1:1	Solvent evaporation	N/A	In vitro	[55]
					Solubility: ~1.6-fold ↑	
					Dissolution rate: 3.78-fold ↑	
					In vivo	

					C_{max}: 3.9-fold ↑	
					AUC: 3.1-fold ↑	
Naringin	Talinolol	1:1, 1:2	Quench cooling	Hydrogen bonds	Solubility: ↑	[56]
					AUC: ~9-fold ↑	
Sodium taurocholate	Carbamazepine	1:1	Ball milling	No intermolecular interactions	Dissolution rate: ↑	[57]
	Indomethacin	1:1			Stability: ↑	
	Mefenamic acid	1:1				
	Sulfamerazine	1:1	Cryomilling	Hydrogen bonds	Dissolution: sulfamerazine ↑	[58]
					Stability: ↑	
Quercetin	Ritonavir	2:1	Solvent evaporation	Hydrogen bonds	Solubility: ~5-fold ↑	[59]
					Bioavailability: ↑	
					Stability: ↑	
Vanillin	Valsartan	1:1	Solution evaporation	Hydrogen bonds	Dissolution rate: valsartan ↑	[60]

N/A not available

11.3 Preparation of Cocrystal and Coamorphous Systems

Selecting appropriate approaches to prepare pharmaceutical cocrystals and coamorphous formulations is crucial to achieve satisfactory performances of the final products. Generally, the properties of both active ingredients and excipients influence the selection of preparation methods. On the other hand, pharmaceutical cocrystals and coamorphous systems prepared by different methods might exhibit differences in their physiochemical properties, such as dissolution behavior and physical stability due to polymorphism and crystal habits.

11.3.1 Preparation of Pharmaceutical Cocrystals

Up to now, effective cocrystal preparation methods in use can be classified into solid-state grinding (grinding and solvent-assisted grinding) and solvent-based method (slurring, solvent evaporation, crystallization from solution, and antisolvent addition). For the solvent-based approaches, the selection of solvent plays a key role, since its addition will potentially alter the intermolecular interactions between components and affect the cocrystal formation.

11.3.1.1 Solvent Evaporation Technique

The solvent evaporation technique is the most commonly used approach to prepare cocrystals. Generally, API and coformer(s) are dissolved in a volatile organic solvent with a certain stoichiometric ratio, and then the solvent is completely evaporated to generate cocrystal [61]. During evaporation of the solvent, noncovalent bonds (commonly hydrogen bonds) form between different functional groups and produce a thermodynamically favored product [62]. Baicalein-nicotinamide cocrystal (molar ratio 1:1) [16] and naringenin-isonicotinamide (molar ratio 1:2) [49] were prepared by solvent evaporation from ethyl acetate in a fume hood. It is worth mentioning that solvent selection is crucial for the creation of cocrystals. If the solubility of two components is not similar, then one with lower solubility will first precipitate followed by the other.

11.3.1.2 Solid-State Grinding Technique

The solid-state grinding technique (also referred to as neat grinding) is used to generate cocrystals without a solvent. API and coformer(s) are admixed in an appropriate stoichiometric ratio and then pressed and crushed together with a mortar and pestle or a ball mill or vibrator mill. Reducing the particle size could increase the specific surface area between components for the development of intermolecular bonds. This technique is simple and quick to investigate the potential of cocrystallization, but the crystallinity is often relatively low by this method.

11.3.1.3 Liquid-Assisted Grinding

Liquid-assisted grinding (also referred to as solvent-drop grinding or wet cogrinding) is a modification of neat grinding by adding a small amount of solvent during the grinding process and has been used to enhance supramolecular selectivity, both polymorphic and stoichiometric, in crystalline systems [63]. The added solvent, as a catalytic agent, could significantly shorten the grinding time. Cocrystals of nutraceutical compound pterostilbene with caffeine (1:1), carbamazepine (1:1), glutaric acid (1:1), or piperazine (2:1) were successfully prepared by liquid-assisted grinding [64]. Besides, selective polymorphic forms of cocrystals may be synthesized via this approach by adding different solvents. For example, form I and form II of caffeine-glutaric acid cocrystals could be prepared via liquid-assisted grinding by adding less polar solvent (e.g., cyclohexane or hexane) and more polar solvent (e.g., water or acetonitrile), respectively [65].

11.3.1.4 Slurring Technique

This technique involves the suspension of API and coformer(s) in a fixed molar ratio, in the solvent with the solid fraction always remaining in excess. In practical terms, API can also be added to a solution or suspension of the coformer in the solvent, after which the resulting suspension is stirred, filtered, and dried. The generation rate of cocrystals depends on the solubility driving force, the relative concentrations of API and coformer, and the nucleation and growth kinetics of the system [66]. Zhang et al. found that the transformation time from theophylline suspension to theophylline-glutaric acid cocrystal ranged from 15 min to 5 h, relying on the solution concentration and solvent selection [67]. Setyawan et al. prepared a cocrystal of artesunate-nicotinamide by mixing artesunate and nicotinamide in water to form a slurry sample [68]. Quercetin-caffeine cocrystal was successfully prepared by overnight slurrying of quercetin dihydrate and caffeine in methanol [17].

11.3.1.5 Antisolvent Cocrystallization

Using this method, a solvent in which the compound is less soluble is often added to the solution of API and coformer(s), favoring the precipitation of the solids. The used solvent and antisolvent should be miscible. Choi et al. investigated the effects of solvents, the antisolvent addition rate, and the agitation speed on the purity and polymorphism of cocrystals. High-purity carbamazepine-saccharin cocrystal was manufactured by adding water to methanol solution, while water addition to acetone/ethanol solution could not obtain any cocrystal [69]. Besides, form I of carbamazepine-saccharin cocrystal preferably formed when increasing the addition rate or agitation speed, whereas form II under the opposite conditions [70].

11.3.1.6 Intermediate Phase or Form Transformations

Sometimes, cocrystals could be obtained through a process of intermediate phase or form transformations (e.g., melt, solution, polymorphic transition, etc.). The required transformation may undergo consecutive intermediate stages, but not all of which are always easily identifiable when the very fast transitions occur, no matter which process is used (e.g., grinding, solvent grinding, melt cooling, moisture sorption). The intermediate forms (such as hydrates, amorphous form, or metastable polymorphic form) act as unstable intermediates in the cocrystallization nucleus [71]. Carbamazepine-saccharin and carbamazepine-nicotinamide cocrystals can be formed from the amorphous phases generated either by quenching the melt of components [71] or by grinding a blend of components [72]. Ma et al. reported that forms I and II of adefovir dipivoxil-saccharin cocrystals could undergo solid-solid transformations to generate form III by heating; on the other hand, form I could be harvested by adding forms II and III in ethanol via solvent-mediated transformation [73].

11.3.2 Preparation of Coamorphous Systems

Based on the mechanism involved, preparation methods of coamorphous systems can also be categorized into two types similar to the preparation of cocrystals as solid-state grinding (grinding, ball milling, cryomilling) and solvent-based method (solvent evaporation, quench cooling, spray-drying, freeze-drying, hot-melt extrusion).

11.3.2.1 Solvent Evaporation

Solvent evaporation technique is a widely used method for preparing coamorphous systems [20, 74–76]. Rapid evaporation connecting vacuum is the most frequently used since the organic solvents could be removed quickly in a short time and drugs precipitate from the solution state without enough time for rearrangement, nucleation, and crystal growth [77]. Suresh et al. successfully generated a curcumin-artemisinin coamorphous system by dissolving two components in ethanol, followed by fast vacuum evaporation [52]. Coamorphous myricetin-docetaxel was obtained by dissolving myricetin and docetaxel (molar ratio of 1:1) in methanol, followed by rotary vacuum evaporation at 55 °C. The difficulty for the solvent evaporation method is to select a suitable solvent for dissolving both drug and coformer [24]. Meanwhile, solvent residues, probably responsible for instability via solvent-mediated recrystallization during storage, should be controlled according to ICH guidance [24, 78, 79].

11.3.2.2 Quench Cooling

Quench cooling is another commonly used method to convert crystalline physical mixture into the coamorphous system [19, 80–82]. Briefly, the physical mixture is heated to a molten liquid state in a heated vessel under agitation for intensive mixing and then quickly cooled by liquid nitrogen or ice [8, 77, 79]. The rapid cooling rate would prevent the nucleation and crystal growth processes, facilitating the formation of coamorphous binary system. Wang et al. prepared coamorphous curcumin-piperine system by quenching the co-melted physical mixture using liquid nitrogen [19]. The obtained coamorphous system with a high yield (~97%) exhibited superior stability without thermal decomposition for at least 3 months under accelerated testing conditions (40 °C/75% RH). Although quench cooling is an easy and fast method to prepare coamorphous systems, it is not applicable for thermosensitive drugs or coformers [77].

11.3.2.3 Spray-Drying

Spray-drying can also be applied to produce coamorphous systems, especially for scale-up production [77, 83, 84]. Two steps including nebulization and drying are involved in the process [79]. The nebulization step sprays a solution of the components as mist droplets into a heated chamber [77–79]. For the drying step, the droplets continue an outward movement and solvent removal, resulting in particles with ideal size and morphology [12]. Lu et al. developed coamorphous budesonide-arginine for inhalation administration by dissolving in ethanol/water binary co-solvent and pumping to a spray dryer with the following conditions, i.e., inlet temperature, 100 °C; feed rate, 4 mL/min; drying air flow rate, 35 m^3/h; and atomization air flow rate, 742 L/h. The obtained coamorphous budesonide-arginine exhibited desired size (less than 5μm in diameter) and morphology (spherical with a smooth surface), which was suitable for inhalation administration.

11.3.2.4 Freeze-Drying

Freeze-drying (also namely lyophilization) is a widely used process for drying and improving the stability of multiple pharmaceutical products including vaccines, proteins, and nano-formulations (such as nanoparticles and nano-emulsions). It could also be used to prepare coamorphous systems with porous and low-density property [79]. Freeze-drying involves three major procedures: freezing, primary drying, and secondary drying. Among them, the primary drying is considered to be the most important procedure, mainly determining the total processing time and the quality of the final product [85–87]. Zhu et al. dissolved ofloxacin and tryptophan (1:1 molar ratio) in water and generated a coamorphous system with excellent physical and chemical stability by freeze-drying [86].

11.3.2.5 Hot-Melt Extrusion

At present, hot-melt extrusion, as a continuous solvent-free technique, has been extensively used in the pharmaceutical industry, especially for preparing ASDs from the laboratory-scale to scale-up production [24, 77]. The materials are mixed and fed with a temperature-controlled barrel and rotating screws through a die and a hot melt extruder. The material properties and process variables involving zone temperatures and speed of screw rotation have marked impacts on properties of the extrudate [77]. Lenz et al. fed a mixed mixture of indomethacin with a little amount of copovidone to the extruder barrel using a powder feeder, and then the arginine solution was added by a peristaltic pump through a nozzle into the extruder barrel to form coamorphous indomethacin-arginine system [88]. Besides, to modify the viscosity of the melts, the addition of copovidone significantly enhanced the physical stability of the prepared coamorphous system. Besides, hot-melt extrusion can conveniently combine with online spectroscopy techniques to monitor mixing efficiency and adjust extrusion parameters in time [24, 89].

11.3.2.6 Ball Milling

Mechanical milling, including ball milling, cryomilling, and liquid-assisted grinding, is a well-known kinetic technique to manufacture the disordered pharmaceutical product [90]. The induced mechanical activation generates crystal lattice defects and causes a transformation from crystalline form to amorphous state. Since neither organic solvents nor high temperatures are involved, ball milling becomes a "green" and high yield approach for the preparation of coamorphous systems [77, 91]. Gniado et al. mixed sodium taurocholate with small molecule drugs (carbamazepine, indomethacin, or mefenamic acid) in a 1:1 molar ratio and then milled the mixture using an oscillatory ball mill. The prepared coamorphous systems with superior physical stability showed significant dissolution advantages over crystalline drugs [57]. It is worth noting that ball milling sometimes produces the highly defective crystals, rather than the real and full amorphous solids. Incomplete crystal defects could trigger nucleation and crystal growth in amorphous formulations [79], which would result in recrystallization during storage.

11.3.2.7 Cryomilling

Conventional ball milling is sometimes inadequate to transform crystals into amorphous solids due to heat generation when milling, which may potentially induce recrystallization. Given the rise of temperature, cryomilling is generally applied to compromise the generated heat during the milling process [33]. For cryomilling, the samples are placed and sealed in milling jars and then immersed in liquid nitrogen, followed by milling. Due to the cryogenic temperature far below T_g of most amorphous drugs, the solids are quite brittle and easily mechanically milled into the disordered state. Gniado et al. successfully prepared the coamorphous combination of sodium taurocholate and sulfamerazine by cryomilling the equimolar mixture [58, 92]. To avoid overheating-assisted recrystallization of amorphous materials, the milling jar containing the mixture was sealed and immersed in liquid nitrogen for 3 min before milling. During the milling process, the milling jar was re-cooled with liquid nitrogen for 2 min every 7.5 min.

11.3.2.8 Liquid-Assisted Grinding

Sometimes, when coamorphous systems cannot be prepared by ball milling or cryomilling, the liquid-assisted grinding, where a drop of solvent is added during milling [77, 79], maybe an alternative approach to prepare coamorphous solid. Here, the liquid serves as a medium for promoting molecular diffusion and facilitating a potential reaction between the drug and coformer. For example, Pang et al. successfully prepared coamorphous curcumin-piperazine (molar ratio of 1:2) via ethanol-assisted grinding rather than dry ball milling [54]. Adding a little amount of ethanol partially dissolved curcumin and piperazine and increased the reaction interfaces, resulting in effective induction of formation of coamorphous systems.

11.4 Improving the Druggability of Chinese Medicines

Although the application of a majority of Chinese medicines or their extracts has achieved decent therapeutic efficacy in the treatment of various diseases, the widespread use of Chinese medicines is severely limited because of druggability issues including poor water solubility, slow dissolution rate, instability under different environmental factors, poor tabletability, poor permeability, and short half-life due to extensive metabolism. Cocrystallization and coamorphization processes change the crystal structure of the original active ingredients without alteration of their chemical structure, which provides potential ways to improve the druggability of Chinese medicines by modulating above issues via selectively perturbing network motifs.

11.4.1 Solubility

The solubility of a drug is one of its most important physicochemical properties. Drug molecules are required to be dissolved in the digestive juice before transport

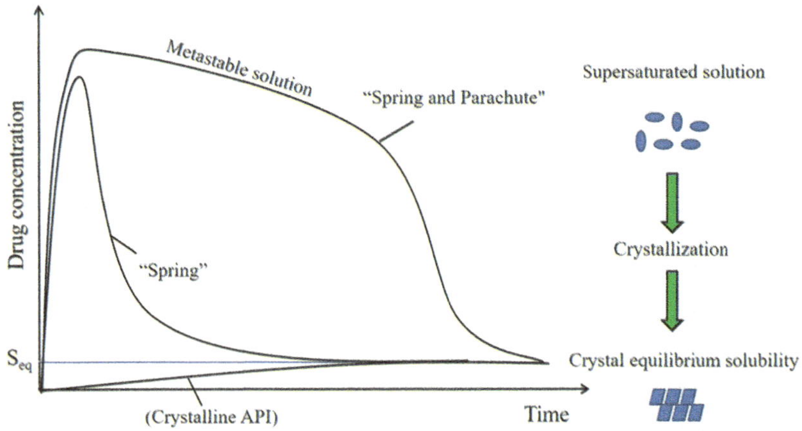

Fig. 11.2 "Spring and parachute" effect illustrating the API dissolution from cocrystals or coamorphous systems in supersaturated conditions. (Adapted and modified from ref. [100])

across biological membranes, and low aqueous solubility (e.g., drugs belonging to Biopharmaceutical Classification System (BCS) Class II or IV) can either delay or limit drug absorption [93]. Therefore, improving drug solubility is an essential topic in pharmaceutical development programs. The solubility of a crystalline drug is highly related to its crystal structure [15] (such as the arrangement of molecules, the intermolecular interactions that hold all molecules together, the chemical environment exposed on the crystal surface, and so on). In the past decades, cocrystallization [94] and coamorphization [24] technologies have been widely studied to improve poor solubility of active ingredients via alteration of the drug crystal structure. Quercetin is an extensively studied flavonoid compound [17] and is known for its numerous biological and pharmacological effects including antioxidant, anticarcinogenic, cardioprotective, bacteriostatic, and antiviral activity [95–98]. However, the in vivo efficacy in pure form is limited by its low solubility and consequent low absorption in the gut [17]. Smith et al. cocrystallized quercetin with caffeine, and the prepared cocrystal increased the solubility of quercetin by 14-fold [17]. Wang et al. prepared coamorphous loratadine-citric acid in a 1:1 molar ratio, which exhibited 53.9-fold higher solubility in water at 37 °C compared to crystalline loratadine [99]. This significant improvement of solubility contributed to the dissolution and oral absorption of loratadine.

During solubility measurement, most of the cocrystal or coamorphous systems usually generate supersaturated concentration concerning the thermodynamic equilibrium solubility of the stable crystalline form in a short period (minutes to an hour), followed by nucleation and crystal growth over time, which is so-called "spring and parachute" effect (Fig. 11.2) [15, 100]. The highest drug concentration that could be measured during the "spring" period is usually regarded as the solubility of the cocrystal or coamorphous system, which is sometimes more accurately called the apparent solubility [15, 101]. Therefore, the strength that the "spring" effect can reach determines the solubility improvement ability of the cocrystal or coamorphous system [15, 102]. The reasons for the peak solubility exhibited by coamorphous systems are reasonably well understood. The higher free energy, randomization of molecules, smaller particle size, larger surface area, higher wettability, and usually a combination of the above effects give the solubility advantage for amorphous drugs [15, 101]. A cocrystal is typically made up of an active ingredient and a more water-soluble coformer (such as nicotinamide, saccharin, caffeine, etc.) connecting together via weak noncovalent bonds (usually hydrogen bond) [102]. During the solubility measurement, dissociation of the hydrogen-bonded cocrystal would occur in a short period (minutes to an hour) in the biological medium. As the cocrystal dissociates, the more water-soluble coformer is extracted out from the crystal lattice into the aqueous medium. The hydrophobic drug molecules, now in their native state, become supersaturated in the aqueous biological solution and immediately precipitate to give loosely aggregated clusters. This sudden "crashing out" of the drug results in supramolecular aggregates or clusters composed of randomly oriented molecules with a lack of long-range order. Such nanosized clusters resemble the amorphous drug phase. This in situ generated amorphous cluster from cocrystal dissociation would exhibit the same kind of spike in drug solubility like the coamorphous system [15, 102].

11.4.2 Dissolution Rate

The dissolution rate refers to the amount of drug dissolved from solid formulations (such as tablets, capsules, or granules) at a given period in the dissolution medium. Dissolution tests run through the whole process of drug development and commercial production. It is not only a key reference index for the research and development of new drug formulations but also an important means for the quality control and evaluation of the production process. The dissolution rate of a solute in a solvent is directly proportional to its solubility, as described by the Noyes-Whitney equation [103].

The true dissolution rate of an active ingredient is usually investigated by its intrinsic dissolution rate (IDR), which is the inherent physical property that is defined as the amount of solid drug dissolved at a unit time from a unit surface area [15]. Before the test, drugs or formulations are pressed into circular tablets and embedded in the polytetrafluoroethylene (PTFE) intrinsic dissolution sample holders with only one flat surface exposed, to avoid the dissolution difference caused by the area change in contact with the medium during dissolution or by disintegration. In general, cocrystallization and coamorphization can enhance the solubility of crystalline drugs, thereby increasing their dissolution rate. For example, curcumin is the active ingredient from *Jianghuang* (*Curcuma longa L.*) with low solubility and IDR. After cocrystallization with pyrogallol, the solubility and IDR of curcumin were significantly enhanced by ~5-fold and ~12-fold, respectively, in comparison to that of crystalline curcumin [38]. Qian et al. studied the IDR of coamorphous lurasidone

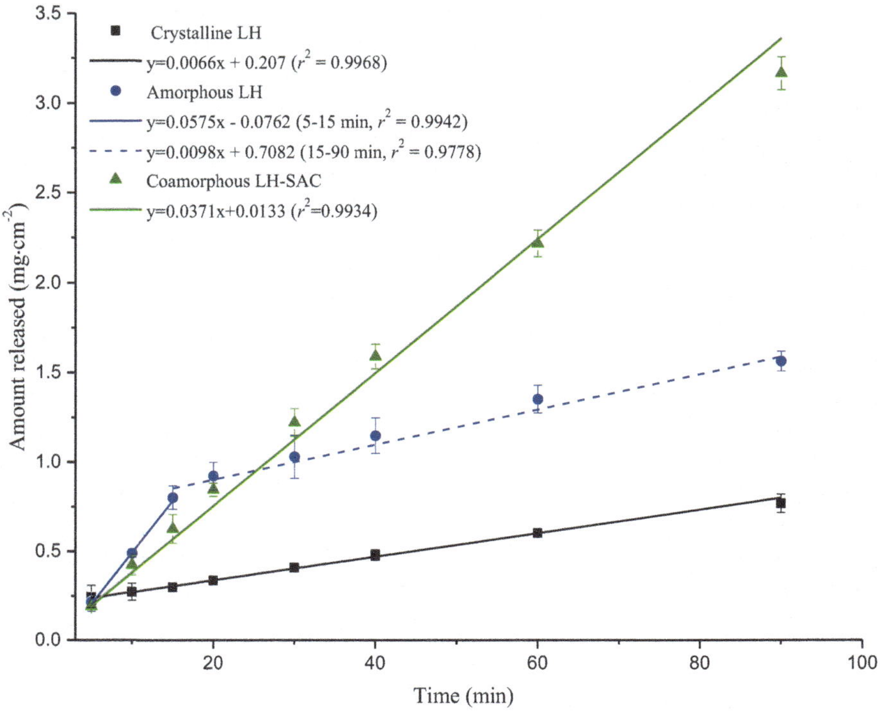

Fig. 11.3 Intrinsic dissolution profiles of crystalline LH, amorphous LH, and coamorphous LH-SAC in 0.2 M PBS 3.8 ($n = 6$). (Adapted from ref. [104])

hydrochloride (LH)-saccharin (SAC) in phosphate buffer (pH 3.8) [104]. In comparison to crystalline LH, the amorphous one exhibited a rapid dissolution behavior and increased by 8.7-fold in the first 15 min, followed by a slow dissolution after 15 min, and subsequently decreased to be similar to that of the crystal due to the occurrence of solution-mediated transformation. However, coamorphous LH-SAC exhibited a linear release profile without a decline, and its IDR was 5.6-fold higher than that of the crystalline form (Fig. 11.3). Besides, Wei et al. found a similar dissolution process occurred in coamorphous myricetin-docetaxel [55]. Such coamorphous system showed a 3.8-fold increase of IDR in comparison with pure crystalline docetaxel.

11.4.3 Stability

11.4.3.1 Physical Stability

Physical stability is extremely important for commercial dosage forms, e.g., low water sorption, the absence of hydration, or polymorphic transformation of the active ingredients [105]. The ability of cocrystals to address physical instability problems of drugs, such as hydrate formation on exposure to high relative humidity, is one of the demonstrated advantages of cocrystallization [106]. For example, both caffeine and theophylline are extracted from plants, whose anhydrous forms readily form hydrates upon exposure to water or water vapor [107, 108]. Trask et al. prepared cocrystals of caffeine and theophylline with oxalic acid and showed superior physical stability in comparison to each anhydrous crystalline form by exposing a high humidity environment (20 °C/98% RH). Berberine is a quaternary ammonium alkaloid, extracted from the Chinese medicine, *Huanglian* (*Coptis chinensis*). Berberine chloride is the most commonly used salt form in commercial tablets and can exist as an anhydrate, monohydrate, dihydrate, and tetrahydrate [109]. The anhydrate and monohydrate would transform into the dihydrate at RH above 12% [110]. The dihydrate can further transform into the tetrahydrate when RH is above 70% [111]. Qi et al. cocrystallized berberine chloride with citric acid, and no hydration process occurred for the prepared cocrystal in the RH range of 0–95% [109]. Such improvement of stability was believed to be achieved through the formation of $O\text{-}H\cdots Cl^-$ halogen bonds between the chloride ion in berberine hydrochloride and citric acid in cocrystal; otherwise, it is very easy to form hydrogen bonds with water molecules and exhibit high hygroscopicity.

Conversion of a crystalline drug to an amorphous form often offers higher apparent solubility and dissolution and leads to the increase in bioavailability. However, amorphous drugs are usually thermodynamically unstable, and their solubility advantage is easily lost due to the recrystallization tendency [24]. Coamorphization of drugs with small molecules has been proven to be a useful method to enhance the physical stability of amorphous API. For example, amorphous simvastatin and amorphous glipizide began to recrystallize at 67 days and 74 days under the condition of 4 °C/0% RH, respectively, whereas the recrystallization occurred at 128 days after the formation of coamorphous simvastatin-glipizide, indicating that physical stability of amorphous drugs was significantly enhanced after coamorphization [112]. Similarly, no crystallization phenomenon occurred in coamorphous curcumin-piperine for at least 3 months at 40 °C/75% RH, while amorphous curcumin started to recrystallize quickly under the same condition [19]. Currently, several mechanisms have been proposed for the stability advantage of coamorphous systems, including good miscibility, higher T_g, reduced molecular mobility, strong intermolecular interactions, as well as intimate mixing under molecular level [24].

11.4.3.2 Chemical Stability

In addition to physical stability, cocrystallization and coamorphization also demonstrated the ability to improve the chemical stability of drugs. Adefovir dipivoxil suffers from chemical instability and undergoes degradation during storage via hydrolysis and dimerization. Gao et al. prepared and compared cocrystals containing adefovir dipivoxil and two different conformers (i.e., acidic coformer saccharin and basic coformer nicotinamide, respectively) [113]. Both cocrystals enhanced the chemical stability of adefovir dipivoxil, with saccharin contained in cocrystal exhibited superior stability. Several factors are involved in the different performances for two coformers, including different micro-environments, intermolecular distances, and packing styles. This study provides a coformer selection strategy based on the degradation pathway of the active ingredients. Ritonavir degrades immediately at 40 °C after their conversion into amorphous form [114]. Dengale et al. found that the prepared coamorphous system of ritonavir with indomethacin showed significantly improved chemical stability.

Many active ingredients of Chinese medicines suffered chemical degradation problems due to specific reactive functional groups in their chemical structures [115]. For example, most of the compounds (e.g., salvianolic acid B, chlorogenic acid, and forsythoside) containing carboxyl ester bonds are prone to hydrolysis; most of the polyphenol compounds (e.g., gallic acid, curcumin, and baicalein) containing phenolic hydroxyl groups are easily oxidized [115]. Encouraged by the above successful cases, it is expected to improve the chemical stability of easily degradable active ingredients from Chinese medicines via cocrystallization and coamorphization techniques.

11.4.4 Mechanical Properties

Mechanical properties of APIs affect various manufacturing processes in the pharmaceutical industry, such as milling and compaction [116, 117]. Deficient mechanical properties often lead problems in tablet formation and manufacture. Tablet tensile strength is controlled by both bonding area and bonding strength between particles [118]. A crystalline drug with low plasticity suffers from poor tabletability because a very small bonding area is developed by compaction. In this case, both cocrystallization and coamorphization have been proven with the capacity to improve plasticity and better tabletability [84, 106].

It is generally believed that the effects of cocrystallization on crystal mechanical properties follow the known structure-property relationships [119–121]. A crystal with a flat-layered structure tends to be plastic, and larger interlayer distance usually leads to higher plasticity. For example, baicalein is one of the major bioactive flavones extracted from the Chinese medicine, *Huangqin* (*Scutellaria baicalensis Georgi*) [122]. Baicalein shows diverse pharmacological activities, including anti-oxidant, anti-inflammatory, anticancer, antibacterial, antifungal, and anti-HIV effects [123]. However, the extremely poor compaction property of the commercial α form of baicalein is one of the main challenges for its successful tablet development since the dose is relatively high (≥200 mg). To overcome this problem, three cocrystals, namely, baicalein-nicotinamide (1:1), baicalein-caffeine (2:1), and baicalein-isonicotinamide (1:1), were developed [123]. Crystal structure analysis revealed that these cocrystals consist of parallel molecular layers linked with weak hydrogen bonds, which promoted plastic deformation with better tabletability

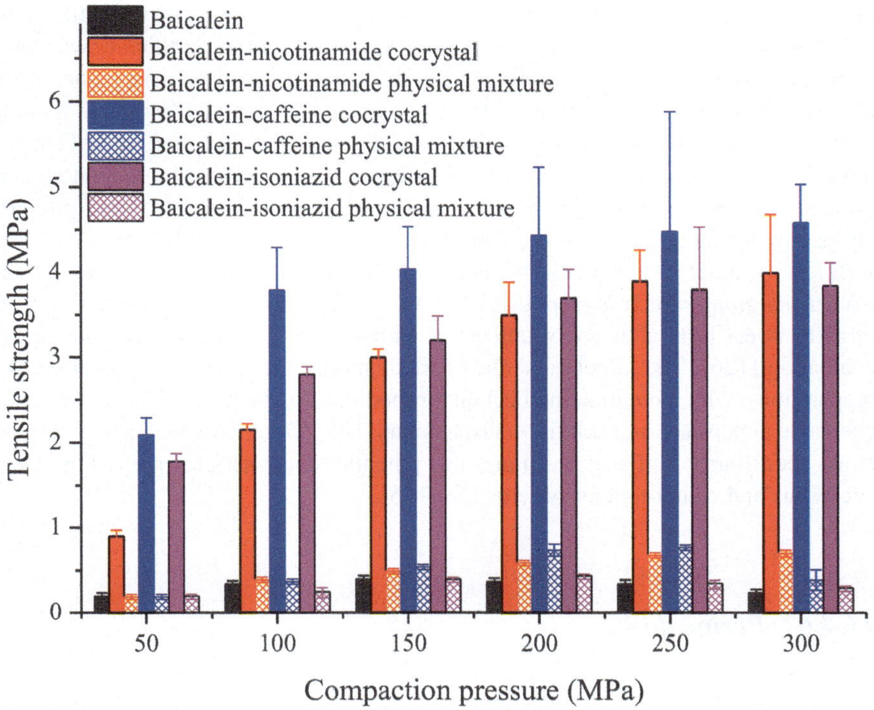

Fig. 11.4 Tabletability of baicalein-nicotinamide, baicalein-caffeine, and baicalein-isoniazid cocrystals

(Fig. 11.4) in comparison to crystalline baicalein or corresponding physical mixtures.

Similarly, the coamorphous system could also tailor the mechanical properties of active ingredients by the destruction of their original crystal structures [84, 124, 125]. Lenz et al. developed an appropriate tablet formulation for spray-dried indomethacin-arginine coamorphous system with excellent mechanical properties. Due to the better plastic deformation of the coamorphous system, its tablet tensile strength was significantly higher in comparison with the physical mixture under the same compaction pressure [84].

11.4.5 Taste Masking

The bitterness or other unpleasant taste of Chinese medicines is another challenge in developing oral products especially for infants and toddlers [106]. Such taste problems are usually overcome by developing either film-/sugar-coated tablets or capsule products [126]. In recent years, cocrystallization and coamorphization are also employed to either mask functional groups of unpleasant taste or modify taste by artificial sweeteners as coformers [66, 106]. Saccharin, an artificial sweetener commonly used in foods and drinks, has been widely used for preparing cocrystals [27, 126–130] and coamorphous systems [74, 75, 104]. Theophylline, with a bitter taste, is a natural compound from cocoa beans. Except for dissolution improvement, theophylline-saccharin cocrystal masked its bitter taste evaluated by the automated sweetness tasting machine [130]. *Huanglian*, as described by a Chinese proverb circulating for thousands of years "Dumb eating *Huanglian* can't tell the pain," is a well-known bitter taste Chinese medicine. Berberine is the major active ingredient from *Huanglian*, which is responsible for such intense bitter taste. Surprisingly, it turns to sweet taste after cocrystallization with saccharin according to volunteers' evaluation [126]. The sweet cocrystals and coamorphous systems, as intermediate preparations with potential intellectual properties, are beneficial for developing chewable tablets and oral solutions/suspensions [106]. Other sweeteners (e.g., aspartame, acesulfame, and sucralose) are also potential coformers for preparing sweet cocrystals and coamorphous systems [66, 106].

11.4.6 Permeability

Permeability across the biological membrane is essential for in vivo drug absorption. The drug candidates with low permeability are classified as BCS class III or IV drugs [93], such as puerarin, ephedrine hydrochloride, scutellarin, and ferulic acid extracted from Chinese medicines. Several aspects including structural features (hydrophilic drugs), active transport, as well as membrane-based efflux mechanisms are related to their poor permeability [131, 132]. For membrane-based efflux issue, cocrystallization or coamorphization with suitable small molecule efflux inhibitors is an effective way to increase their permeability. For instance, docetaxel is a BCS class IV drug [93], with quite low intestinal permeability (absorptive permeability on the Caco-2 cell model, ~0.07×10^{-5} cm/s). The multidrug efflux transporter P-glycoprotein (P-gp) plays an important role in the transport process crossing intestinal epithelia. Wei et al. simultaneously enhanced the dissolution (~3.8-fold) and permeability (~3.5-fold) of docetaxel by coamorphization with a natural P-gp inhibitor myricetin [55]. Several other cocrystals, such as hydrochlorothiazide cocrystals with nicotinic acid, nicotinamide, 4-aminobenzoic acid, and resorcinol [133], acyclovir cocrystals with fumaric and glutaric acids [134], theophylline cocrystals with isomeric aminobenzoic acids, and entacapone cocrystal with theophylline [135], have also shown significantly enhanced permeability benefit from the incorporated functional coformers.

11.4.7 In Vivo Performance

As discussed above, cocrystals or coamorphous systems offer an opportunity to enhance druggability-related properties (solubility, dissolution rate, and permeability) of active ingredients from Chinese medicine, hence resulting in improved in vivo performances. For example, quercetin-caffeine cocrystal increased the solubility of quercetin by 14-fold, thereby exhibiting superior pharmacokinetic performance than quercetin itself (~10-fold higher bioavailability) [17]. For another flavonoid baicalein, a 2.5-fold higher C_{max} and a 2.8-fold higher oral bioavailability were achieved after cocrystallization with nicotinamide [16], which was more effective than nanocrystallization of baicalein [131]. Wei et al. successfully improved the IDR, supersaturated dissolution, and oral bioavailability of a BCS IV drug docetaxel by coamorphization with a natural P-gp inhibitor myricetin [55]. As shown in Fig. 11.5, compared to crystalline docetaxel, the physical mixture of crystalline docetaxel and myricetin exhibited 1.7- and 1.8-fold increase in the C_{max} and $AUC_{0-\infty}$, suggesting that the addition of myricetin as a P-gp efflux pump inhibitor could effectively increase the absorption of docetaxel. After coamorphization, the highest plasma concentration curve was observed over that of others (i.e., crystalline docetaxel, amorphous docetaxel, and physical mixture of docetaxel and myricetin).

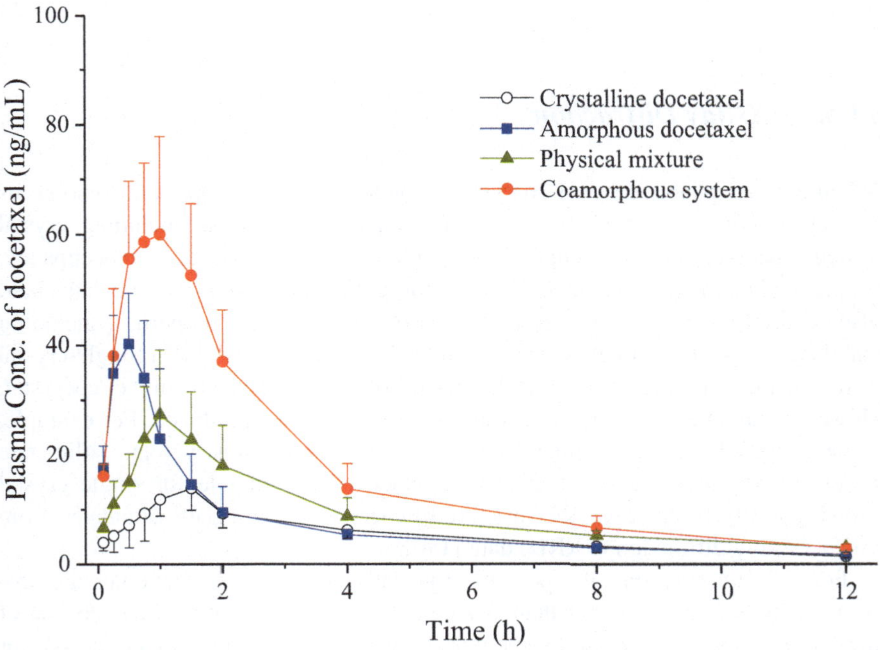

Fig. 11.5 Plasma concentration-time curves of docetaxel after oral administration of crystalline docetaxel, amorphous docetaxel, physical mixture of docetaxel and myricetin, and coamorphous docetaxel-myricetin in rats. (Adapted from ref. [55])

Curcumin is a BCS IV drug with low aqueous solubility, extensive glucuronidase metabolism, and poor membrane permeability, Wang et al. designed a coamorphous system of curcumin using piperine, an inhibitor of glucuronidation with permeation modulator properties, as the coformer [136, 137]. The prepared coamorphous system exhibited a significant increase in C_{max} (2.64-fold) and AUC_{0-24h} (2.16-fold) over crystalline curcumin [19].

11.5 Characterizations of Cocrystal and Coamorphous Systems

It is necessary to characterize cocrystals and coamorphous systems by appropriate analytical methods (e.g., X-ray diffraction (XRD), thermal analysis including differential scanning calorimetry (DSC) and thermogravimetric analysis (TGA), Fourier-transform infrared spectroscopy (FTIR), Raman spectroscopy, and solid-state nuclear magnetic resonance (ssNMR)) to achieve the following objectives: to determine whether the cocrystal or coamorphous system has been successfully generated; whether the prepared system is a pure phase; and to identify basic structure information and characterize physical properties of the cocrystal and coamorphous systems.

11.5.1 X-Ray Diffraction

When a novel pharmaceutical cocrystal is synthesized, it is important to solve its crystal structure to get its basic crystallographic information, including crystal system, space group, bond length, bond angle, cell dimensions, atomic occupancy, intermolecular interaction, etc. [106, 138]. Moreover, the crystal structure data could also be used to model and/or predict a variety of solid-state properties, including stability, morphology, hygroscopicity, tabletability, and so on [119]. Single-crystal X-ray diffraction is the preferred technique to solve the crystal structure of cocrystal. However, suitable X-ray quality crystals cannot always be produced. For example, some cocrystals could be obtained only via mechanochemistry (e.g., solid-state grinding and solvent assisted grinding), which is not suitable for single crystal growing [139]. In this case, the structure of cocrystals was usually simulated from powder X-ray diffraction (PXRD) data [140].

For most pharmaceutical processes, especially at large scale, materials are produced as bulk powders rather than as single crystals. Cocrystal powders consist of imperfect cocrystals, and may sometimes contain traces of pure crystalline API or coformer or even amorphous phases. PXRD has been used to analyze the powder sample of cocrystals and is generally considered as the "gold standard" to identify the cocrystal formation. If the cocrystal powder is phase pure, the diffraction peaks in its experimental PXRD pattern would match well with a "calculated" or "simulated" pattern generated from the corresponding single-crystal data in positions. For instance, baicalein-caffeine (1:1) cocrystal has been prepared through various methods (e.g., slowly evaporation [141], slurry [141], and rotary evaporation [123]), and their phase purity was all confirmed through comparing their experimental PXRD patterns with the calculated one. In this process, the intensity of the diffraction peaks is usually not included in the comparison category, since the peak height is also affected by the particle size and morphology in addition to the crystal structure.

PXRD can also be used to examine coamorphous systems, which do not have the long-range order observed in crystalline materials, but rather have short-range order molecular packing involving eight to ten molecules [24]. Coamorphous systems will exhibit broad peaks called "halos" in their PXRD patterns [142]. In many cases, small crystalline peaks will be observed on top of an amorphous halo when a mixture of crystalline and amorphous materials is present in a sample. Therefore, PXRD can be used to distinguish a small amount of crystalline API or coformer that may exist in the coamorphous powders, no matter they are the residual starting materials or the crystallization products of the coamorphous system. For example, PXRD was used to evaluate the physical stability of coamorphous curcumin-artemisinin under accelerated storage conditions. The crystallization process during storage was identified by the diffraction peak appearances in its PXRD patterns, which matched well with that of crystalline curcumin and artemisinin [52].

11.5.2 Thermal Analysis

DSC and TGA are recognized as the most common thermal methods for analyzing thermal behaviors of cocrystals or coamorphous systems. DSC analysis has been used to detect thermal transitions relative to a reference pan. Transitions that absorb heat, such as melting or desolvation, have produced peaks called "endotherms." Transitions that release heat, such as crystallization or decomposition, have produced peaks called "exotherms." Baseline shifts attributed to a T_g have been observed for amorphous materials. TGA, a technique wherein the mass change of a substance is measured as a function of temperature or time in a controlled atmosphere, is frequently conducted simultaneously with DSC, providing valuable information on the nature of desolvation processes and subsequent transformations.

Characterizing the melting point of cocrystal is particularly important since pharmaceutical-related processes (such as grinding or micronization) would generate considerable heat which is intolerable for some cocrystals with a low melting point. The melting process of cocrystals can be observed in the form of an endothermic peak in DSC curves. Generally, the onset temperature of the endothermic transition is recognized as the melting point of the eutectic instead of the peak temperature, because unlike the peak temperature, the onset temperature of melting will be independent of the heating rate. In most cases, the melting point of the cocrystal is different from corresponding crystalline active ingredients or coformers [105]. Therefore, DSC can also be used to confirm the phase purity of the cocrystal. Moreover, if the cocrystal exists in the form of a solvate, desolvation may occur before the melting point, and an endothermic peak would appear in its DSC trace. Sometimes, the desolvation-related endothermic peak may be mistakenly recognized as a melting peak. In such cases, the desolvation process can be distinguished from the melting point by the weight loss in the TGA profiles.

For coamorphous systems, thermal analysis helps to characterize their T_g, desolvation, degradation, crystallization, and degradation transitions. It is generally believed that coamorphous materials have good physical stability when stored at temperatures below T_g [24], so it is very important to measure their T_g by DSC. Furthermore, experimental T_g can also be used to predict whether there is intermolecular interaction in coamorphous systems by comparing with the predicted T_g calculated by the Gordon-Taylor equation [143, 144].

11.5.3 Vibrational Spectroscopy

Vibrational spectroscopy is typically used to characterize the fundamental vibrational modes of organic molecules either directly by their absorption of infrared (IR or mid-IR) radiation over the range of 4000–400 cm^{-1} or through an inelastic scattering of radiation (producing Raman shifts from the excitation laser wavelength) of 3500–50 cm^{-1}. Historically, definitive fingerprints of an organic compound provided by vibrational spectroscopy (mid-IR and Raman) based on characteristic bond stretching and bending frequencies have been used to identify functional groups in chemical structures. As for cocrystals or coamorphous systems, both Raman and IR spectroscopies have been used to identify functional groups corresponding to the individual components, to characterize proton transfer in the solid-state, and to confirm the presence of new binary phases based on unique IR/Raman fingerprints.

11.5.3.1 Fourier-Transform Infrared Spectroscopy

FTIR, a reliable technique to characterize hydrogen bonding since a change in hydrogen bonds at the intermolecular level would result in distinct vibrational frequency shifts, has been employed to identify the formation of cocrystal or coamorphous system during the discovery process. For example, myricetin showed peaks at 3415 cm^{-1} (corresponding to O-H stretching vibration) and 1618 cm^{-1} (-C=O stretching vibration) in its FTIR spectrum [145]. After formation of cocrystal with nicotinamide, the O-H group and C=O group in myricetin participate in the formation of hydrogen bonds, and the O-H and C=O stretching frequency shifted from their original positions in myricetin to 3470 cm^{-1} and 1661 cm^{-1}, respectively. It is worth noting that in some coamorphous systems, no hydrogen bond is formed between the API and coformer, with no significant difference in the FTIR spectrum between the coamorphous system and the corresponding amorphous physical mixture. For example, in FTIR spectra of quercetin-ritonavir 1:1 and 1:2 coamorphous systems [59], peaks did not undergo any significant shift despite of certain attenuation in transmittance.

11.5.3.2 Raman Spectroscopy

Raman spectroscopy, complementary to IR spectroscopy, involves a change in polarizability of symmetric nonpolar groups (aromatic rings, carbon double bonds) with strong signals. Typically, the Raman spectrum of a cocrystal or coamorphous system will exhibit different vibrational frequencies compared with those of API and the coformer. For example, in the Raman spectrum of daidzein, an intense peak near 1620 cm^{-1} was observed, which was attributed to the C=O stretch and -OH bend in combination with either C=C stretch or ring quinoidal stretches [146], while in the spectrum of daidzein-theophylline cocrystal, the peak is shifted to a lower wavenumber by ~10 cm^{-1}.

11.5.4 Solid-State Nuclear Magnetic Resonance

Solid-state nuclear magnetic resonance (ssNMR) spectroscopy is another tool to characterize the intermolecular interactions in a cocrystal or coamorphous system in addition to vibrational spectroscopies. This nondestructive technique has the unique ability to probe electronic environments and the dipolar connectivity of NMR-active nuclei (e.g., ^{13}C, ^{15}N, ^{19}F, ^{31}P, ^{23}Na, and ^{1}H) in the solid state without the requirement of the single crystal. It does not rely on long-range order to determine structures and is an outstanding approach for specific studies of amorphous materials, which usually display vital line broadening owing to their conformational distribution [147].

Typically, the API and coformer in a cocrystal are held together by intermolecular interactions such as hydrogen bonding. Thus, it is of particular importance to identify the intermolecular interactions that direct the self-assembly in the solid state, which is usually achieved by determining a three-dimensional structure using single crystal or PXRD. However, it may be difficult to grow a suitable single crystal or to solve the structure from the PXRD pattern. In these cases, ssNMR is an excellent complement to X-ray technology. For example, Maruyoshi et al. identified the specific intermolecular $COOH{\cdots}N_{arom}$ and $CH_{arom}{\cdots}O{=}C$ hydrogen bonding interactions in the solid-state structure of indomethacin-nicotinamide cocrystal using multi-nuclear two-dimensional solid-state magic-angle spinning NMR method [148].

For the coamorphous system, ssNMR is also very sensitive to short-range changes in chemical structure. For example, Heng et al. found that the resonance signals of the benzene ring at 152.39, 131.03, 128.72, 127.24, 123.81, and 121.98 ppm in the ss ^{13}C NMR spectrum of amorphous lurasidone hydrochloride transformed into one broad resonance signal with a peak at 133.31 ppm after coamorphization with L-cysteine hydrochloride [149]. Such signal shifts were attributed to the formation of hydrogen bond interactions between the nitrogen atom in the benzisothiazole ring of lurasidone hydrochloride and the NH_3^+ group of L-cysteine hydrochloride in the coamorphous system.

11.5.5 Others

In addition to above characterization methods, there are other analytical methods to investigate the physicochemical properties of cocrystal or coamorphous systems, such as polarized light microscope and scanning electron microscope for depicting micro-morphology [24], dynamic vapor sorption for evaluating hygroscopicity [138], nanoindentation technology for assessing mechanical properties including Young's elastic modulus and hardness [150], powder Brillouin light scattering for exploring the anisotropy of cocrystals [151], and broadband dielectric spectroscopy for determining the relaxation time of the coamorphous systems. Moreover, increasing computational modeling is also applied for the simulation and characterization of the properties of cocrystal or coamorphous systems, such as density functional theory calculation [152], Hirshfeld surface analysis [153], elastic constants calculation [154], energy framework calculation [155], and so on.

11.6 Concluding Remarks and Future Perspectives

Nowadays, around 90% of active ingredients from Chinese medicines suffer from low solubility/dissolution, low permeability, low stability, or/and poor mechanical properties, which are related to formulation issues and their in vivo performances. The number of drug candidates from Chinese medicines is expected to increase significantly due to the research extension and deep excavation in TCM with the support from national policies of China. Therefore, there is an urgent need to improve the druggability of Chinese medicines. Cocrystallization and coamorphization, with alteration of crystal structure but not the chemical structure of active ingredients by incorporation of a suitable coformer, have a great potential to enhance the druggability of Chinese medicines via addressing above issues from formulation and manufacture to in vivo pharmacokinetic performances.

In recent decade years, although significant progress is achieved in cocrystal formation theories and product development, a current challenge in the wide application of the cocrystallization technique is still empiric in the discovery and production of cocrystals. It is highly desired to move cocrystal discovery from screening against a large number of coformers to the reliable design of new cocrystals. Besides, a strategic shift from property enhancement to specific property tailoring, and from simple case reports of novel cocrystals, sometimes discovered serendipitously, to the systematic design of cocrystals, will greatly benefit the druggability improvement for both Chinese medicines and new chemical entities. To achieve this goal, a clearer understanding of the structure-property-performance relationship of cocrystals is critical, which is relied on big data mining and analysis as well as computer-based cocrystal design with desired pharmaceutical properties.

The situation of appropriate coformer selection for coamorphous systems is similar to that of cocrystals. A reasonable screening approach based on a comprehensive understanding of the physicochemical properties of APIs and coformers should be applied. Currently, it is still difficult to predict the stability of the prepared coamorphous systems, and the recrystallization of amorphous APIs may occur in the solid state (e.g., during processing, handling, and storage) or/and during dissolution, resulting in the loss of the solubility/dissolution advantage of coamorphous systems. The enhancement in stability relative to pure amorphous drugs and the complicated stabilization mechanisms of coamorphous systems should be explored, paving the way for further stability prediction in early development stage based on several measurable parameters, like T_g, relaxation time, enthalpic recovery, fragility, as well as the binding energy of intermolecular interactions between components. To date, the dry condition under room temperature is usually used to evaluate the physical stability of coamorphous systems in laboratory-scale screening. It is worth to assess both physical and chemical stabilities under long-term storage condition, accelerated storage condition, as well as stress testing conditions.

For both cocrystals and coamorphous systems containing two active ingredients, except for modification of formulation-related properties by various in vitro characterizations, the in vivo pharmacokinetic and pharmacodynamic interactions should be considered and evaluated, which is also crucial for their further development to commercial products.

References

1. Cheung, F. (2011). TCM: Made in China. *Nature, 480*, S82–S83.
2. Li, P., Feng, B., Jiang, H., Han, X., Wu, Z., Wang, Y., Lin, J., Zhang, Y., Yang, M., Han, L., & Zhang, D. (2018). A novel forming method of traditional Chinese medicine dispersible tablets to achieve rapid disintegration based on the powder modification principle. *Scientific Reports, 8*(1), 10319.
3. Xu, H., Zhang, Y., Liu, Z., Chen, T., Lv, C., Tang, S., Zhang, X., Zhang, W., Li, Z., Zhou, R., Yang, H., Wang, X., & Huang, L. (2019). ETCM: An encyclopaedia of traditional Chinese medicine. *Nucleic Acids Research, 47*, D976–D982.
4. D'Arrigo, G., Navarro, G., Meo, C. D., Matricardi, P., & Torchilin, V. (2014). Gellan gum nanohydrogel containing anti-inflammatory and anti-cancer drugs: A multi-drug delivery system for a combination therapy in cancer treatment. *European Journal of Pharmaceutics and Biopharmaceutics, 87*(1), 208–216.
5. Serajuddin, A. T. (2007). Salt formation to improve drug solubility. *Advanced Drug Delivery Reviews, 59*(7), 603–616.

6. Hsu, C. M., Yu, S. C., Tsai, F. J., & Tsai, Y. (2019). Characterization of in vitro and in vivo bioactivity of a ferulic acid-2-hydroxypropyl-beta-cyclodextrin inclusion complex. *Colloids and Surfaces. B, Biointerfaces, 180*, 68–74.
7. Ahmed, S., Corvis, Y., Gahoual, R., Euan, A., Lai-Kuen, R., Couillaud, B. M., Seguin, J., Alhareth, K., & Mignet, N. (2019). Conception of nanosized hybrid liposome/poloxamer particles to thicken the interior core of liposomes and delay hydrophilic drug delivery. *International Journal of Pharmaceutics, 567*, 118488.
8. Vasconcelos, T., Marques, S., das Neves, J., & Sarmento, B. (2016). Amorphous solid dispersions: Rational selection of a manufacturing process. *Advanced Drug Delivery Reviews, 100*, 85–101.
9. Abdulkarim, M., Sharma, P. K., & Gumbleton, M. (2019). Self-emulsifying drug delivery system: Mucus permeation and innovative quantification technologies. *Advanced Drug Delivery Reviews, 142*, 62–74.
10. Hou, G., Wang, Z., Ma, H., Ji, Y., Yu, L., Xu, J., & Chen, K. (2019). High-temperature stable plasmonic and cavity resonances in metal nanoparticle-decorated silicon nanopillars for strong broadband absorption in photothermal applications. *Nanoscale, 11*(31), 14777–14784.
11. Trubitsyn, G., Nguyen, V. N., Di Tommaso, C., Borchard, G., Gurny, R., & Moller, M. (2019). Impact of covalently Nile Red and covalently Rhodamine labeled fluorescent polymer micelles for the improved imaging of the respective drug delivery system. *European Journal of Pharmaceutics and Biopharmaceutics, 142*, 480–487.
12. Sverdlov Arzi, R., & Sosnik, A. (2018). Electrohydrodynamic atomization and spray-drying for the production of pure drug nanocrystals and co-crystals. *Advanced Drug Delivery Reviews, 131*, 79–100.
13. Bak, A., Gore, A., Yanez, E., Stanton, M., Tufekcic, S., Syed, R., Akrami, A., Rose, M., Surapaneni, S., Bostick, T., King, A., Neervannan, S., Ostovic, D., & Koparkar, A. (2008). The co-crystal approach to improve the exposure of a water-insoluble compound: AMG 517 sorbic acid co-crystal characterization and pharmacokinetics. *Journal of Pharmaceutical Sciences, 97*(9), 3942–3956.
14. Good, D. J., & Rodríguez-Hornedo, N. (2009). Solubility advantage of pharmaceutical cocrystals. *Crystal Growth & Design, 9*(5), 2252–2264.
15. Babu, N. J., & Nangia, A. (2011). Solubility advantage of amorphous drugs and pharmaceutical cocrystals. *Crystal Growth & Design, 11*(7), 2662–2679.
16. Huang, Y., Zhang, B., Gao, Y., Zhang, J., & Shi, L. (2014). Baicalein-nicotinamide cocrystal with enhanced solubility, dissolution, and oral bioavailability. *Journal of Pharmaceutical Sciences, 103*(8), 2330–2337.
17. Smith, A. J., Kavuru, P., Wojtas, L., Zaworotko, M. J., & Shytle, R. D. (2011). Cocrystals of quercetin with improved solubility and oral bioavailability. *Molecular Pharmaceutics, 8*(5), 1867–1876.
18. Chadha, K., Karan, M., Chadha, R., Bhalla, Y., & Vasisht, K. (2017). Is failure of cocrystallization actually a failure? Eutectic formation in cocrystal screening of hesperetin. *Journal of Pharmaceutical Sciences, 106*(8), 2026–2036.
19. Wang, R., Han, J., Jiang, A., Huang, R., Fu, T., Wang, L., Zheng, Q., Li, W., & Li, J. (2019). Involvement of metabolism-permeability in enhancing the oral bioavailability of curcumin in excipient-free solid dispersions co-formed with piperine. *International Journal of Pharmaceutics, 561*, 9–18.
20. Shi, X., Song, S., Ding, Z., Fan, B., Huang, W., & Xu, T. (2019). Improving the solubility, dissolution, and bioavailability of ibrutinib by preparing it in a coamorphous state with saccharin. *Journal of Pharmaceutical Sciences, 108*(9), 3020–3028.
21. Kasten, G., Lobmann, K., Grohganz, H., & Rades, T. (2019). Co-former selection for co-amorphous drug-amino acid formulations. *International Journal of Pharmaceutics, 557*, 366–373.

22. Wu, W., Lobmann, K., Rades, T., & Grohganz, H. (2018). On the role of salt formation and structural similarity of co-formers in co-amorphous drug delivery systems. *International Journal of Pharmaceutics, 535*(1–2), 86–94.
23. Fung, M. H., DeVault, M., Kuwata, K. T., & Suryanarayanan, R. (2018). Drug-excipient interactions: Effect on molecular mobility and physical stability of ketoconazole-organic acid coamorphous systems. *Molecular Pharmaceutics, 15*(3), 1052–1061.
24. Chavan, R. B., Thipparaboina, R., Kumar, D., & Shastri, N. R. (2016). Co amorphous systems: A product development perspective. *International Journal of Pharmaceutics, 515*(1–2), 403–415.
25. Li, B., Konecke, S., Wegiel, L. A., Taylor, L. S., & Edgar, K. J. (2013). Both solubility and chemical stability of curcumin are enhanced by solid dispersion in cellulose derivative matrices. *Carbohydrate Polymers, 98*(1), 1108–1116.
26. Korhonen, O., Pajula, K., & Laitinen, R. (2017). Rational excipient selection for co-amorphous formulations. *Expert Opinion on Drug Delivery, 14*(4), 551–569.
27. Gao, Y., Zu, H., & Zhang, J. (2011). Enhanced dissolution and stability of adefovir dipivoxil by cocrystal formation. *The Journal of Pharmacy and Pharmacology, 63*(4), 483–490.
28. Thakuria, R., Delori, A., Jones, W., Lipert, M. P., Roy, L., & Rodriguez-Hornedo, N. (2013). Pharmaceutical cocrystals and poorly soluble drugs. *International Journal of Pharmaceutics, 453*(1), 101–125.
29. Ong, T. T., Kavuru, P., Nguyen, T., Cantwell, R., Wojtas, L., & Zaworotko, M. J. (2011). 2:1 cocrystals of homochiral and achiral amino acid zwitterions with Li+ salts: Water-stable zeolitic and diamondoid metal-organic materials. *Journal of the American Chemical Society, 133*(24), 9224–9227.
30. Velaga, S. P., Basavoju, S., & Bostrom, D. (2008). Norfloxacin saccharinate-saccharin dihydrate cocrystal - A new pharmaceutical cocrystal with an organic counter ion. *Journal of Molecular Structure, 889*(1–3), 150–153.
31. Aitipamula, S., Banerjee, R., Bansal, A. K., Biradha, K., Cheney, M. L., Choudhury, A. R., Desiraju, G. R., Dikundwar, A. G., Dubey, R., Duggirala, N., Ghogale, P. P., Ghosh, S., Goswami, P. K., Goud, N. R., Jetti, R. R. K. R., Karpinski, P., Kaushik, P., Kumar, D., Kumar, V., . . . Zaworotko, M. J. (2012). Polymorphs, salts, and cocrystals: What's in a name? *Crystal Growth & Design, 12*(5), 2147–2152.
32. Lu, W., Rades, T., Rantanen, J., & Yang, M. (2019). Inhalable co-amorphous budesonide-arginine dry powders prepared by spray drying. *International Journal of Pharmaceutics, 565*, 1–8.
33. Moinuddin, S. M., Ruan, S., Huang, Y., Gao, Q., Shi, Q., Cai, B., & Cai, T. (2017). Facile formation of co-amorphous atenolol and hydrochlorothiazide mixtures via cryogenic-milling: Enhanced physical stability, dissolution and pharmacokinetic profile. *International Journal of Pharmaceutics, 532*(1), 393–400.
34. Zhang, D. J., Zhou, C., Lv, P., Zhao, Y. L., Liang, J., Liao, X. L., & Yang, B. (2018). Preparation and characterization of a novel host-guest complex based on folate-modified beta-cyclodextrin and artesunate. *Materials Science and Engineering: C, 86*, 48–55.
35. Deng, C., & Jiang, C. (2018). Preparation and characterization of a curcumin-catechol cocrystal. *Journal of Zhejiang University of Science, 30*(1), 16–21.
36. Xuan, B., Zhang, Y., & Chow, S. F. (2019). Design and characterization of a new drug-herb isoniazid-curcumin cocrystal for potentially improving tuberculosis treatment. In *2019 AAPS PharmSci 360. San Antonio, Texas*.
37. Mannava, M. K. C., Suresh, K., Kumar Bommaka, M., Bhavani Konga, D., & Nangia, A. (2018). Curcumin-artemisinin coamorphous solid: Xenograft model preclinical study. *Pharmaceutics, 10*(1), 7.
38. Sanphui, P., Goud, N. R., Khandavilli, U. B. R., & Nangia, A. (2011). Fast dissolving curcumin cocrystals. *Crystal Growth & Design, 11*(9), 4135–4145.

39. Deng, Y. P., Zhang, Y. J., Huang, Y. L., Zhang, M., & Lou, B. Y. (2018). Preparation, crystal structures, and oral bioavailability of two cocrystals of emodin with berberine chloride. *Crystal Growth & Design, 18*(12), 7481–7488.
40. Sowa, M., Slepokura, K., & Matczak-Jon, E. (2013). Cocrystals of fisetin, luteolin and genistein with pyridinecarboxamide coformers: Crystal structures, analysis of intermolecular interactions, spectral and thermal characterization. *CrystEngComm, 15*(38), 7696–7708.
41. Sowa, M., Slepokura, K., & Matczak-Jon, E. (2013). A 1:2 cocrystal of genistein with isonicotinamide: Crystal structure and Hirshfeld surface analysis. *Acta Crystallographica. Section C, 69*(Pt 11), 1267–1272.
42. Zhang, Y. N., Yin, H. M., Zhang, Y., Zhang, D. J., Su, X., & Kuang, H. X. (2017). Preparation of a 1:1 cocrystal of genistein with 4,4′-bipyridine. *Journal of Crystal Growth, 458*, 103–109.
43. Chadha, K., Karan, M., Bhalla, Y., Chadha, R., Khullar, S., Mandal, S., & Vasisht, K. (2017). Cocrystals of hesperetin: Structural, pharmacokinetic, and pharmacodynamic evaluation. *Crystal Growth & Design, 17*(5), 2386–2405.
44. He, M. Y. (2017). *Synthesis and properties of natural pharmaceutical cocrystals of polyhydroxy flavonoids*. Jiamusi University.
45. Zhang, Y. N., Yin, H. M., Zhang, Y., Zhang, D. J., Su, X., & Kuang, H. X. (2017). Cocrystals of kaempferol, quercetin and myricetin with 4,4′-bipyridine: Crystal structures, analyses of intermolecular interactions and antibacterial properties. *Journal of Molecular Structure, 1130*, 199–207.
46. Hu, C., Cheng, H., Xu, J., Qian, S., Zhang, J., & Gao, Y. (2017). Formation thermodynamics of myricetin-caffeine cocrystal in different organic solvents. *Journal of Central South University, 15*, 567–572.
47. Xu, J., Wei, Y., Qian, S., & Zhang, J. (2016). Preparation of myricetin-caffeine cocrystal and its single crystal analysis. *Journal of China Pharmaceutical University, 47*, 324–328.
48. Sowa, M., Slepokura, K., & Matczak-Jon, E. (2014). A 1:1 pharmaceutical cocrystal of myricetin in combination with uncommon piracetam conformer: X-ray single crystal analysis and mechanochemical synthesis. *Journal of Molecular Structure, 1058*, 114–121.
49. Luo, C., Liang, W. D., Chen, X., Wang, J. M., Deng, Z. W., & Zhang, H. L. (2018). Pharmaceutical cocrystals of naringenin with improved dissolution performance. *CrystEngComm, 20*(22), 3025–3033.
50. Schultheiss, N., Bethune, S., & Henck, J. O. (2010). Nutraceutical cocrystals: Utilizing pterostilbene as a cocrystal former. *CrystEngComm, 12*(8), 2436–2442.
51. Bethune, S. J., Schultheiss, N., & Henck, J. O. (2011). Improving the poor aqueous solubility of nutraceutical compound pterostilbene through cocrystal formation. *Crystal Growth & Design, 11*(7), 2817–2823.
52. Suresh, K., Mannava, M. K. C., & Nangia, A. (2014). A novel curcumin-artemisinin coamorphous solid: Physical properties and pharmacokinetic profile. *RSC Advances, 4*(102), 58357–58361.
53. Skieneh, J. M., Sathisaran, I., Dalvi, S. V., & Rohani, S. (2017). Co-amorphous form of curcumin-folic acid dihydrate with increased dissolution rate. *Crystal Growth & Design, 17*(12), 6273–6280.
54. Pang, W., Lv, J., Du, S., Wang, J., Wang, J., & Zeng, Y. (2017). Preparation of curcumin-piperazine coamorphous phase and fluorescence spectroscopic and density functional theory simulation studies on the interaction with bovine serum albumin. *Molecular Pharmaceutics, 14*(9), 3013–3024.
55. Wei, Y. F., Zhou, S. Y., Hao, T. Y., Zhang, J. J., Gao, Y., & Qian, S. (2019). Further enhanced dissolution and oral bioavailability of docetaxel by coamorphization with a natural P-gp inhibitor myricetin. *European Journal of Pharmaceutical Sciences, 129*, 21–30.
56. Teja, A., Musmade, P. B., Khade, A. B., & Dengale, S. J. (2015). Simultaneous improvement of solubility and permeability by fabricating binary glassy materials of talinolol with naringin: Solid state characterization, in-vivo in-situ evaluation. *European Journal of Pharmaceutical Sciences, 78*, 234–244.

57. Gniado, K., MacFhionnghaile, P., McArdle, P., & Erxleben, A. (2018). The natural bile acid surfactant sodium taurocholate (NaTC) as a coformer in coamorphous systems: Enhanced physical stability and dissolution behavior of coamorphous drug-NaTc systems. *International Journal of Pharmaceutics, 535*(1–2), 132–139.
58. Gniado, K., Lobmann, K., Rades, T., & Erxleben, A. (2016). The influence of co-formers on the dissolution rates of co-amorphous sulfamerazine/excipient systems. *International Journal of Pharmaceutics, 504*(1–2), 20–26.
59. Dengale, S. J., Hussen, S. S., Krishna, B. S., Musmade, P. B., Gautham Shenoy, G., & Bhat, K. (2015). Fabrication, solid state characterization and bioavailability assessment of stable binary amorphous phases of Ritonavir with Quercetin. *European Journal of Pharmaceutics and Biopharmaceutics, 89*, 329–338.
60. Hashim Ali, K., Mohsin Ansari, M., Ali Shah, F., Ud Din, F., Abdul Basit, M., Kim, J. K., & Zeb, A. (2019). Enhanced dissolution of valsartan-vanillin binary co-amorphous system loaded in mesoporous silica particles. *Journal of Microencapsulation, 36*(1), 10–20.
61. Weyna, D. R., Shattock, T., Vishweshwar, P., & Zaworotko, M. J. (2009). Synthesis and structural characterization of cocrystals and pharmaceutical cocrystals: Mechanochemistry vs slow evaporation from solution. *Crystal Growth & Design, 9*(2), 1106–1123.
62. Karagianni, A., Malamatari, M., & Kachrimanis, K. (2018). Pharmaceutical cocrystals: New solid phase modification approaches for the formulation of APIs. *Pharmaceutics, 10*(1), 18.
63. Jones, W., Motherwell, S., & Trask, A. V. (2006). Pharmaceutical cocrystals: An emerging approach to physical property enhancement. *MRS Bulletin, 31*(11), 875–879.
64. Schultheiss, N. C., & Bethune, S. J. (2011). *Pterostilbene cocrystals*. US20110189275 A1.
65. Trask, A. V., Motherwell, W. D. S., & Jones, W. (2004). Solvent-drop grinding: Green polymorph control of cocrystallisation. *Chemical Communications, 7*, 890–891.
66. Karimi-Jafari, M., Padrela, L., Walker, G. M., & Croker, D. M. (2018). Creating cocrystals: A review of pharmaceutical cocrystal preparation routes and applications. *Crystal Growth & Design, 18*(10), 6370–6387.
67. Zhang, S., & Rasmuson, A. C. (2013). Thermodynamics and crystallization of the theophylline-glutaric acid cocrystal. *Crystal Growth & Design, 13*(3), 1153–1161.
68. Setyawan, D., Sari, R., Yusuf, H., & Primaharinastiti, R. (2014). Preparation and characterization of artesunate-nicotinamide cocrystal by solvent evaporation and slurry method. *Asian Journal of Pharmaceutical and Clinical Research, 7*(Suppl 1), 62–65.
69. Wang, I. C., Lee, M. J., Sim, S. J., Kim, W. S., Chun, N. H., & Choi, G. J. (2013). Anti-solvent co-crystallization of carbamazepine and saccharin. *International Journal of Pharmaceutics, 450*(1–2), 311–322.
70. Lee, M. J., Wang, I. C., Kim, M. J., Kim, P., Song, K. H., Chun, N. H., Park, H. G., & Choi, G. J. (2015). Controlling the polymorphism of carbamazepine-saccharin cocrystals formed during antisolvent cocrystallization using kinetic parameters. *Korean Journal of Chemical Engineering, 32*(9), 1910–1917.
71. Jayasankar, A., Somwangthanaroj, A., Shao, Z. J., & Rodriguez-Hornedo, N. (2006). Cocrystal formation during cogrinding and storage is mediated by amorphous phase. *Pharmaceutical Research, 23*(10), 2381–2392.
72. Seefeldt, K., Miller, J., Alvarez-Nunez, F., & Rodriguez-Hornedo, N. (2007). Crystallization pathways and kinetics of carbamazepine-nicotinamide cocrystals from the amorphous state by in situ thermomicroscopy, spectroscopy, and calorimetry studies. *Journal of Pharmaceutical Sciences, 96*(5), 1147–1158.
73. Ma, K., Wang, N., Cheng, L., Wei, Y., Zhang, J., Gao, Y., & Qian, S. (2019). Identification of novel adefovir dipivoxil-saccharin cocrystal polymorphs and their thermodynamic polymorphic transformations. *International Journal of Pharmaceutics, 566*, 361–370.
74. Gao, Y., Liao, J., Qi, X., & Zhang, J. (2013). Coamorphous repaglinide-saccharin with enhanced dissolution. *International Journal of Pharmaceutics, 450*(1–2), 290–295.

75. Maher, E. M., Ali, A. M., Salem, H. F., & Abdelrahman, A. A. (2016). In vitro/in vivo evaluation of an optimized fast dissolving oral film containing olanzapine co-amorphous dispersion with selected carboxylic acids. *Drug Delivery, 23*(8), 3088–3100.
76. Bi, Y., Xiao, D., Ren, S., Bi, S., Wang, J., & Li, F. (2017). The binary system of ibuprofen-nicotinamide under nanoscale confinement: From cocrystal to coamorphous state. *Journal of Pharmaceutical Sciences, 106*(10), 3150–3155.
77. Karagianni, A., Kachrimanis, K., & Nikolakakis, I. (2018). Co-amorphous solid dispersions for solubility and absorption improvement of drugs: Composition, preparation, characterization and formulations for oral delivery. *Pharmaceutics, 10*(3), 98.
78. Singh, A., & Van den Mooter, G. (2016). Spray drying formulation of amorphous solid dispersions. *Advanced Drug Delivery Reviews, 100*, 27–50.
79. Shi, Q., Moinuddin, S. M., & Cai, T. (2019). Advances in coamorphous drug delivery systems. *Acta Pharmaceutica Sinica B, 9*(1), 19–35.
80. Cruz-Angeles, J., Videa, M., & Martinez, L. M. (2019). Highly soluble glimepiride and irbesartan co-amorphous formulation with potential application in combination therapy. *AAPS PharmSciTech, 20*(4), 144.
81. Martinez-Jimenez, C., Cruz-Angeles, J., Videa, M., & Martinez, L. M. (2018). Co-amorphous simvastatin-nifedipine with enhanced solubility for possible use in combination therapy of hypertension and hypercholesterolemia. *Molecules, 23*(9), 2161.
82. Anand, V. S. K., Sakhare, S. D., Navya Sree, K. S., Nair, A. R., Raghava Varma, K., Gourishetti, K., & Dengale, S. J. (2018). The relevance of co-amorphous formulations to develop supersaturated dosage forms: In-vitro, and ex-vivo investigation of ritonavir-lopinavir co-amorphous materials. *European Journal of Pharmaceutical Sciences, 123*, 124–134.
83. Jensen, K. T., Blaabjerg, L. I., Lenz, E., Bohr, A., Grohganz, H., Kleinebudde, P., Rades, T., & Lobmann, K. (2016). Preparation and characterization of spray-dried co-amorphous drug-amino acid salts. *The Journal of Pharmacy and Pharmacology, 68*(5), 615–624.
84. Lenz, E., Jensen, K. T., Blaabjerg, L. I., Knop, K., Grohganz, H., Lobmann, K., Rades, T., & Kleinebudde, P. (2015). Solid-state properties and dissolution behaviour of tablets containing co-amorphous indomethacin-arginine. *European Journal of Pharmaceutics and Biopharmaceutics, 96*, 44–52.
85. Ali, A. M., & Al-Remawi, M. M. (2016). Freeze dried quetiapine-nicotinamide binary solid dispersions: A new strategy for improving physicochemical properties and ex vivo diffusion. *Journal of Pharmaceutics, 2016*, 2126056.
86. Zhu, S., Gao, H., Babu, S., & Garad, S. (2018). Co-amorphous formation of high-dose zwitterionic compounds with amino acids to improve solubility and enable parenteral delivery. *Molecular Pharmaceutics, 15*(1), 97–107.
87. Ohori, R., Akita, T., & Yamashita, C. (2019). Mechanism of collapse of amorphous-based lyophilized cake induced by slow ramp during the shelf ramp process. *International Journal of Pharmaceutics, 564*, 461–471.
88. Lenz, E., Lobmann, K., Rades, T., Knop, K., & Kleinebudde, P. (2017). Hot melt extrusion and spray drying of co-amorphous indomethacin-arginine with polymers. *Journal of Pharmaceutical Sciences, 106*(1), 302–312.
89. Hitzer, P., Bauerle, T., Drieschner, T., Ostertag, E., Paulsen, K., van Lishaut, H., Lorenz, G., & Rebner, K. (2017). Process analytical techniques for hot-melt extrusion and their application to amorphous solid dispersions. *Analytical and Bioanalytical Chemistry, 409*(18), 4321–4333.
90. Descamps, M., & Willart, J. F. (2016). Perspectives on the amorphisation/milling relationship in pharmaceutical materials. *Advanced Drug Delivery Reviews, 100*, 51–66.
91. Krupa, A., Descamps, M., Willart, J. F., Strach, B., Wyska, E., Jachowicz, R., & Danede, F. (2016). High-energy ball milling as green process to vitrify tadalafil and improve bioavailability. *Molecular Pharmaceutics, 13*(11), 3891–3902.
92. Willart, J. F., & Descamps, M. (2008). Solid state amorphization of pharmaceuticals. *Molecular Pharmaceutics, 5*(6), 905–920.

93. Amidon, G. L., Lennernas, H., Shah, V. P., & Crison, J. R. (1995). A theoretical basis for a biopharmaceutic drug classification: The correlation of in vitro drug product dissolution and in vivo bioavailability. *Pharmaceutical Research, 12*(3), 413–420.
94. Dai, X. L., Chen, J. M., & Lu, T. B. (2018). Pharmaceutical cocrystallization: An effective approach to modulate the physicochemical properties of solid-state drugs. *CrystEngComm, 20*(36), 5292–5316.
95. Formica, J. V., & Regelson, W. (1995). Review of the biology of quercetin and related bioflavonoids. *Food and Chemical Toxicology, 33*(12), 1061–1080.
96. Murakami, A., Ashida, H., & Terao, J. (2008). Multitargeted cancer prevention by quercetin. *Cancer Letters, 269*(2), 315–325.
97. Spencer, J. P., Kuhnle, G. G., Williams, R. J., & Rice-Evans, C. (2003). Intracellular metabolism and bioactivity of quercetin and its in vivo metabolites. *The Biochemical Journal, 372*(Pt 1), 173–181.
98. Bakay, M., Mucsi, I., Beladi, I., & Gabor, M. (1968). Effect of flavonoids and related substances. II. Antiviral effect of quercetin, dihydroquercetin and dihydrofisetin. *Acta Microbiologica Academiae Scientiarum Hungaricae, 15*(3), 223–227.
99. Wang, J., Chang, R., Zhao, Y., Zhang, J., Zhang, T., Fu, Q., Chang, C., & Zeng, A. (2017). Coamorphous loratadine-citric acid system with enhanced physical stability and bioavailability. *AAPS PharmSciTech, 18*(7), 2541–2550.
100. Brouwers, J., Brewster, M. E., & Augustijns, P. (2009). Supersaturating drug delivery systems: The answer to solubility-limited oral bioavailability? *Journal of Pharmaceutical Sciences, 98*(8), 2549–2572.
101. Laitinen, R., Lobmann, K., Grohganz, H., Priemel, P., Strachan, C. J., & Rades, T. (2017). Supersaturating drug delivery systems: The potential of co-amorphous drug formulations. *International Journal of Pharmaceutics, 532*(1), 1–12.
102. Bavishi, D. D., & Borkhataria, C. H. (2016). Spring and parachute: How cocrystals enhance solubility. *Progress in Crystal Growth and Characterization of Materials, 62*(3), 1–8.
103. Noyes, A. A., & Whitney, W. R. (1897). The rate of solution of solid substances in their own solutions. *Journal of the American Chemical Society, 19*(12), 930–934.
104. Qian, S., Heng, W., Wei, Y., Zhang, J., & Gao, Y. (2015). Coamorphous lurasidone hydrochloride-saccharin with charge-assisted hydrogen bonding interaction shows improved physical stability and enhanced dissolution with pH-independent solubility behavior. *Crystal Growth & Design, 15*(6), 2920–2928.
105. Schultheiss, N., & Newman, A. (2009). Pharmaceutical cocrystals and their physicochemical properties. *Crystal Growth & Design, 9*(6), 2950–2967.
106. Sun, C. C. (2013). Cocrystallization for successful drug delivery. *Expert Opinion on Drug Delivery, 10*(2), 201–213.
107. Trask, A. V., Motherwell, W. D., & Jones, W. (2006). Physical stability enhancement of theophylline via cocrystallization. *International Journal of Pharmaceutics, 320*(1–2), 114–123.
108. Trask, A. V., Motherwell, W. D. S., & Jones, W. (2005). Pharmaceutical cocrystallization: Engineering a remedy for caffeine hydration. *Crystal Growth & Design, 5*(3), 1013–1021.
109. Lu, Q., Dun, J. N., Chen, J. M., Liu, S. Y., & Sun, C. C. (2019). Improving solid-state properties of berberine chloride through forming a salt cocrystal with citric acid. *International Journal of Pharmaceutics, 554*, 14–20.
110. Nakagawa, H., Miyata, T., Mohri, K., Sugimoto, I., & Manabe, H. (1978). Water of crystallization of berberine chloride. *Yakugaku Zasshi, 98*(8), 981–985.
111. Yoshimatsu, K., Nakabayashi, S., Ogaki, J., Kimura, M., & Horikoshi, I. (1981). Dielectric study on the water of crystallization of berberine chloride. *Yakugaku Zasshi, 101*(12), 1143–1148.
112. Lobmann, K., Strachan, C., Grohganz, H., Rades, T., Korhonen, O., & Laitinen, R. (2012). Co-amorphous simvastatin and glipizide combinations show improved physical stability

without evidence of intermolecular interactions. *European Journal of Pharmaceutics and Biopharmaceutics, 81*(1), 159–169.
113. Gao, Y., Gao, J., Liu, Z., Kan, H., Zu, H., Sun, W., Zhang, J., & Qian, S. (2012). Coformer selection based on degradation pathway of drugs: A case study of adefovir dipivoxil-saccharin and adefovir dipivoxil-nicotinamide cocrystals. *International Journal of Pharmaceutics, 438*(1–2), 327–335.
114. Dengale, S. J., Ranjan, O. P., Hussen, S. S., Krishna, B. S., Musmade, P. B., Gautham Shenoy, G., & Bhat, K. (2014). Preparation and characterization of co-amorphous ritonavir-indomethacin systems by solvent evaporation technique: Improved dissolution behavior and physical stability without evidence of intermolecular interactions. *European Journal of Pharmaceutical Sciences, 62*, 57–64.
115. Meng, W., Xiaoliang, R., Xiumei, G., Vincieri, F. F., & Bilia, A. R. (2009). Stability of active ingredients of traditional Chinese medicine (TCM). *Natural Product Communications, 4*(12), 1761–1776.
116. Duncan-Hewitt, W. C., & Weatherly, G. C. (1990). Modeling the uniaxial compaction of pharmaceutical powders using the mechanical properties of single crystals. I: Ductile materials. *Journal of Pharmaceutical Sciences, 79*(2), 147–152.
117. Meier, M., John, E., Wieckhusen, D., Wirth, W., & Peukert, W. (2009). Influence of mechanical properties on impact fracture: Prediction of the milling behaviour of pharmaceutical powders by nanoindentation. *Powder Technology, 188*(3), 301–313.
118. Sun, C. C. (2011). Decoding powder tabletability: Roles of particle adhesion and plasticity. *Journal of Adhesion Science and Technology, 25*(4–5), 483–499.
119. Sun, C. C. (2009). Materials science tetrahedron--A useful tool for pharmaceutical research and development. *Journal of Pharmaceutical Sciences, 98*(5), 1671–1687.
120. Sun, C., & Grant, D. J. (2001). Influence of crystal structure on the tableting properties of sulfamerazine polymorphs. *Pharmaceutical Research, 18*(3), 274–280.
121. Bag, P. P., Chen, M., Sun, C. C., & Reddy, C. M. (2012). Direct correlation among crystal structure, mechanical behaviour and tabletability in a trimorphic molecular compound. *CrystEngComm, 14*(11), 3865–3867.
122. Zhao, Q., Zhang, Y., Wang, G., Hill, L., Weng, J. K., Chen, X. Y., Xue, H. W., & Martin, C. (2016). A specialized flavone biosynthetic pathway has evolved in the medicinal plant, Scutellaria baicalensis. *Science Advances, 2*(4), e1501780.
123. Liu, L. L., Wang, C. G., Dun, J. N., Chow, A. H. L., & Sun, C. C. (2018). Lack of dependence of mechanical properties of baicalein cocrystals on those of the constituent components. *CrystEngComm, 20*(37), 5486–5489.
124. Ojarinta, R., Saarinen, J., Strachan, C. J., Korhonen, O., & Laitinen, R. (2018). Preparation and characterization of multi-component tablets containing co-amorphous salts: Combining multimodal non-linear optical imaging with established analytical methods. *European Journal of Pharmaceutics and Biopharmaceutics, 132*, 112–126.
125. Petry, I., Lobmann, K., Grohganz, H., Rades, T., & Leopold, C. S. (2017). Solid state properties and drug release behavior of co-amorphous indomethacin-arginine tablets coated with Kollicoat(R) Protect. *European Journal of Pharmaceutics and Biopharmaceutics, 119*, 150–160.
126. Wang, C. G., Perumalla, S. R., Lu, R. L., Fang, J. G., & Sun, C. C. (2016). Sweet berberine. *Crystal Growth & Design, 16*(2), 933–939.
127. Aitipamula, S., Chow, P. S., & Tan, R. B. H. (2009). Dimorphs of a 1:1 cocrystal of ethenzamide and saccharin: Solid-state grinding methods result in metastable polymorph. *CrystEngComm, 11*(5), 889–895.
128. Basavoju, S., Bostrom, D., & Velaga, S. P. (2008). Indomethacin-saccharin cocrystal: Design, synthesis and preliminary pharmaceutical characterization. *Pharmaceutical Research, 25*(3), 530–541.

129. Bhatt, P. M., Ravindra, N. V., Banerjee, R., & Desiraju, G. R. (2005). Saccharin as a salt former. Enhanced solubilities of saccharinates of active pharmaceutical ingredients. *Chemical Communications, 8*, 1073–1075.
130. Lu, E., Rodriguez-Hornedo, N., & Suryanarayanan, R. (2008). A rapid thermal method for cocrystal screening. *CrystEngComm, 10*(6), 665–668.
131. Bolla, G., & Nangia, A. (2016). Pharmaceutical cocrystals: Walking the talk. *Chemical Communications, 52*, 8342–8360.
132. Fong, S. Y., Liu, M., Wei, H., Lobenberg, R., Kanfer, I., Lee, V. H., Amidon, G. L., & Zuo, Z. (2013). Establishing the pharmaceutical quality of Chinese herbal medicine: A provisional BCS classification. *Molecular Pharmaceutics, 10*(5), 1623–1643.
133. Sanphui, P., Devi, V. K., Clara, D., Malviya, N., Ganguly, S., & Desiraju, G. R. (2015). Cocrystals of hydrochlorothiazide: Solubility and diffusion/permeability enhancements through drug-coformer interactions. *Molecular Pharmaceutics, 12*(5), 1615–1622.
134. Yan, Y., Chen, J. M., & Lu, T. B. (2013). Simultaneously enhancing the solubility and permeability of acyclovir by crystal engineering approach. *CrystEngComm, 15*(33), 6457–6460.
135. Bommaka, M. K., Mannava, M. K. C., Suresh, K., Gunnam, A., & Nangia, A. (2018). Entacapone: Improving aqueous solubility, diffusion permeability, and cocrystal stability with theophylline. *Crystal Growth & Design, 18*(10), 6061–6069.
136. Khajuria, A., Thusu, N., & Zutshi, U. (2002). Piperine modulates permeability characteristics of intestine by inducing alterations in membrane dynamics: Influence on brush border membrane fluidity, ultrastructure and enzyme kinetics. *Phytomedicine, 9*(3), 224–231.
137. Di, X., Wang, X., Di, X., & Liu, Y. (2015). Effect of piperine on the bioavailability and pharmacokinetics of emodin in rats. *Journal of Pharmaceutical and Biomedical Analysis, 115*, 144–149.
138. Izutsu, K. I., Koide, T., Takata, N., Ikeda, Y., Ono, M., Inoue, M., Fukami, T., & Yonemochi, E. (2016). Characterization and quality control of pharmaceutical cocrystals. *Chemical & Pharmaceutical Bulletin, 64*(10), 1421–1430.
139. Shemchuk, O., Esposti, L. D., Grepioni, F., & Braga, D. (2017). Ionic co-crystals of enantiopure and racemic histidine with calcium halides. *CrystEngComm, 19*(42), 6267–6273.
140. Harris, K. D. M., Tremayne, M., & Kariuki, B. M. (2001). Contemporary advances in the use of powder X-ray diffraction for structure determination. *Angewandte Chemie. International Edition, 40*(9), 1626–1651.
141. Zhu, B. Q., Zhang, Q., Wang, J. R., & Mei, X. F. (2017). Cocrystals of baicalein with higher solubility and enhanced bioavailability. *Crystal Growth & Design, 17*(4), 1893–1901.
142. Bates, S., Zografi, G., Engers, D., Morris, K., Crowley, K., & Newman, A. (2006). Analysis of amorphous and nanocrystalline solids from their X-ray diffraction patterns. *Pharmaceutical Research, 23*(10), 2333–2349.
143. Qian, S., Li, Z., Heng, W., Liang, S., Ma, D., Gao, Y., Zhang, J., & Wei, Y. (2016). Charge-assisted intermolecular hydrogen bond formed in coamorphous system is important to relieve the pH-dependent solubility behavior of lurasidone hydrochloride. *RSC Advances, 6*(108), 106396–106412.
144. Forster, A., Hempenstall, J., Tucker, & Rades, T. (2001). The potential of small-scale fusion experiments and the Gordon-Taylor equation to predict the suitability of drug/polymer blends for melt extrusion. *Drug Development and Industrial Pharmacy, 27*(6), 549–560.
145. Hong, C., Xie, Y., Yao, Y. S., Li, G. W., Yuan, X. R., & Shen, H. Y. (2015). A novel strategy for pharmaceutical cocrystal generation without knowledge of stoichiometric ratio: Myricetin cocrystals and a ternary phase diagram. *Pharmaceutical Research, 32*(1), 47–60.
146. Huang, S., Xue, Q., Xu, J., Ruan, S. D., & Cai, T. (2019). Simultaneously improving the physicochemical properties, dissolution performance, and bioavailability of apigenin and daidzein by co-crystallization with theophylline. *Journal of Pharmaceutical Sciences, 108*(9), 2982–2993.

147. Vogt, F. G., Clawson, J. S., Strohmeier, M., Edwards, A. J., Pham, T. N., & Watson, S. A. (2009). Solid-state NMR analysis of organic cocrystals and complexes. *Crystal Growth & Design, 9*(2), 921–937.
148. Maruyoshi, K., Iuga, D., Antzutkin, O. N., Alhalaweh, A., Velaga, S. P., & Brown, S. P. (2012). Identifying the intermolecular hydrogen-bonding supramolecular synthons in an indomethacin-nicotinamide cocrystal by solid-state NMR. *Chemical Communications, 48*(88), 10844–10846.
149. Heng, W. L., Su, M. L., Cheng, H., Shen, P. Y., Liang, S. J., Zhang, L. H., Wei, Y. F., Gao, Y., Zhang, J. J., & Qian, S. (2020). Incorporation of complexation into a coamorphous system dramatically enhances dissolution and eliminates gelation of amorphous lurasidone hydrochloride. *Molecular Pharmaceutics, 17*(1), 84–97.
150. Ghosh, S., Mondal, A., Kiran, M. S. R. N., Ramamurty, U., & Reddy, C. M. (2013). The role of weak interactions in the phase transition and distinct mechanical behavior of two structurally similar caffeine co-crystal polymorphs studied by nanoindentation. *Crystal Growth & Design, 13*(10), 4435–4441.
151. Joshi, T. V., Singaraju, A. B., Shah, H. S., Morris, K. R., Stevens, L. L., & Haware, R. V. (2018). Structure-mechanics and compressibility profile study of flufenamic acid:nicotinamide cocrystal. *Crystal Growth & Design, 18*(10), 5853–5865.
152. Darwish, S., Zeglinski, J., Krishna, G. R., Shaikh, R., Khraisheh, M., Walker, G. M., & Croker, D. M. (2018). A new 1:1 drug-drug cocrystal of theophylline and aspirin: Discovery, characterization, and construction of ternary phase diagrams. *Crystal Growth & Design, 18*(12), 7526–7532.
153. Malecka, M., Checinska, L., Kusz, J., Biernacka, M., & Kupcewicz, B. (2020). Interactions in flavanone and chalcone derivatives: Hirshfeld surface analysis, energy frameworks and global reactivity descriptors. *Acta Crystallographica Section C: Structural Chemistry, 76*(Pt 3), 212–224.
154. Wang, C., & Sun, C. C. (2019). Computational techniques for predicting mechanical properties of organic crystals: A systematic evaluation. *Molecular Pharmaceutics, 16*(4), 1732–1741.
155. Turner, M. J., Thomas, S. P., Shi, M. W., Jayatilaka, D., & Spackman, M. A. (2015). Energy frameworks: Insights into interaction anisotropy and the mechanical properties of molecular crystals. *Chemical Communications, 51*(18), 3735–3738.

Chapter 12
Application of Insoluble Excipients in Solid Dispersion of Chinese Medicines

Hangyi Wu, Huixia Lv, and Zhenhai Zhang

Abstract In recent years, as the great success of arteannuin in the area of antimalarial treatment and commercial benefit, traditional Chinese medicine (TCM) has received great attention. However, most of the active pharmaceutical ingredients (API) of Chinese medicines are hydrophobic, which causes the low oral bioavailability of Chinese medicine and extremely limits their application. To ameliorate the solubility of the hydrophobic ingredients, many strategies have been developed. Solid dispersion is considered as dosage forms with good industrial feasibility, and some of the solid dispersions have been already commercially available. In the technologies/researches of solid dispersions, excipients play a vital role by affecting the interaction of excipients-drugs and the in vitro and in vivo fate of preparations by influencing the preparation process, stability, dissolution, and finally absorption and then enhancing the oral bioavailability. Most of the researches and commercially available productions of solid dispersion focused on the hydrophilic excipients such as PEG, PVP, etc. However, some of the hydrophobic excipients used in the solid dispersions could lead to unexpected result such as improvement of the dissolution rate, the fluidity, and the storage stability of the powder and then increase the feasibility of further industrial processing into solid dosage form of tablets or capsules. Thus, here we focus on the application of hydrophobic excipients in solid dispersion of Chinese medicine and elaborate it from three aspects including excipient types, preparation methods, and application forms.

Keywords Solid dispersion · Insoluble excipients · Chinese medicine · Preparation method · Application form

---

H. Wu · H. Lv
Department of Pharmaceutics, China Pharmaceutical University, Nanjing, China

Z. Zhang (✉)
Jiangsu Province Academy of Traditional Chinese Medicine, Nanjing, China

Affiliated Hospital of Integrated Traditional Chinese and Western Medicine, Nanjing University of Chinese Medicine, Nanjing, China
e-mail: 1020040766@cpu.edu.cn

N. Feng, Z. Yang (eds.), *Novel Drug Delivery Systems for Chinese Medicines*,
https://doi.org/10.1007/978-981-16-3444-4_12

12.1 Introduction

The Chinese medicine is mainly composed of botanical medicine (root, stem, leaf, and fruit), animal medicine (viscera, skin, bone, organ, etc.), and mineral medicine. Its API with pharmacological effects generally has already been extracted and purified for the treatment of diseases. In recent years, TCM has been recognized internationally and got extensive research, benefiting from the in-depth studies and clinical application of some API such as arteannuin, hydroxycamptothecin, resveratrol, berberine, curcumin, etc. (TCM-related commercial products such as dihydroartemisinin tablets). Chinese medicine is derived from natural products and generally considered as low toxicity. However, compared with chemical compounds, the components of Chinese medicine are more complex, which increases the difficulty of new medical research and development. Furthermore, patients generally need to take larger doses because of the lower purity, solubility, and absorption of Chinese medicines. All of these restrictions prevent Chinese medicine from clinical application worldwide. Therefore, it is an urgent need to apply modern formulation technology to solve those problems.

With the development of pharmaceutics of Chinese medicine, TCM products are not only limited to traditional dosage forms of Chinese medicines such as powders and decoctions but also have been successively prepared into modern ones. Liposomes, micelles, microemulsions, nanoparticles, solid lipid nanoparticles, nanostructure lipid carriers, inorganic nanoparticles, etc. have been reported to process the API. Active targeting strategies and even biomimetic methods are developed. These efforts can significantly improve the solubility of API, ameliorate the bioavailability of drugs, extend the systemic circulation time, promote the cellular uptake, as well as reduce systemic toxicity. In this chapter, we will introduce the application of solid dispersion technology in Chinese medicine preparations.

Solid dispersions have been defined as dispersion form with one or more API in an inert matrix or carrier at the solid state. The API in solid dispersions can be detached into separate molecules, amorphous particles, or crystalline particles by the carrier in the crystalline or amorphous state. Extensive research on solid dispersions has been published, showing significant advantages in reducing particle size, enhancing wettability and porosity, as well as changing drug crystalline state preferably into an amorphous state, which in turn lead to improved solubility and dissolution rate of poorly water-soluble API and improved stability of drugs. Moreover, compared with other novel drug carrier systems such as nano-preparation, the preparation process of solid dispersion is more simple and feasible in the commercial process.

Despite solid dispersions have multiple advantages, the number of commercially available products prepared by solid dispersion technology is not as many as expected. This is mainly due to the challenges in the scale-up preparation process, physicochemical instability of drugs, and excipients with aging during the period of storage. In addition, the amount of hydrophilic excipients as carriers in solid dispersion is large, which might make an already large dosage of Chinese medicine even larger and low compliance even lower, while the necessary amount of insoluble excipients in solid dispersions is less than that of aqueous ones. Thus, compared with hydrophilic excipients, the hydrophobic excipients used in solid dispersion may lead to a better solution to industrialization and compliance problems.

At present, water-insoluble excipients have been also applied in the solid dispersion of Chinese medicines, and some of them have been proved to have potential, such as mesoporous silica and hydroxyapatite. Water-insoluble excipients versatilely improve the dissolution of poorly soluble drugs, including by increasing the specific surface area and attaching apparent groups. They can also ameliorate the feasibility of industrial preparation by reducing the viscosity and optimizing the fluidity of the powder. Many conventional methods for preparing solid dispersions are also suitable for the application of insoluble excipients in solid dispersion of Chinese medicine. This article will introduce the insoluble excipients, preparation technologies, and application forms of Chinese medicine solid dispersions.

12.2 Insoluble Excipients of Solid Dispersions

Some water-insoluble excipients have been used in solid dispersions including silica, hydroxyapatite, calcium carbonate, cellulose, and super disintegrate.

12.2.1 Silica

Silica is primarily used as an excipient for improving powder fluidity in solid dosage forms such as tablets, capsules, and granules [1]. But in recent years, it was utilized in solid dispersions owing to its brilliant capacity for improving the formed solid dispersion's dispersibility, fluidity, and stability.

Silica is generally considered as a safe excipient in oral administration (LD50 oral rat, 3.16 g/kg) [2, 3]. Silica has a nano-sized particle with a large specific surface area [1, 4]. Meanwhile, many silanol groups are present on the surface of silica nanoparticles, which enable to form hydrogen bonds with the drug molecules [4]. Furthermore, silica can increase the wettability of drug particles to achieve a high drug dissolution rate [2]. Using silica as a carrier of solid dispersion could enhance API's dispersion ability and decrease its particle size even to the molecular level [3]. Furthermore, silica can prevent drugs from recrystallization and then improve the physical stability of solid dispersions [5]. Yan et al. [4] reported that solid dispersion with porous silica presented much more stability than the tanshinone IIA alone, showing no significant decrease in either the in vitro dissolution or the drug content during the stability study at room temperature for 12 months. Furthermore, the formed solid dispersion with silica can significantly enhance oral bioavailability, compared to the crystalline drug [3]. Jiang et al. [3] approximately doubled the dissolution rate of tanshinone IIA by the solid dispersion with silica and significantly improved oral bioavailability. Moreover, commercial silica has different types with different particle size, pore structure, and degree of hydrophilicity and hydrophobicity, which can regulate the dissolution rate as a carrier of solid dispersion [6, 7].

Compared with the water-soluble excipients such as polyvinyl pyrrolidone (PVP) and polyethylene glycol (PEG) [8], silica can reduce the stickiness of intermediate materials of solid dispersion, which can decrease the amount of other excipients and obtain good flowability of powders and then facilitate the subsequent processing of final dosage form such as capsules and tablets [3, 8].

12.2.2 Hydroxyapatite

Hydroxyapatite (HA), a weakly alkaline calcium phosphate, is the main component of bones and teeth of vertebrates, showing excellent biocompatibility as the excipient of solid dispersions [9]. The surface of HA can be fully bonded to human tissues, which makes HA partially or completely absorbed by the human body. And when it was used in the oral administration, part of the HA can be degraded, while the other will be excreted in the form of nanoparticle. Herein, HA is considered non-toxic and can possibly be used as a safe and effective drug carrier [9, 10].

Nano-porous HA has a large specific surface area with linking the hydrophilic groups such as phosphate and hydroxyl groups [11, 12], which endows itself a strong adsorption capacity for drugs and also makes it easy to introduce the other molecules to form HA derivatives for achieving special functions [13, 14]. When solid dispersions are prepared by nano-porous HA, the particle size of the insoluble drug can be significantly reduced, and its dispersibility will be greatly improved. The drug exists in the solid dispersion as a molecular, amorphous, or microcrystalline state, which can accelerate the dissolution rate in the gastrointestinal tract. Furthermore, solid dispersions with HA have good adhesion, which can prolong the residence time in the gastrointestinal tract, thereby improving the bioavailability of the drug. HA also can be used to enhance the stability of solid dispersions [10, 13]. Hu et al. [10] reported that solid dispersions with HA could significantly improve the stability and dissolution rate of andrographolide and prevent the solid dispersion from aging. This is because its large specific surface area and the hydroxyl groups on the surface of HA which can form hydrogen bonds with drugs or biological tissues bring itself better adsorption and bioadhesion. Yan et al. [13] also enhanced the properties of the dissolution rate and stability of tanshinone IIA by solid dispersion-employed nano-hydroxyapatite. Similar to silica, the size, morphology, and shape of nano-porous HA can be controlled by different preparation methods and reaction conditions [15]. Benefiting from this, different kinds of nano-porous HA can be screened to meet the different requirements and to regulate drug release up to our expectation. Moreover, HA is worth developing as an excipient of solid dispersions because it is cheap and easy to prepare for solid dispersions.

12.2.3 Calcium Carbonate

Calcium carbonate is widely used in the medical field as an inexpensive dietary calcium supplement for a gastric antacid. It is also applied for the pharmaceutical industry as an inert excipient for tablets and other pharmaceuticals. There are three types of calcium carbonate used as a carrier of solid dispersion, precipitated calcium carbonate (PCC), ground calcium carbonate (GCC), and mesoporous calcium carbonate (MCC).

PCC is an inorganic chemical product. It is regarded as a monodisperse powder due to its relatively regular particle shape and small particle size with narrow particle size distribution. Commonly water-soluble solid dispersion excipients such as PVP and pluronic F68 are mostly from chemical synthesis, which cause the concern of residual reagents. However, PCC has not this worry. In addition, PCC is cheap, easy to obtain, and mature in production technology. It can be applied as a neutralizer, buffer, and solubilizer for pharmaceutical products, as well as a supplement for fillers [16]. Yan et al. [17] reported that the accumulated dissolution rate of oleanolic acid in solid dispersion with PCC as a carrier was up to 90% at 45 min and the release profit was not reduced after storing over 6 months. These reports proved that PCC, as an excipient of solid dispersion, can enhance the dissolution rate and has favorable store stability.

GCC has been widely used as an adjuvant in solid dosage forms, especially as a diluent in dissolution for dispersible tablets [18]. It is a natural and economic element with a bright potential for pharmaceutical drug use in developing countries. Ana et al. [19] reported that GCC in the solid dispersion could provoke a conformational change in the praziquantel molecule which was tentatively assigned into a disordered pseudoracemate solid phase. This is due to the interaction of the carbonyl groups of praziquantel with calcium carbonate. The solvation water of Ca^{2+} probably forms hydrogen bonds with the carbonyl group. Then, the hydrated cyclohexyl-carbonyl group can connect to another praziquantel molecule to form the hemihydrate enantiomer crystal. The conformational change might lead to a supernumerary bonus in the dissolution.

In recent years, mesoporous inorganic materials have obtained considerable attention as prospective oral drug carriers to improve the solubility and dissolution properties of hydrophobic drugs. After adsorption to the nano-pores or conjunction to the surface of inorganic carriers, the drug was loaded as an amorphous state, leading to an enhanced in vitro dissolution rate. The mesoporous silica is struggling with high manufacturing costs and environmental concerns due to the use of expensive and/or toxic surfactants. Similar to mesoporous silica, mesoporous calcium carbonate (MCC) is also considered as a prospective drug carrier for oral administration due to its porous structure and relatively large specific surface area, ability to protect encapsulated drugs, and especially excellent biocompatibility and biodegradability [20, 21]. Moreover, the synthesis of MCC is economically applicable and environmentally friendly. Zhang et al. [22] reported that solid dispersion with hydroxypropyl-β-cyclodextrin functionalized MCC could improve the solubility and oral bioavailability of irbesartan. The mean peak plasma concentration and the area under the mean plasma concentration-time curve for 48 h of irbesartan-loaded hydroxypropyl-β-cyclodextrin functionalized MCC were 1.56-fold and 1.52-fold higher than that of the commercial product, respectively.

12.2.4 Cellulose and Cellulose Derivatives

Cellulose, as the chief structural component of plants, is the most abundant biopolymer in the world. Cellulose is highly hydrophilic. However, it is insoluble in water due to its strong inter-molecular and intra-molecular hydrogen bonding between chains and the high degree of crystallinity.

Cellulose and its derivatives play an important role in the stabilization of amorphous solid dispersions due to the polymeric matrix which can hold the drug in an amorphous form and inhibit its crystallization [23]. This remarkable property may also benefit from their high molecular weights and resistance to hydrolysis, which limits the absorption of the most cellulose derivatives from the GI tract. Even if the derivatives were hydrolyzed by chemical or lipase-catalyzed hydrolysis, the obtained by-products would be endogenous or dietary. Herein, the cellulose derivatives are considered safer compared with the synthetic excipients. Moreover, the strong interactions between drugs and polymers and the high glass transition temperatures make cellulose and its derivatives more credible as the stabilizers for amorphous solid dispersion [24].

In recent years, cellulose derivatives with a special function of pH-responsive drug release have been considered attractive. Cellulose containing carboxyl groups can remain unionized at the acidic pH, which prevents drug release in gastric [25]. The derivatives structurally modified with pendent carboxylic acids enable the drug to be triggered release in the intestine. Hydroxypropylmethylcellulose acetylsuccinate (HPMCAS) is the most widely studied derivative in this category as an amorphous solid dispersion excipient. For example, Bin et al. [26] reported that solid dispersion with HPMCAS could stabilize resveratrol against crystallization and trigger the drug release in the small intestine. Compared with poly (vinylpyrrolidinone), HPMCAS leaks less at pH 1.2, making it an attractive candidate for preparing solid dispersions.

12.2.5 Superdisintegrant

Disintegrants can facilitate dispersion or breakup of tablets and capsules into smaller fragments, which significantly improves the dissolution of cargos [27]. Compared with common disintegrants, superdisintegrants show stronger disintegration effects with low doses, which can resolve the compliance issues caused by large doses of Chinese medicine. Those superdisintegrants now were developed and applied for

Table 12.1 Insoluble excipients of solid dispersions

Insoluble excipients	Functions and advantages	Reference
Silica	Large specific surface area, abundant silanol groups, increasing the wettability and dispersion ability of drugs, improving powder fluidity, reducing the stickiness of intermediate materials, facilitating the subsequent processing of final dosage form	[1–8]
Hydroxyapatite	Excellent biocompatibility, large specific surface area, abundant phosphate and hydroxyl groups, good adhesion in the gastrointestinal tract	[9–15]
Calcium carbonate	Excellent biocompatibility, no residual reagents, cheap, easy to obtain, mature in production technology, able to be applied as a neutralizer, buffer, and solubilizer	[16–22]
Cellulose	Safe, stable, endogenous, or dietary by-products, be able to functionalized and controlled release	[23–26]
Superdisintegrant	Significantly improve dissolution, low doses, swelling and water absorption synergy, promoting the wettability and dispersibility, not irritating to the GI tract, advantages of flowability and crushing	[27–34]
Eudragit S100	Sustained release, colonic delivery, protect gastric mucosa from drug irritation	[36]

Chinese medicine solid dispersions including porous starch [28], sodium starch glycolate (SSG) [29, 30], low-substituted hydroxypropyl cellulose [31, 32], acid-polyvinylpolypyrrolidone (PVPP) [33], croscarmellose sodium (CCS), and crospovidone (CP) [34].

Superdisintegrants perform quick disintegration due to the synergy of swelling and water absorption. They can increase the wetted surface of the carrier to promote the wettability and dispersibility of the system, thus facilitating the disintegration and dissolution rate [27]. In addition, superdisintegrants are not irritating to the GI tract. And utilized as the carriers of solid dispersion, they can help disperse the drug into an amorphous state and inhibit drug recrystallization. Moreover, there are certain superiorities in the subsequent processing of shaping into tablets due to the bonus of outstanding flowability and the advantage of crushing.

In addition to the above terms, insoluble excipients such as hydrogenated phosphatidylcholine (HPC) [35], Eudragit S100 [36], etc. have also been made into solid dispersions efficiently.

In summary, water-insoluble excipients can (1) effectively disperse the drugs to form amorphous solid dispersions, increase the solubility and dissolution rate of drugs, and thereby improve the oral bioavailability. (2) Furthermore, they can reduce the viscosity of the solid dispersions, increase the flowability of the intermediate powder, and then be beneficial to the subsequent industrial processing of solid preparations. (3) Moreover, these insoluble ingredients as the carrier of solid dispersions can improve the storage stability of the formulation so as to partly dissolve the problem of aging of solid preparations. The advantages of water-insoluble excipients are summarized in Table 12.1.

12.3 Preparation Methods of Solid Dispersion with Insoluble Excipients

The methods for preparing solid dispersions can be roughly divided into the following categories: melting method, solvent method, melting-solvent method, and some specific methods.

12.3.1 Melting Method

When using the melting method, the drug and the carrier are firstly heated over the eutectic point temperature to fuse, and then cool them down by putting into ice bath, agitation, or immersing in liquid nitrogen to quickly freeze. Next, the resultant mixture is crushed and sieved to reduce its particle size for subsequent processing. An important prerequisite for this method is that the drug and the carrier are miscible under heating conditions to obtain a homogeneous mixture. Herein, a rational carrier should have similar physicochemical properties to the cargos. The advantage of this method is that it works without any solvents.

Despite being frequently used, the melting method has some significant limitations. This method struggles with the compatibility and miscibility of the drug and the carrier. The incompatibility may cause phase separation, and the high viscosity of the mixture under melting may obstruct the mixing, leading to inhomogeneous dispersion. Fortunately, this phenomenon can partly be solved by using a surfactant. The phase separation can also be minimized by rapidly cooling to make the resultant into amorphous solid dispersion rather than a mild mode related to the crystalline one. Spray congealing technology is often used in conjunction with the melting method for rapidly cooling [37]. Another limitation worth pondering is the thermal stability of drugs at high temperatures. It may be a way out by dispersing the drug into a previously molten carrier due to the reduction of the drug's healing time and the process temperature.

Hot-melt extrusion is one of the most popular melting methods developed in the recent year because of its "one-step" feature. By this method, the drug and the excipient can be mixed, melted, homogenized, and extruded into the pre-set form programmatically [38]. During the preparation process, the stirring of rotating screw accompanied by extra heat disperses the mixture uniformly, making it inclined to form an amorphous solid dispersion. Compared with the traditional melting method, the hot-melt extrusion method can shorten the exposure time of the mixture at elevated temperature, hence reducing the degradation of thermolabile drugs. Furthermore, this method is considered continuous and efficient, while it does well in easy scale-up [39].

12.3.2 Solvent Method

It is named solvent method that the drug and carrier are dissolved in a solvent and then the solvent is removed to obtain a solid phase resultant which is ready for subsequent processing. This method was developed mainly for the thermolabile API because the drug and carrier are dissolved by a solvent instead of heating as in the melting method. Compositions with a high melting point can also be applied in this method.

This method also has its prerequisite manifested as the sufficient solubility of the drug and carrier in a volatile solvent for homogeneous mixing [40]. Sometimes, it is difficult to find a suitable non-toxic solvent due to the difference in physicochemical properties of the compositions [41]. Surfactants can be used as an additive to improve solubility. However, the amount of additives needs to be carefully considered because excess dosage may mutate the matrix structure. Another limitation of this method is the residual solvent problem as it is nearly impossible to remove the solvent completely which may cause toxicity. In addition, the residual solvent may lower the glass transition temperature and plasticize the system, further leading to phase separation. Furthermore, the solvent method is a little dim due to its large environmental issues and high production cost. Herein, melting method especially hot-melt extrusion is more advantageous to prepare solid dispersions, compared with the solvent method, if the thermal stability of compositions is ensured during the process.

Similarly, the solidification rate in the solvent method affects the crystalline state of API, showing that a rapid solidification process symbolizes the formation of an amorphous solid dispersion [42]. Several drying technologies for removing volatile solvents are introduced below.

12.3.2.1 Rotary Evaporation and Vacuum Drying

Rotary evaporation and vacuum drying are commonly used in drying technologies. Rotary evaporation removes most of the solvent, while vacuum drying is a response to the residual part. These methods are easy to perform, but their processes are all quite long and might easily result in phase separation and recrystallization.

12.3.2.2 Spray Drying Technology

Spray drying technology can effectively shorten the drying time. In this technology, the solution is sprayed from the nozzle and forms countless fine droplets, which increases the specific surface area and thus improves the drying rate. The resultants prepared by the spray drying method are often in an amorphous state. In addition, customizable particle size and size distribution, continuity, and stability of manufacturing, as well as cost-effectiveness, are all achieved by the spray drying method [43–45].

12.3.2.3 Freeze-Drying

Freeze-drying is a potential drying method because of its gift in controlling phase separation and reducing the degradation of thermolabile drugs. This method consists of freezing and lyophilization. There are also several disadvantages. Most organic solvents have low freezing temperatures and can't be frozen during sublimation. In addition, if glass formation is required, the sample temperature must be maintained below the glass transition temperature of the frozen concentrated fraction. The drying process is long and takes even a few days. Fortunately, some cryogenic processing technologies such as spray freeze-drying (SFD) and ultra-rapid freezing (URF) can significantly enhance the freezing rate compared with freeze-drying technology.

SFD, as a potential drying technique, is the process of spraying the solution of the drug and polymer into/on liquid nitrogen or cold-dry air and lyophilizing the frozen droplets subsequently [46]. The large specific surface area and direct contact with the cooling agents lead to rapid freezing rate and prevent molecular arrangement into crystalline domains [47–49]. SFD can also customize the particle size to satisfy the further processing or applications. Van Drooge et al. [50] proved that the stability of tetrahydrocannabinol-inulin solid dispersion prepared by SFD was significantly better than that of freeze-drying solid dispersion due to the higher cooling rate of SFD, especially at high drug loads.

12.3.2.4 Electrostatic Spinning

Electrostatic spinning (electrospinning) can be considered as a combination of solid dispersion technology and nanotechnology. In this method, a polymeric fluid is jetted through a millimeter-scale nozzle, and solid fibers are produced by a strong electric field [51]. The main benefit of this technology is the extremely high ratio of surface area to fiber mass, which facilitates solvent evaporation and leads to the formation of amorphous dispersions [52]. The dissolution of the resultant is significantly improved by nanosizing and amorphization [53]. It is worth mentioning that electrospinning process is simple and inexpensive. The schematic of electrostatic spinning is shown in Fig. 12.1.

12.3.3 Solubility Adjustment Method

Co-precipitation is a suitable technology for preparing solid dispersions of poorly water-soluble drugs with high melting points and low solubility in organic solvents,

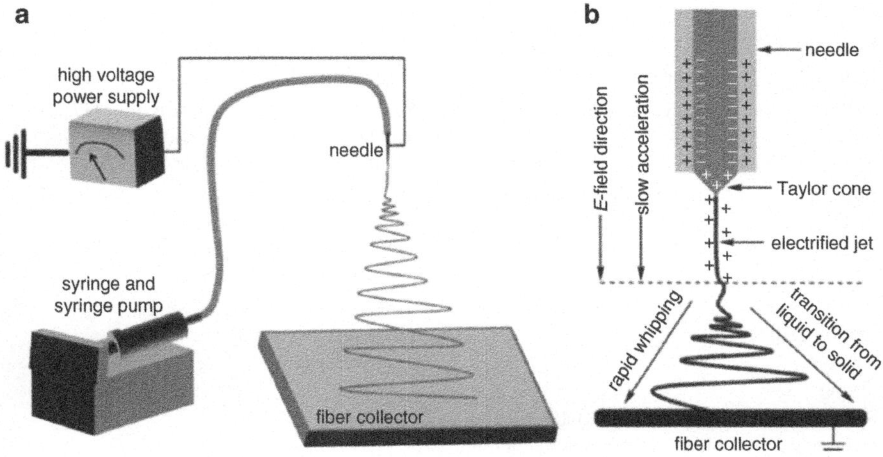

Fig. 12.1 A schematic of (**a**) basic setup and (**b**) process of electrospinning. (Reprinted with permission from Ref. [54]. Copyright 2014 Springer Publishing Company)

which can't be produced by melting methods and other solvent methods [55]. In this method, the drug and carrier are firstly dissolved in an organic solvent, and an anti-solvent which causes simultaneous precipitation of the compositions is added. Then, the resultant is filtered and washed to remove the residual solvent. The solvents selected in this method can be less volatile and removed by aqueous solutions. However, the solvent and anti-solvent mixture may act as plasticizers causing high molecular mobility and crystallization [56].

Another solubility adjustment method is supercritical fluid (SCF) technology. A supercritical fluid is used as a solvent to dissolve the drug and carrier and sprayed through a nozzle into an expanded state with lower solubility, leading to rapid nucleation of the precipitation with a desirable size distribution. Supercritical carbon dioxide (CO_2) is generally used in the SCF method. Supercritical CO_2 has a low critical temperature (31.04 °C) and critical pressure (7.38 MPa) that gives great SCF prominence to eco-friendliness and non-toxicity for environment [57]. In addition, SCF can also be used as an anti-solvent to extract solvent from other solutions to form solid dispersion.

12.3.4 Melting-Solvent Method

The melting-solvent method is a hybrid of the melting method and solvent method first reported by Goldberg et al. [58]. This method is suitable for drugs with a high melting point. Here, drugs are firstly dissolved in a suitable solvent and then mixed with a molten carrier followed by removing solvent and solidification into solid dispersions. This method can reduce the temperature and time of mixing in comparison with the melting method, efficiently protecting drugs from thermal

Table 12.2 The preparation methods of solid dispersion with insoluble excipients

Preparation methods	Advantages	Disadvantages	Reference
Melting method	No solvents, convenience, low cost	Possible to be phase separation or inhomogeneous dispersion, unsuitable for thermolabile API	[37]
Solvent method	Mainly for the thermolabile API	Difficult to find a suitable non-toxic solvent, residual solvent, large environmental issues, and high production cost	[40–47]
Rotary evaporation and vacuum drying	Easy to perform and have few restrictions	Time consuming, possible to be phase separation and recrystallization	
Spray drying technology	Complete in seconds, customizable particle property, continuity and stability of manufacturing, cost-effectiveness		
Freeze-drying	Control phase separation and reduce the degradation of thermolabile drugs	Low freezing temperatures of most organic solvents and disable to be frozen during sublimation, time-consuming	
Electrostatic spinning	Easy to the formation of amorphous dispersions, significantly improve dissolution, simple and low cost		
Solubility adjustment method			[48–50]
Co-precipitation	Suitable for poorly water-soluble drugs with high melting points and low solubility in organic solvents	Possible to cause high molecular mobility and crystallization	
Supercritical fluid technology	Environmentally friendly, lack of toxicity, and inflammability	Non-economic applicability	
Melting-solvent method	Reduce the temperature and time of mixing and efficiently protect drugs from thermal degradation compared with the melting method; the carrier in the molten state can be dispersed and dissolved in the solvent more easily compared with the solvent method	Both in melting method and solvent method	[51]

degradation. Furthermore, the carrier in the molten state can be dispersed and dissolved in the solvent more easily compared with the solvent method.

The preparation methods of solid dispersion with insoluble excipients are summarized in Table 12.2.

12.4 Application Form of Wxcipients

Excipients applied in solid dispersions can be generally divided into three forms: individual applications, auxiliary applications, and combined applications. Among them, the individual application form is the most common form, in which excipients utilizing their specific physicochemical properties affect the state of drugs through the excipient-drug interaction, thereby determining the in vivo fate of the drugs. The major purpose of most excipients in solid dispersions is to ameliorate the solubility and dissolution. However, not all the excipients are so perfect to fully upgrade the solid dispersions. Therefore, the resultants are frequently accompanied by in vivo and in vitro instability and/or difficulty in subsequent processing.

Auxiliary application refers to the application with two or more excipients simultaneously applied in one preparation, while the excipients are playing the same role. Despite working synergistically, the excipients may still feel weak in making up the deficiencies. For example, both sodium starch glycolate (Primojel®) and croscarmellose sodium (Ac-Di-Sol®) were used as superdisintegrants in the solid dispersion tablets, significantly improving the dissolution of fenofibrate, while the stability is not always satisfactory [30].

In contrast, the combined application is the most promising form, in which the most common rewards are increased drug stability and/or improved feasibility of industrial production. In the amorphous solid dispersion, carriers and drugs are highly dispersed with high Gibbs free energy, which tends to transform into a more stable crystalline state. Therefore, solid dispersions often face storage stability issues. Yan et al. [59] prepared tanshinone IIA solid dispersions with nano-$CaCO_3$ and poloxamer 188 as excipients. The results showed that solid dispersions with nano-$CaCO_3$ represented stable drug content and dissolution behavior over 6 months in comparison with freshly prepared SDs. In addition, despite excipients with the ability to enhance solubility and dissolution of drugs, the large stickiness, poor fluidity, and unsatisfactory tablet formability are still adverse to the manufacturing process. Insoluble excipients are sometimes added into the combined application preparations for solving these problems. For example, it was hypothesized that low-substituted hydroxypropyl cellulose dispersed into hypromellose acetate succinate-based solid dispersion tablets would improve the compressibility of the resultant, while the dissolution rate of nifedipine was extremely improved [31]. Apart from these, there are many other benefits of combined applications. Adding silica to the total *Epimedium* flavonoid (TEF) powder before being prepared into solid dispersion can effectively increase the dispersibility of TEF and make the solid dispersion more uniform, further enhancing the dissolution of the drug [28]. Zhang et al. reported that berberine solid dispersion composed of soybean lecithin (SPC), d-α-tocopheryl polyethylene glycol 1000 succinate (TPGS 1000), and silica gained significant improvement in cumulative dissolution percentages and relative bioavailability. In the study, SPC was employed to enhance the liposolubility of berberine, and TPGS 1000 played a dual role as improving the dissolution rate of SPC-berberine complex and as a P-gp inhibitor to increase the intestinal absorption of berberine, while silica was used to erase the side effect of poor flowability followed by TPGS 1000 [8].

In summary, both individual applications and auxiliary applications are committed to overcome one of the most critical barriers. The only difference is that auxiliary applications apply two or more excipients to collaboratively solve the problem more effectively, but auxiliary applications are still mediocre in other aspects. Unlike the above methods, combined applications utilize the advantages of several excipients to improve the formulation comprehensively, giving the solid dispersion increased solubility and dissolution, improved drug stability, and/or enhanced feasibility of industrial production. Herein, the combined application is considered as a potential method to ameliorate the properties of solid dispersions.

12.5 Conclusion

TCM is being recognized internationally, in which the pharmaceutics of Chinese medicine has played a key role. Up to now, there are not too much novel pharmaceutical technologies applied in this field. We still need to do much deeper work against the problem of Chinese medicine preparations such as overdose, low bioavailability, etc. Solid dispersion is an effective strategy to resolve the poor solubility and low bioavailability of Chinese medicines. Meanwhile, insoluble excipients used in the solid dispersions could stand out for their abilities in improving the solubility, dissolution, and stability of drugs, reducing the amount of auxiliary materials and the feasibility of the subsequence process. Thus, insoluble excipients and their applications in solid dispersions are worth doing further study and evaluation.

References

1. PlaninsEk, O., KovacIc, B., & VrecEr, F. (2011). Carvedilol dissolution improvement by preparation of solid dispersions with porous silica. *International Journal of Pharmaceutics, 406*(1–2), 41–48.
2. Cai, C., Liu, M., Li, Y., et al. (2016). A silica-supported solid dispersion of bifendate using supercritical carbon dioxide method with enhanced dissolution rate and oral bioavailability. *Drug Development and Industrial Pharmacy, 42*(3), 412–417.
3. Jiang, Y. R., Zhang, Z. H., Liu, Q. Y., et al. (2013). Preparation, characterization, and in vivo evaluation of tanshinone IIA solid dispersions with silica nanoparticles. *International Journal of Nanomedicine, 8*, 2285–2293.
4. Yan, H. M., Sun, E., Cui, L., et al. (2015). Improvement in oral bioavailability and dissolution of tanshinone IIA by preparation of solid dispersions with porous silica. *Journal of Pharmacy and Pharmacology, 67*(9), 1207–1214.
5. Yannian, H., Xiuhua, Z., Yuangang, Z., et al. (2019). Enhanced solubility and bioavailability of apigenin via preparation of solid dispersions of mesoporous silica nanoparticles. *Iranian Journal of Pharmaceutical Research, 18*(1), 168–182.

6. Chen, B., Wang, Z., et al. (2012). In vitro and in vivo evaluation of ordered mesoporous silica as a novel adsorbent in liquisolid formulation. *International Journal of Nanomedicine, 2012*, 199.
7. Du, X., & He, J. (2011). Spherical silica micro/nanomaterials with hierarchical structures: Synthesis and applications. *Nanoscale, 3*(10), 3984.
8. Zhang, Z., Chen, Y., Deng, J., et al. (2014). Solid dispersion of berberine–phospholipid complex/TPGS 1000/SiO2: Preparation, characterization and in vivo studies. *International Journal of Pharmaceutics, 465*(1–2), 306–316.
9. Curtin, C. M., Cunniffe, G. M., Lyons, F. G., et al. (2012). Innovative collagen nano-hydroxyapatite scaffolds offer a highly efficient non-viral gene delivery platform for stem cell-mediated bone formation. *Advanced Materials, 24*(6), 749–754.
10. Hu, S. Y., Zhang, Z. H., & Jia, X. B. (2013). [Study on andrographolide solid dispersion vectored by hydroxyapatite]. *Zhongguo Zhong Yao Za Zhi, 38*(3), 341–345.
11. Zhang, C., Li, C., Huang, S., et al. (2010). Self-activated luminescent and mesoporous strontium hydroxyapatite nanorods for drug delivery. *Biomaterials, 31*(12), 3374–3383.
12. Biomaterialia, A. (2010). In situ generation of sodium alginate/hydroxyapatite nanocomposite beads as drug-controlled release matrices. *Acta Biomaterialia, 6*(2), 445–454.
13. Jiang, Y. R., Zhang, Z. H., Huang, S. Y., et al. (2014). Enhanced dissolution and stability of Tanshinone IIA base by solid dispersion system with nano-hydroxyapatite. *Pharmacognosy Magazine, 10*(39), 332.
14. Mohsen-Nia, M., Bidgoli, M. M., Behrashi, M., et al. (2012). Human serum protein adsorption onto synthesis nano-hydroxyapatite. *Protein Journal, 31*(2), 150–157.
15. Yang, P., Quan, Z., Li, C., et al. (2008). Bioactive, luminescent and mesoporous europium-doped hydroxyapatite as a drug carrier. *Biomaterials, 29*(32), 4341–4347.
16. Fatehi, P., Hamdan, F. C., & Ni, Y. (2013). Adsorption of lignocelluloses of pre-hydrolysis liquor on calcium carbonate to induce functional filler. *Carbohydrate Polymers, 94*(1), 531–538.
17. Yan, H. M., Zhang, Z. H., Jia, X. B., et al. (2015) [Study on solid dispersion of precipitated calcium carbonate-based oleanolic acid]. *Zhongguo Zhong yao za zhi = Zhongguo zhongyao zazhi = China Journal of Chinese Materia Medica, 40*(10), 1935–1938.
18. Rowe, R. C., Sheskey, P. J., & Weller, P. J. (2009). *Handbook of pharmaceutical excipients* (6th ed.). Pharmaceutical Press.
19. Borrego-Sánchez, A., Carazo, E., Albertini, B., et al. (2018). Conformational polymorphic changes in the crystal structure of the chiral antiparasitic drug praziquantel and interactions with calcium carbonate. *European Journal of Pharmaceutics and Biopharmaceutics, 132*, 180–191.
20. Preisig, D., Haid, D., Varum, F. J. O., et al. (2014). Drug loading into porous calcium carbonate microparticles by solvent evaporation. *European Journal of Pharmaceutics and Biopharmaceutics, 87*(3), 548–558.
21. Svenskaya, Y., Parakhonskiy, B., Haase, A., et al. (2013). Anticancer drug delivery system based on calcium carbonate particles loaded with a photosensitizer. *Biophysical Chemistry, 182*, 11–15.
22. Zhang, L., Zhu, W., Lin, Q., et al. (2015). Hydroxypropyl-β-cyclodextrin functionalized calcium carbonate microparticles as a potential carrier for enhancing oral delivery of water-insoluble drugs. *International Journal of Nanomedicine, 10*, 3291–3302.
23. Brough, C., & Williams, R. O. (2013). Amorphous solid dispersions and nano-crystal technologies for poorly water-soluble drug delivery. *International Journal of Pharmaceutics, 453*(1), 157–166.
24. Chavan, R. B., Rathi, S., & Shastri, N. R. (2019). Cellulose based polymers in development of amorphous solid dispersions. *Asian Journal of Pharmaceutical Sciences, 14*, 248.
25. Liu, H., Taylor, L. S., & Edgar, K. J. (2015). The role of polymers in oral bioavailability enhancement; a review. *Polymer, 77*, 399.
26. Li, B., Wegiel, L. A., Taylor, L. S., et al. (2013). Stability and solution concentration enhancement of resveratrol by solid dispersion in cellulose derivative matrices. *Cellulose, 20*(3), 1249–1260.

27. Deshmkh, H., Nagesh, C., Murade, A., & Usgaunkar, S. (2012). Superdisintegrants: A recent investigation and current approach. *Asian Journal of Pharmacy and Technology, 2*, 19–25.
28. Yan, H.-M., Jia, X.-B., Zhang, Z.-H., Sun, E., & Xu, Y.-H. (2015). [Study on porous starch as solid dispersion carrier of total Epimedium flavonoids]. *China Journal of Materia Medica, 40*(9), 1723–1726.
29. Chaud, M. V., Lima, A. C., Vila, M. M. D. C., et al. (2013). Development and evaluation of praziquantel solid dispersions in sodium starch glycolate. *Tropical Journal of Pharmaceutical Research, 12*(2), 163–168.
30. Srinarong, P., Faber, J. H., Visser, M. R., et al. (2009). Strongly enhanced dissolution rate of fenofibrate solid dispersion tablets by incorporation of superdisintegrants. *European Journal of Pharmaceutics and Biopharmaceutics, 73*(1), 154–161.
31. Hughey, J. R., Keen, J. M., Bennett, R. C., et al. (2015). The incorporation of low-substituted hydroxypropyl cellulose into solid dispersion systems. *Drug Development and Industrial Pharmacy, 41*(8), 1294–1301.
32. Tascon-Otero, E., Torre-Iglesias, P., Garcia-Rodriguez, J. J., et al. (2019). Enhancement of the dissolution rate of indomethacin by solid dispersions in low-substituted hydroxypropyl cellulose. *Indian Journal of Pharmaceutical Sciences, 81*(5), 824–833.
33. Wang, W., Cui, C., Li, M., et al. (2017). Study of a novel disintegrable oleanolic acid-polyvinylpolypyrrolidone solid dispersion. *Drug Development and Industrial Pharmacy, 43*(7), 1178–1185.
34. Suthar, R. M., Chotai, N. P., Patel, H. K., Patel, S. R., Shah, D. D., & Jadeja, M. B. (2013). In vitro dissolution enhancement of ondansetron by solid dispersion in superdisintegrants. *Dissolution Technologies, 20*(4), 34–38.
35. Shi, C., Tong, Q., Fang, J., et al. (2015). Preparation, characterization and in vivo studies of amorphous solid dispersion of berberine with hydrogenated phosphatidylcholine. *European Journal of Pharmaceutical Sciences, 74*, 11–17.
36. Guo, S., Wang, G., Wu, T., et al. (2017). Solid dispersion of berberine hydrochloride and Eudragit® S100: Formulation, physicochemical characterization and cytotoxicity evaluation. *Journal of Drug Delivery Science and Technology, 40*, 21.
37. Passerini, N., Albertini, B., Perissutti, B., & Rodriguez, L. (2006). Evaluation of melt granulation and ultrasonic spray congealing as techniques to enhance the dissolution of praziquantel. *International Journal of Pharmaceutics, 318*, 92–102.
38. Verhoeven, E., De Beer, T., Schacht, E., Van den Mooter, G., Remon, J. P., & Vervaet, C. (2009). Influence of polyethylene glycol/polyethylene oxide on the release characteristics of sustained-release ethylcellulose mini-matrices produced by hot-melt extrusion: In vitro and in vivo evaluations. *European Journal of Pharmaceutics and Biopharmaceutics, 72*, 463–470.
39. Williams, M., Tian, Y., Jones, D. S., & Andrews, G. P. (2010). Hot-melt extrusion technology: Optimizing drug delivery. *European Journal of Parenteral and Pharmaceutical Sciences, 15*, 61.
40. Leuner, C., & Dressman, J. (2000). Improving drug solubility for oral delivery using solid dispersions. *European Journal of Pharmaceutics and Biopharmaceutics, 50*, 47–60.
41. Sahoo, N. G., Kakran, M., Li, L., Judeh, Z., & Müller, R. H. (2011). Dissolution enhancement of a poorly water-soluble antimalarial drug by means of a modified multi-fluid nozzle pilot spray drier. *Materials Science & Engineering, C: Materials for Biological Applications, 31*, 391–399.
42. Vo, L. N., Park, C., & Lee, B. J. (2013). Current trends and future perspectives of solid dispersions containing poorly water-soluble drugs. *European Journal of Pharmaceutics and Biopharmaceutics, 85*, 799–813.
43. Srinarong, P., de Waard, H., Frijlink, H. W., & Hinrichs, W. L. (2011). Improved dissolution behavior of lipophilic drugs by solid dispersions: The production process as starting point for formulation considerations. *Expert Opinion on Drug Delivery, 8*, 1121–1140.

44. Bikiaris, D. N. (2011). Solid dispersions, Part I: Recent evolutions and future opportunities in manufacturing methods for dissolution rate enhancement of poorly water-soluble drugs. *Expert Opinion on Drug Delivery, 8*, 1501–1519.
45. Dan Smithey, P. G., & Taylor, L. (2013). Amorphous solid dispersions: An enabling formulation technology for oral delivery of poorly water soluble drugs. *AAPS Newsmagazine, 16*, 11–14.
46. Purvis, T., Mattucci, M. E., Crisp, M. T., Johnston, K. P., & Williams, R. O. (2007). Rapidly dissolving repaglinide powders produced by the ultra-rapid freezing process. *AAPS PharmSciTech, 8*, E52–E60.
47. Hu, J. H., Rogers, T. L., Brown, J., Young, T., Johnston, K. P., & Williams, R. O. (2002). Improvement of dissolution rates of poorly water soluble APIs using novel spray freezing into liquid technology. *Pharmaceutical Research, 19*, 1278–1284.
48. Hu, J. H., Johnston, K. P., & Williams, R. O. (2003). Spray freezing into liquid (SFL) particle engineering technology to enhance dissolution of poorly water soluble drugs: Organic solvent versus organic/aqueous co-solvent systems. *European Journal of Pharmaceutical Sciences, 20*, 295–303.
49. Tong, H., Du, Z., Wang, G. N., Chan, H. M., Chang, Q., Lai, L., et al. (2011). Spray freeze drying with polyvinylpyrrolidone and sodium caprate for improved dissolution and oral bioavailability of oleanolic acid, a BCS Class IV compound. *International Journal of Pharmaceutics, 404*, 148–158.
50. Drooge, D. V., Hinrichs, W., Dickhoff, B., Elli, M., Visser, M., Zijlstra, G. S., et al. (2005). Spray freeze drying to produce a stable-tetrahydrocannabinol containing inulin-based solid dispersion powder suitable for inhalation, Spray freeze drying to produce a stable Δ9-tetrahydrocannabinol containing inulin-based solid dispersion powder suitable for inhalation. *European Journal of Pharmaceutical Sciences, 26*, 231.
51. Yu, D.-G., Li, J.-J., Williams, G. R., & Zhao, M. (2018). Electrospun amorphous solid dispersions of poorly water-soluble drugs: A review. *Journal of Controlled Release, 292*, 91–110.
52. Yu, D. G., Shen, X. X., Branford-White, C., White, K., Zhu, L. M., & Bligh, S. W. (2009). Oral fast-dissolving drug delivery membranes prepared from electrospun polyvinylpyrrolidone ultrafine fibers. *Nanotechnology, 20*, 055104.
53. Kawakami, K. (2012). Miscibility analysis of particulate solid dispersions prepared by electrospray deposition. *International Journal of Pharmaceutics, 433*, 71–78.
54. Wang, C., & Wang, M. (2014). Electrospun Multifunctional Tissue Engineering Scaffolds. *Frontiers of Materials Science, 8*, 3–19.
55. Shah, N., Iyer, R. M., Mair, H. J., Choi, D. S., Tian, H., Diodone, R., Fahnrich, K., Pabst-Ravot, A., Tang, K., Scheubel, E., Grippo, J. F., Moreira, S. A., Go, Z., Mouskountakis, J., Louie, T., Ibrahim, P. N., Sandhu, H., Rubia, L., Chokshi, H., . . . Malick, W. (2013). Improved human bioavailability of vemurafenib, a practically insoluble drug, using an amorphous polymer-stabilized solid dispersion prepared by a solvent-controlled coprecipitation process. *Journal of Pharmaceutical Sciences, 102*, 967–981.
56. Sertsou, G., Butler, J., Scott, A., Hempenstall, J., & Rades, T. (2002). Factors affecting incorporation of drug into solid solution with HPMCP during solvent change co-precipitation. *International Journal of Pharmaceutics, 245*, 99–108.
57. Abuzar, S. M., Hyun, S.-M., Kim, J.-H., Park, H. J., Kim, M.-S., Park, J.-S., & Hwang, S.-J. (2018). Enhancing the solubility and bioavailability of poorly water-soluble drugs using supercritical antisolvent (SAS) process. *International Journal of Pharmaceutics, 538*, 1–13.
58. Goldberg, A. H., Gibaldi, M., & Kanig, J. L. (1966). Increasing dissolution rates and gastrointestinal absorption of drugs via solid solutions and eutectic mixtures III. *Journal of Pharmaceutical Sciences, 55*, 487–492.
59. Jia, X. B., Yan, H. M., Zhang, Z. H., et al. (2014). An attempt to stabilize tanshinone IIA solid dispersion by the use of ternary systems with nano-$CaCO_3$ and poloxamer 188. *Pharmacognosy Magazine, 10*(38), 311.

Chapter 13
3D Printed Drug Delivery: An Appealing Trend for Chinese Medicines

Haiyan Zhao, Qin Nie, and Shaobing Wang

Abstract Drug delivery based on 3D printing technology is a rapidly growing area of research, as 3D printing can tailor dosage forms according to individual need. This review introduces several commonly used 3D printing technologies in the pharmaceutical preparations and summarizes the advantages and disadvantages of each 3D printing technique. Also, we provide a timely perspective on potential applications and challenges of 3D printing technology in the field of Chinese medicine preparation, which will give much inspiration to the researchers of Chinese medicine.

Keywords 3D printing technology · Drug delivery system · Chinese medicine

13.1 Introduction

Three-dimensional (3D) printing is an additive manufacturing process built by depositing or binding materials layer by layer to produce a 3D structure [1, 2]. As a subset of rapid prototyping to quickly fabricate models and prototypes, additive manufacturing is now being considered as a scalable manufacturing process [3]. With the rapid development of computer science and material science, 3D printing and other additive manufacturing techniques have been widely applied in aviation [4, 5], mold [6], food [7], pharmaceutics [8–10], and many other fields.

During years of drug therapy, the inappropriate dose frequently results in a high incidence of side effects [11]. With the penetration of rapid prototyping technologies in the pharmaceutical field, 3D printing technology gains growing attention to develop personalized-dose medicines [12, 13]. Personalized medicine refers to a way of delivering medicines to meet patient's individual needs regarding their ages, weights, organ functions, and severity of diseases. Personalized medicine is distinct from popular delivery systems and relies on genetic testing and targeted drug delivery [14]. 3D printing technology provides a new approach to quickly

H. Zhao · Q. Nie · S. Wang (✉)
School of Pharmaceutical Sciences, South-Central University for Nationalities, Wuhan, China
e-mail: pharm_wang@scuec.edu.cn

N. Feng, Z. Yang (eds.), *Novel Drug Delivery Systems for Chinese Medicines*,
https://doi.org/10.1007/978-981-16-3444-4_13

manufacture personalized pharmaceutical formulations with the tailored shape or dose using computer-aided design (CAD) file [15].

3D printing technology is very interdisciplinary in nature. It brings together the fields of information technology, polymer chemistry, precision machinery, biology, and basic and clinical medicines [2]. Of course, it has become a research hotspot and an important development direction in the pharmaceutical field. Future drug design and manufacturing are likely to shift from mass production of limited doses of tablets (or capsules) to just-in-time manufacturing of limited doses for individual patients [16]. Various pharmaceutical technologies were employed in the past to manufacture the dosage of active pharmaceutical ingredients (APIs) to satisfy the patient's individual needs [11]. The concept of individualized dosing was put into effect by implementing inkjet printing of APIs onto different substrates such as dispersible films [17]. 3D printing technology can produce novel pharmaceutical preparations with specific drug release from simple to complex models, which enhances medication compliance of patients and improves the effect of treatment [18–20]. In addition, personalized patient care is an emerging trend in medicine and pharmacy today. In this context, the traditional mass production and mass market approach has been challenged in allowing tailored doses to meet patient's individual needs in a direct and effective manner [21].

In the face of huge drug market demand, the application of 3D printing also promotes the development of pharmaceutical preparations. From 3D printing technology application in 2000 to the marketing of "Levetiracetam instant tablet," the first 3D printed pharmaceutical product was approved by the FDA in 2015, and 3D printing has triggered a new round of research upsurge among scientists at home and abroad [22, 23].

At present, there are few pieces of investigations focusing on the application of 3D printing technology in Chinese medicine preparations. Professor Chen's team applied 3D printing technology to prepare and evaluate the quick-acting *Suxiao Jiuxin* orally disintegrating tablets, which provided a good idea for 3D printing technology in the research and development of innovative Chinese medicine preparations [24]. Based on the overall principle and characteristics of 3D printing technology, this review discusses its advantages, challenges, and applications in the solid preparations of Chinese medicines, aiming to provide insights on the research and development of innovative Chinese medicine preparations.

13.2 3D Printing Technology

3D printing or additive manufacturing is a highly appealing technology that produces three-dimensional objects by constructing the used materials layer by layer with the aid of computer software. Among the 3D printing technologies introduced to the market in the recent decades, the commonly used 3D printers in the pharmaceutical formulations are stereolithography (SLA), selective laser sintering (SLS), fused deposition modeling (FDM), and inkjet-based printers [25]. Figure 13.1

illustrates the main building parts and working principle of the four types of 3D printers, and Table 13.1 summarizes the advantages, limitation, and typical materials of the four types of 3D printing technologies.

13.2.1 Stereolithography Apparatus (SLA)

SLA printing depends on the solidification of a liquid containing a drug and photosensitive resin into the designed 3D objects by the exposure to a high energy initiating polymerization (schematically shown in Fig. 13.1a). Commonly, SLA 3D printers use laser beam as a source of ultraviolet light, and the photosensitive resin acts as a cross-linker. During the printing process, the liquid resin is placed in a bath, which was integrated on movable building platform. The focused UV laser is vector scanned over the top of the bath of a photopolymerizable polymer and leads to a radical polymerization at the selected coordinates. After the first layer is formed, the building platform is lowered to a depth equivalent to the layer thickness, and the laser scanning is repeated until 3D object is printed completely [45]. Once the printing process is completed, the excess of unpolymerized resin is washed off using solvents like isopropanol. Such a structure has poor mechanical properties, since the conversion of reactive groups is usually incomplete. The mechanical properties can be improved by the post-curing with ultraviolet light [46]. In SLA printing, the thickness of the cured layer is the most important parameter and can be controlled by the energy of the light to which the resin is exposed. The energy of the laser is influenced by several factors, including the power of the light source, the scanning speed, the exposure time, and the amount of polymer and photoinitiator [47]. The prominent advantage of SLA printing is its outstanding resolution (down to 0.2μm) and smooth surfaces compared to other printing techniques [46]. On the other hand, SLA printing has some limitations. The number of biocompatible/biodegradable polymers suitable for SLA is very small, which hampers the use of such polymers for human. Besides, the residual photo-initiator is cytotoxic and liable to result in side effects, upon leaching out of the structure, so that the post-curing process is essential for the removal of uncured resin and avoiding toxicity [47, 48].

13.2.2 Selective Laser Sintering (SLS)

SLS printing is accomplished by curing liquid resin and polymer on a movable platform using high-power laser beam. In this technique, polymer powders are placed on a stage and preheated close to the melting point of the polymer. A laser beam scans over the powder bed, and the preheated powders are heated to melt. Thereafter, the first layer of the printed object is formed upon the fusion of the molten powder particles takes place, which is called as sintering process. After the first layer is formed, the powder stage moves down by the thickness of one layer. The

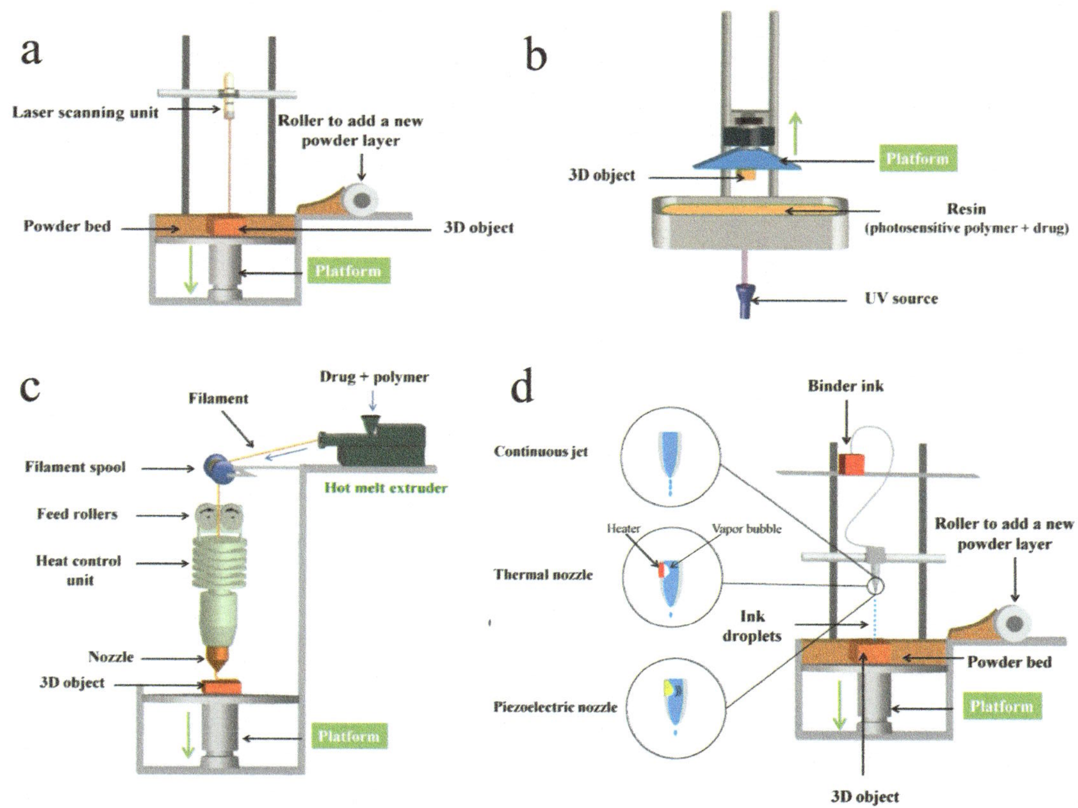

Fig. 13.1 Schematic parts and working principle of four types of 3D printers: (**a**) stereolithography (SLA), (**b**) selective laser sintering (SLS), (**c**) fused deposition modeling (FDM), and (**d**) inkjet-based printers. (Modified with permission from Ref. [26], Copyright 2020 Elsevier)

Table 13.1 Summary of advantages, limitations, and typical materials of common 3D printing technologies

Technology	Advantages	Limitations	Typical materials
SLA	High accuracy and outstanding resolution	Costly equipment and long printing time	Polyhydroxyethyl methacrylate and polyethylene glycol diacrylate [27], polyethylene glycol dimethacrylate [28], diethyl fumarate/poly(propylene fumarate) [29]
	Low thermal stress	Require post-printing curing	
		Slow printing process	
SLS	Don't require additional support structure and drying step	Material-consuming	Kollidon VA [30], PCL [31]
	High printing resolution	Require post-printing process	Eudragit L [32], Eudragit RL [33], Kollicoat IR [32]
	Internal porosity is controllable	Possible API degradation caused by high energy of laser	
FDM	Widely available and low cost	Restricted to thermoplastic polymers	PLA [34], PCL [35], polyvinyl alcohol (PVA) [36], polyethylene oxides (PEO) [37], hydroxypropyl cellulose (HPC) [38], hydroxypropylmethylcellulose (HPMC) [39, 40], Soluplus [41], and Eudragit polymers [40, 42]
	High drug uniformity	Comparably high temperature	
	Solvent-free process	Only suitable for thermo-stable APIs	
Inkjet printing	Various materials available	Use of organic solvents	Microcrystalline cellulose (MCC) [22], mannitol [43], beeswax [44]
	Room temperature process	Potential material waste	HPMC and PVPK30 [9], Eudragit E and Eudragit RL [22]
	Suitable for thermosensitive APIs	Printed objects can be fragile	

sintering process is repeated by spreading new powder layers until the designed 3D object is finished (Fig. 13.1b). The unsintered powder serves as the physical support for the part throughout the process, and the free powder can be removed at the end of the build cycle. The important parameters associated with SLS printing include laser energy and scanning speed [49, 50]. The resolution of the printed product is dependent on the precision of the laser and the particle size of the powder, while the mass variation of the product is determined by the laser speed [51]. The properties of SLS printing materials should be stable at the melting point, usually using metal powders, polyamides, polystyrene, polypropylene, and thermoplastic elastomers [52]. The advantage of SLS technology lies in its solvent-free process, which means there is no need for an additional drying step [53]. Compared with FDM, SLS is a step-by-step process that does not require hot-melt extrusion to the pre-produce suitable filament and produce objects. However, the heating of the powder bed and the high energy input of laser are liable to cause the degradation of APIs. The degradation can be reduced by increasing the laser scanning speed to a certain extent [54].

13.2.3 Fused Deposition Modeling Printing

Fused deposition modeling, a most widely used 3D printing technique, is based on the hot-melt extrusion process. In FDM printing, API powder and a thermoplastic polymer are mixed and extruded in the form of filament, which is fed into a nozzle and then heated above the glass transition temperature of the polymer. The extruder head deposits the semi-molten filament onto a printing platform forming consecutive layers, and the designed 3D structure is fabricated upon all layers are finished (Fig. 13.1c).

The important parameters for successful FDM printing include filling density, extrusion speed, layer height, and the temperature of nozzle and building plate [33, 55]. The materials used in FDM printing are usually composed of the modeling material and the supporting material, the modeling material used to form the final product and the support material used as the scaffold. Due to their relatively low melting point, they can be fused to a low viscosity with a low melting point and thus can be used to make hot fuses, such as polylactic acid (PLA) and polycaprolactone (PCL) [34, 35]. Besides, various hot-fusing polymer mixtures are commonly used to prepare wires as printing materials. The advantages of this technology involve low cost, technical feasibility, and high availability of materials, ranging from small printers to large industrial machines. The disadvantage lies in the high operating temperature, which is not suitable for the preparation of thermally unstable objects [56]. Compared with other solid free-form fabrication methods, FDM printing can easily fabricate produce dosage forms with appropriate shapes in favor of improving patient compliance [57]. The need for high temperature to produce polymer substrates allows the formation of amorphous structures, which may be suitable for insoluble drugs. However, the technology is limited to the use of thermally stable low-dose APIs and a limited number of biodegradable thermoplastic polymers, limiting the flexibility of the application.

13.2.4 Inkjet Printing

Inkjet printing is an overall term to describe the systems that are able to digitally break a liquid stream or jet into droplets. The print droplet is directly sprayed to a specific position on the surface of the medium through small holes to solidify and form a section image. Inkjet printing is usually classified as continuous inkjet printing (CIJ) and drop-on-demand (DoD) inkjet, both of which are used in traditional desktop printing but distinguished by the physical process by which the drops are generated [58].

CIJ printing utilizes a pressured flow of liquid to pass through an orifice (nozzle) producing a continuous stream of droplets. Liquid flows tend to break up naturally with a characteristic wavelength of surface distortion, whereafter the final droplets are spaced about 4.5 times the initial diameter of the stream. In actual CIJ devices, the flow through the nozzle is regulated at an appropriate frequency by a piezoelectric sensor behind the orifice, thus enhancing the natural breakup under surface tension force [58]. The curing mode of CIJ printing can be divided into two categories, thermally induced phase transition and UV light curing [59]. The printing material for thermally induced phase transition (such as wax) can be ejected after being heated to a liquid state and be molded after being cooled to a solid state. The printing material for UV light curing (such as gel photosensitive resin) can be deposited at the rear of the inkjet and cured under UV light.

In DoD printing, the liquid is ejected from the printhead once the production of each drop is triggered by a current or an acoustic pulse. A DoD printhead usually contains several hundreds of nozzles which is classified as thermal printhead and piezoelectric printhead. Thermal printhead is restricted to volatile liquids, whereas piezoelectric printhead can be used with a larger variety of inks. Thermal printhead utilizes resistive elements to create a current which leads to the evaporation of liquid and imparts the energy to eject droplet. In the piezoelectric method, the sudden deformation of the piezoelectric crystal generates an acoustic pulse which produces sufficient pressure to eject droplet. [26]. Both printhead can produce droplets with a diameter range from 10 to 50μm, which is similar to the diameter of the nozzle and corresponds to a volume between 1 and 70 pL [58]. In view of the precise control of droplet volume, DOD printing is considered less wasteful than CIJ printing [1].

13.3 Advantages of 3D Printing in Chinese Medicine Preparations

Under the guidance of the traditional Chinese medicine (TCM) theory for disease prevention, treatment, diagnosis, and rehabilitation, Chinese medicines include crude materials, decoction pieces, herbs, ethnic medicine and its products, extracts of Chinese herbal medicines, and natural medicine and its effective parts or its active ingredients. Since ancient times, it has made an indelible contribution to the health of Chinese people. "Evidence-based medicine, with different cure disease" is the soul of TCM to treat disease, but individualized medication is hard to realize for the industrialized production of Chinese medicines. 3D rapid printing and the characteristics of the precise dose control can not only resolve the problems existing in Chinese medicines but also provide a simple and fast preparation technology. Thus, 3D printing technology combined with the treatment of Chinese medicines provides a promising implementation of TCM "evidence-based medicine."

13.3.1 Simplify the Preparation Process of Chinese Medicines

Generally, Chinese medicine preparation procedures include the extraction, concentration, granulation and drying, and it is difficult to granulate for Chinese medicine extracts due to its high viscosity and hygroscopicity [60]. Abundant excipients need to be added for the granulation of Chinese medicines, which results in the large doses for patients and the difficulty in drug dissolution. The 3D printed Chinese medicine preparation is controlled by a computer CAD model, and the adhesive is sprayed onto Chinese medicine powders according to the digital information of the discrete layer of the solid model, so that Chinese medicine powders are superimposed layer by layer to print a loose porous tablet. For the Chinese medicine extract, it can be mixed with suitable materials and printed via melt deposition technology. It does not need to add a large number of auxiliary materials and omit many procedures such as granulation, drying, and spheronization, which can not only solve the above problems of Chinese medicine preparations but also achieve individualized administration of Chinese medicines.

13.3.2 Improve Stability and Taste Masking of Volatile Materials

Many Chinese medicine preparations contain volatile materials, such as borneol, bezoar, daphne, and volatile oil, which play an important role in the gastrointestinal system, central nervous system, and respiratory system diseases [61]. These volatile materials are liable to gradually dissipate with the prolongation of storage time. To minimize the loss of volatile materials during the preparation process, several techniques are commonly used, including adsorption method [62], inclusion technology [63], and microcapsule/microsphere technology [64]. 3D printing technology can achieve the entrapment or encapsulation of the volatile materials of Chinese medicines through the dual-nozzle device. According to the set program and 3D graphics, the product can be designed as tablet with a shell-core structure [36], and volatile materials of Chinese medicines can be directly printed in the center of the tablet. The tailored functional structure is able to reduce the volatilization and increase the stability of Chinese medicines, thus ensuring the curative effect. The functional structures can be customized as multiple dosing regimens, which play an important role in improving patient adherence in case of multi-drug therapy [65].

13.3.3 Realize Precise Medication and Individualized Administration

Chinese medicine preparations are mostly complicated with complex components and exert a comprehensive therapeutic effect on the disease. The soul of TCM lies in treating diseases by syndrome differentiation. The dosage of medicine depends on the person, the time, and the syndrome. The prescription for some patients with different diseases may include precious or toxic Chinese medicines. Materials such as donkey-hide gelatin, tortoiseshell gum, antler gum, ganoderma lucidum, and arsenic have excellent curative effects in balancing *Yin* and *Yang*, compensating the internal organs, relieving the pathogen, and reconciling *Qi* and blood. In the process of solid preparation of Chinese medicines, the raw materials and auxiliary materials are made into the designed dosage form through the steps of powdering, mixing, screening, drying, and molding, which affect the uniformity of the drug content of the preparation [66]. Uneven dosage will cause the waste of precious medicinal materials and even lead to drug inefficiency or poisoning. Furthermore, there is an obvious correlation between the dosage and efficacy. For example, a small amount of *Rheum officinale* can clear heat and dampness, but a high dosage has a laxative effect [67]. *Guizhi* soup is often used for exogenous diseases, but the flexible addition and subtraction of *Guizhi* soup successfully treated allergic rhinitis and children with pneumonia [68]. It can be seen that the dosage of Chinese medicines is very flexible and must be treated and determined according to different situations. These characteristics of Chinese medicines are not suitable for industrialized production of modern dosage forms such as tablets and capsules. Namely, modern preparation technology is difficult to adapt to the characteristics of Chinese medicines. 3D printing is a promising strategy to solve the backwardness of Chinese medicine clinical dosage forms because of its miniaturization and convenience. The supply of medicine can be controlled by a quantitative pump and a high-precision stepper motor to ensure the accuracy of medicament dose according to the requirements of the individualized dose. Furthermore, 3D printed products can be fabricated immediately on the demand of the patient's actual condition or the doctor's prescription, and the printing raw material formula can be customized at any time with the prescription. The printed preparation is easy to carry, which is in line with the trend of future personalized medical services and realizes the perfect combination of Chinese medicines and modern medical models.

13.4 Application of 3D Printing Technology in Innovative Chinese Medicines

13.4.1 New Preparations of Chinese Medicines

With the continuous development of 3D printing technology, this technology has shown an attractive trend toward the research of Chinese medicine preparations. Compound *Danshen* oral disintegrating tablets were prepared by 3D printing technology, choosing Danshen (*salvia miltiorrhiza*), Sanqi (*Panax notoginseng*), borneol, lactose, PVP K30, mannitol, aspartame, and micronized silica gel as the layering powder and ethanol solution containing 2% PVP K30 as the binder

[69]. The printed tablets had an ODT radius of 5.1 ± 0.1 mm and a thickness of 3.2 ± 0.2 mm, with average weight of 167.6 mg and hardness of 1.72 ± 0.2 kg. The printed tablets disintegrated within 1.0 min with high porosity and good appearance. Scanning electron microscope observation results suggested that the internal microstructure of the tablet was relatively uniform. This study showed that the binder jet 3D printing technology for Chinese medicine preparation is simple, reliable, and easy to control, and it is expected to be widely used in the research of new drug formulations.

Yan et al. [70] chose snake gourd fruit and astragalus polysaccharides as carriers and prepared polysaccharide-astragalus polysaccharide-carboxymethyl chitosan hydrogel with different shapes (round, rod, and square) by melt extrusion. Bovine serum albumin (BSA) was chosen as a model protein to investigate the in vitro release activity of carriers with different shapes. The results of the release activity showed that there was significant difference among different shapes of composite hydrogels, and the cumulative release rate of BSA ranged from 49% to 89%. It indicated that the shape of the preparation was significantly related to the activity of drug release, which provided a favorable reference for the research and development of 3D printing innovative Chinese medicine preparation.

A sandwich oral preparation containing both ibuprofen and ganoderma lucidum polysaccharides was prepared by 3D printing and electrostatic spinning, and the complete fiber-membrane sandwich can be folded to form capsules to enhance the oral compliance of the drug [71]. The bottom layer and the top layer are ibuprofen acetic acid fiber membrane, and the middle layer is ganoderma polysaccharides polyvinylpyrrolidone. In vitro release experiments showed that the drug had a distinct release activity in step. First, the ganoderma lucidum polysaccharide was released in the gastric juice, and then 60% of the ibuprofen was released within the subsequent 1 h. The remaining ibuprofen was released and absorbed slowly in the small intestine. This new 3D drug preparation technology combining Chinese medicines with chemical drug provided a useful reference for the development of slow-release and controlled-release preparations as well as personalized drug preparation technologies.

Integration of Chinese medicine ingredients into biological tissue scaffolds using 3D printing technology is conducive to exert the therapeutic effect of Chinese medicine ingredients and promote tissue repair. Peng et al. [72] fabricated epimedium glycoside-loaded β-tricalcium phosphate stents by 3D printing technology and investigated its repair function of femoral head necrosis in rabbit, compared with the autologous bone and the blank β-tricalcium phosphate stents. Results indicated that 3D printed β-tricalcium phosphate stents containing epimedium glycoside were able to promote osteoblast proliferation and differentiation, inhibit the activity of osteoclasts, promote the new angiogenesis, and repair the rabbit femoral head necrosis.

13.4.2 Functional Foods of Chinese Medicines

The application of 3D printing in food manufacturing opened a new era of food customization, which could provide consumers with customized food in terms of nutrition, taste, appearance, and other aspects, reduce food waste, and create more brandnew food structures [73]. Zhu et al. investigated the correlation between rheological properties and proposed a more “rational approach” for food formulation and printing design development (Fig. 13.2), based on the investigation in the effect of rheological properties on the printing behavior during extrusion-based 3D printing [74]. Cornell University scientific research team used 3D printing technology to realize the specific configuration and composition of the special food, meeting the demand of personal customized personalized rheological highly edible food and materials [75]. Xiao et al. [76] printed a health active chocolate containing ganoderma lucidum, medlar, and *Radix ophiopogonis* compound polysaccharide with 3D technology, followed by evaluating its oil content, thermal properties, viscosity, and rheological properties, which demonstrated 3D printing preparation was a feasible method for Chinese medicine health food. Wang et al. [77] used the extrusion process to prepare gel jelly containing complex polysaccharides. The printing raw materials include 1.2 g gellan, 12 g agar-agar, 12 g gelatin, 4 g starch, 50 g liquid maltitol, 44 g erythritol, 0.5 g polyglycerol ricinol, 0–0.05 g newsweet, 0–0.5 g peppermint powder, and 0–20 g complex polysaccharides. Boil end solid content was optimized for 70–76% (w/w). The procedure not only masked the bitter taste of the drug but also effectively adjusted the elasticity and gel strength of gel jelly, which greatly improved the compliance of Chinese medicine products. 3D food printing technology has great application prospects in the development of functional foods rich in Chinese medicines for the elderly and children. 3D printing technology can provide a variety of shapes of products easy to swallow and realize the flexible adjustment of the ingredients and the types of food. The application of 3D printing technology can integrate Chinese medicinal materials into modern food manufacturing, combining Chinese medicines with Western-style desserts and developing a new “medicinal diet” model. It has extremely broad market potential and can promote the transformation of the traditional Chinese functional food industry.

13.4.3 Medical Devices of Chinese Medicines

Facial mask as a kind of skincare product is commonly respected and trusted by consumers. The Chinese medicine mask is widely used in the medical cosmetology industry because of its convenience and satisfactory effect. Cao et al. [78] prepared a hydrogel mask containing cryptotanshinone by 3D printing technology and found that it had a good anti-acne effect and higher skin safety for external use. Using 3D technology to customize Chinese medicine masks, the most suitable product can be

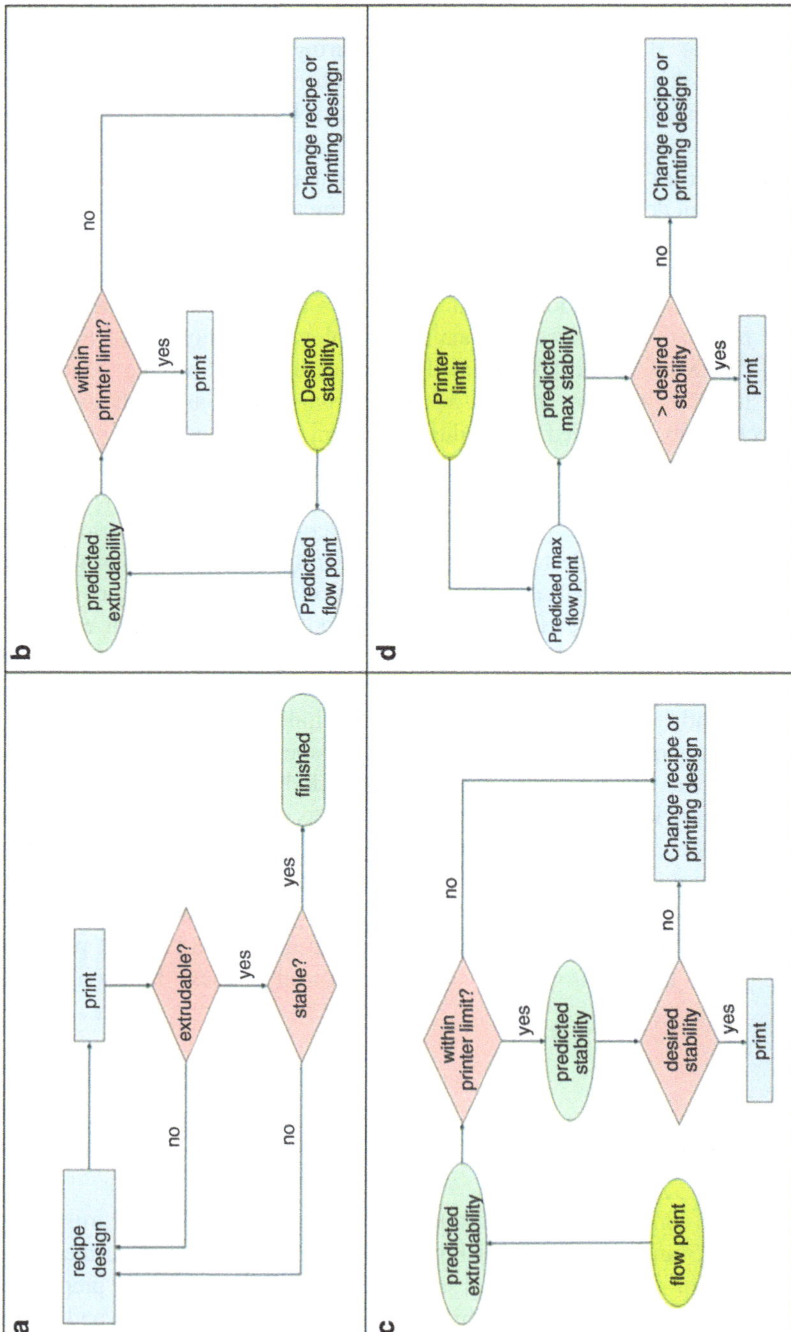

Fig. 13.2 Decision flowchart of 3D food printing design and formula selection. (**a**: the traditional "fault law"; **b–d**: follow the new guidelines of the "rational approach"). (Reprinted with permission from Ref [74], Copyright 2020 Elsevier)

prepared according to the skin state of consumers, which is completely consistent with today's customized beauty service concept. Innovative medical devices containing Chinese medicines are effective in disease treatment and prevention. Chen et al. [79] investigated the changes in peak plantar pressure, peak arterial systolic flow velocity, and the incidence of foot ulcers in diabetic foot patients before and after treatment with 3D-printed diabetic foot decompression insole. The results indicated that 3D printed decompression insole was able to distribute plantar pressure evenly, correct the abnormal stress of diabetic patients with high foot pressure, and reduce the incidence of foot ulcers and amputation rate, which ensured the quality of life of diabetic patients and provided an economical and effective way to prevent the occurrence of diabetic foot disease in diabetic patients. Huang et al. [80] also developed a Chinese medicine insole based on 3D printing for the prevention and treatment of plantar fasciitis. The insole was composed of a 3D printed layer, a shock-absorbing layer, a breathable layer, and a vinyl acetate copolymer (EVA) polymer layer. The therapeutic drug distributed on the upper surface of the EVA polymer layer, which was able to directly stimulate the foot acupoints of patients, eliminate inflammation and achieve the purpose of auxiliary treatment. These researches are following the concept of curing diseases in China and highly unified with the idea of "prevention and treatment first" and "combination of medical care." In the future, these products will truly enter into people's lives and improve people's physical fitness.

13.5 Challenges of 3D Printing in Chinese Medicine Preparation

13.5.1 More Printing Materials for Chinese Medicine Are Needed

Due to the complex for the composition of Chinese medicines and the characteristics for viscosity and hygroscopicity of Chinese medicine extracts, more suitable ingredients and printing materials need to be developed to achieve the purpose of its rapid disintegration and successful printing [81]. The mechanism of 3D printing drug forming is mainly the droplet-powder bonding 3D drug printing technology, which uses liquid adhesives to bind drug particles together and form dosage forms after the adhesives solidify. Therefore, the continuous development of adhesives with excellent performance is crucial to produce various dosage forms and improve the physical properties of 3D printed drugs. In the raw material requirements of each 3D printing technology, the rheological properties of materials are extremely important, which indicates that it is necessary for the development of appropriate flow aids. The innovation of 3D printing technology is closely related to the innovation of printing materials. To upgrade the 3D printing technology in Chinese medicine pharmaceutical industry, the research and development of innovative materials are essential, especially the development of some new materials of Chinese medicines. Some macromolecules in Chinese medicines such as polysaccharides, proteins, tannins, and other components can be used as natural 3D printing materials for the new dosage forms, which cannot only ensure the safety of innovative Chinese medicines but also facilitate the combination with the medicinal components of Chinese medicines. Besides, for some special active substances in Chinese medicines such as volatile oil, printing materials and methods should be creatively selected to effectively ensure the stability and effectiveness of Chinese medicines.

13.5.2 Improve Quality Control and Production Supervision

Although 3D printing is a highly promising technology for manufacturing dosage form, there are several technical and regulatory challenges need to be overcome before it is widely applied in the pharmaceutical field. The most significant limitation of 3D printed products is their appearance and surface imperfections which resulted from the stacking of polymeric beads or powders particularly for powder- or extrusion-based technology [82]. The surface imperfections are also affected by post-treatment processes such as drying method, rate, and duration. Furthermore, the quality of 3D printed products is commonly different from that of the conventional tablets. 3D printing frequently produces the products with a porous morphology or structure, which results into higher friability values and faster release characteristics compared to the conventional tablets [83].

To control the quality of 3D printed products and ensure human's health, the printed products should be manufactured according to appropriate quality standards, and relevant evaluations should be worked out. Like the conventional tablets, printed products require pharmaceutical tests such as content uniformity, disintegration, and other characterization procedures [25]. The quality standard of the printed products should be modified to satisfy 3D-printed formulations, and the modifications should be set according to the type of printing technology. For example, less than 1% weight loss in friability test is too stringent for the products printed by powder-based jet due to their poor mechanical strength [20, 84].

Since the first 3D printing product was approved in August 2015, the FDA established Additive Manufacturing Working Group, who is responsible for the discussion and clarification of the uncertainties and other questions about the additive manufacturing of medical products [85]. Thereafter, the FDA issued the technical guideline on 3D printing for medical applications, which provide initial regulatory insight and guidance for the production and manufacture of 3D printed products [86]. The guideline specified that all aspects of 3D printing process must undergo thorough inspection and evaluation to ensure the final product quality, including hardware, software, raw materials, operation training, post-processing, and quality controls.

As far as the current drug supervision and administration in China is concerned, there are no additional regulations on 3D printing equipment and quality control of

3D printing drugs, let alone putting the approval of 3D printing drugs on the agenda for discussion. The market development process of 3D printing of Chinese medicines is still quite backward. This makes the traditional pharmaceutical companies dare not rush the reform, which also affects the promotion of this technology to some extent.

13.5.3 Insufficient Investment in 3D Printing Technology

3D drug printing technology is still stayed at the laboratory research stage in China. Despite of several patents focusing on 3D printed tablet [87–89], no 3D printed product has been successfully developed so far. Additionally, the fact that only a few domestic hospitals are equipped with 3D printing devices restricts the progress and popularization of 3D printed products to a large extent. The 3D printed products are limited to use within the hospital rather than on the market. Although 3D printing technologies are cost-effective for mass production, they are not widely used in hospitals or pharmaceutical companies for their time-consuming and labor-intensive properties. In the future, abundant research is needed to focus on the feasibility, diversification, and manufacture process of 3D printing technology in Chinese medicines' pharmaceuticals.

13.6 Conclusion

3D printing technology is a very attractive tool for drug delivery systems, and its application in Chinese medicines is still in the beginning stage of research. The preparation technology, auxiliary printing materials, drug delivery devices, printing equipment, and packaging materials still need further optimization and innovation. To further promote the development of 3D printed pharmaceuticals of Chinese medicine, relevant research input should be strengthened, high-level research teams should be trained, and the combination of materials science, chemistry, pharmaceutical engineering, pharmaceutical equipment, and pharmacy should be promoted to achieve the further clinical transformation of research results. With the change of the 3D-printed pharmaceutical model, in the future, doctors can use 3D printers to flexibly prepare drugs needed by patients in hospitals according to their conditions and flexibly adjust the shape, color, and taste of drugs according to patients' preferences. Even at home, patients can purchase the corresponding printing materials and active ingredients of the drug according to the doctor's prescription and print the medicine suitable for their preference and dose. Such a pharmaceutical model cannot only effectively improve patients' recognition of Chinese medicines but also greatly promote the technological upgrading of the Chinese medicine industry. Besides, the future 3D drug printing mode will gradually transform the drug production process from intensification to miniaturization, from factory to family, and from mechanization to digitalization, which will put forward new requirements for the whole drug regulatory concept and system. In the future, more efforts should be made to build and improve these aspects.

References

1. Prasad, L. K., & Smyth, H. (2016). 3D printing technologies for drug delivery: A review. *Drug Development and Industrial Pharmacy, 42*(7), 1019–1031.
2. Goole, J., & Amighi, K. (2016). 3D printing in pharmaceutics: A new tool for designing customized drug delivery systems. *International Journal of Pharmaceutics, 499*(1–2), 376–394.
3. Sachs, E. M., Haggerty, J. S., Cima, M. J., et al. (1993). *Three-dimensional printing techniques*. US, 005204055A.
4. Gisario, A., Kazarian, M., Martina, F., et al. (2019). Metal additive manufacturing in the commercial aviation industry: A review. *Journal of Manufacturing Systems, 53*(1), 124–149.
5. Junfan, S., Xiaoyong, T., Meng, L., et al. (2020). Controllable inter-line bonding performance and fracture patterns of continuous fiber reinforced composites by sinusoidal-path 3D printing. *Composites Science and Technology, 192*(1), 108096.
6. Yan, Y., Haichao, L., Yingying, X., et al. (2019). Fabrication and evaluation of dental fillers using customized molds via 3D printing technology. *International Journal of Pharmaceutics, 562*(1), 66–75.
7. Mantihal, S., Kobun, R., & Lee, B. B. (2020). 3D food printing of as the new way of preparing food: A review. *International Journal of Gastronomy and Food Science, 22*(1), 100260.
8. Nadagouda, M. N., Rastogi, V., & Ginn, M. (2020). A review on 3D printing techniques for medical applications. *Current Opinion in Chemical Engineering, 28*(1), 152–157.
9. Mary, K., Aremu, A., Morgan, R. A., et al. (2017). 3D inkjet printing of tablets exploiting bespoke complex geometries for controlled and tuneable drug release. *Journal of Controlled Release, 261*(1), 207–215.
10. Khaled, S. A., Burley, J. C., Alexander, M. R., et al. (2015). 3D printing of five-in-one dose combination polypill with defined immediate and sustained release profiles. *Journal of Controlled Release, 217*(1), 308–314.
11. Ilias, E. A., Hanna, P., & Julian, Q. (2018). A critical review on 3D-printed dosage forms. *Current Pharmaceutical Design, 24*(42), 4957–4978.
12. Niklas, S., & Maren, P. (2016). Printed drug-delivery systems for improved patient treatment. *Trends in Pharmacological Sciences, 37*(1), 1070–1080.
13. Alomari, M., Mohamed, F. H., Basit, A. W., et al. (2015). Personalised dosing: Printing a dose of one's own medicine. *International Journal of Pharmaceutics, 494*(2), 568–577.
14. Reidenberg, M. M. (2003). Evolving ways that drug therapy is individualized. *Clinical Pharmacology and Therapeutics, 74*(3), 197–202.
15. Van Riet-Nales, D. A., Doeve, M. E., Nicia, A. E., et al. (2014). The accuracy, precision and sustainability of different techniques for tablets subdivision: Breaking by hand and the use of tablets splitters or a kitchen knife. *International Journal of Pharmaceutics, 466*(1–2), 44–51.
16. Goyanes, A., Robles, M. P., Buanz, A., et al. (2015). Effect of geometry on drug release from 3D printed tablets. *International Journal of Pharmaceutics, 494*(2), 657–663.
17. Sandler, N., Määttänen, A., Ihalainen, P., et al. (2011). Inkjet printing of drug substances and use of porous substrates-towards individualized dosing. *Journal of Pharmaceutical Sciences, 100*(8), 3386–3395.
18. Wang, Z. H., Li, Y. F., & Zhang, M. Y. (2013). The current situation and development ideas of China 3D printing industry. *Econometric Reviews, 10*(1), 90–94.

19. Ursan, I. D., Chiu, L., & Pierce, A. (2013). Three-dimensional drug printing: A structured review. *Journal of the American Pharmacists Association, 53*(2), 136–144.
20. Yu, D. G., Zhu, L. M., Branford-White, C., et al. (2008). Three-dimensional printing in pharmaceutics-promises and problems. *Journal of Pharmaceutical Sciences, 97*(9), 3666–3690.
21. Sophia, N. E., Dimitrios, A. L., & Dennis, D. (2018). 3D printing applications for transdermal drug delivery. *International Journal of Pharmaceutics, 544*(2), 415–424.
22. Rowe, C. W., Katstra, W. E., Palazzolo, R. D., et al. (2000). Multimechanism oral dosage forms fabricated by three dimensional printing™. *Journal of Controlled Release, 66*(1), 11–17.
23. Buanz, A. B. M., Saunders, M. H., Basit, A. W., et al. (2011). Preparation of personalized-dose salbutamol sulphate oral films with thermal ink-jet printing. *Pharmaceutical Research, 28*(10), 2386–2392.
24. Lin, Q. F., Yang, F., Fang, G. Y., et al. (2016). Study on preparation of 3D printing instant relief tablet. *Journal of Guangdong Pharmaceutical University, 32*(1), 1–4.
25. Trenfield, S. J., Awad, A., & Goyanes, A. (2018). 3D printing pharmaceuticals: Drug development to frontline care. *Trends in Pharmacological Sciences, 39*(5), 440–451.
26. Elkasabgy, N. A., Mahmoud, A. A., & Maged, A. (2020). 3D printing: An appealing route for customized drug delivery systems. *International Journal of Pharmaceutics, 588*(1), 119732.
27. Hanson Shepherd, J. N., Parker, S. T., Shepherd, R. F., et al. (2011). 3D microperiodic hydrogel scaffolds for robust neuronal cultures. *Advanced Functional Materials, 21*(1), 47–54.
28. Arcaute, K., Mann, B. K., & Wicker, R. B. (2006). Stereolithography of three dimensional bioactive poly(ethylene glycol) constructs with encapsulated cells. *Annals of Biomedical Engineering, 34*(9), 1429–1441.
29. Fisher, J. P., Dean, D., & Mikos, A. G. (2002). Photocrosslinking characteristics and mechanical properties of diethyl fumarate/poly(propylene fumarate) biomaterials. *Biomaterials, 23*(22), 4333–4343.
30. Allahham, N., Fina, F., Marcuta, C., et al. (2020). Selective laser sintering 3D printing of orally disintegrating printlets containing ondansetron. *Pharmaceutics, 12*(2), 110.
31. Fu, J., Yu, X., & Jin, Y. (2018). 3D printing of vaginal rings with personalized shapes for controlled release of progesterone. *International Journal of Pharmaceutics, 539*(1–2), 75–82.
32. Fina, F., Goyanes, A., Gaisford, S., et al. (2017). Selective laser sintering (SLS) 3D printing of medicines. *International Journal of Pharmaceutics, 529*(1–2), 285–293.
33. Korpela, J., Kokkari, A., Korhonen, H., et al. (2012). Biodegradable and bioactive porous scaffold structures prepared using fused deposition modeling. *Journal of Biomedical Materials Research. Part B, Applied Biomaterials, 101B*, 610–619.
34. Cuiffo, M. A., Snyder, J., Elliott, A. M., et al. (2017). Impact of the fused deposition (FDM) printing process on polylactic acid (PLA) chemistry and structure. *Applied Sciences, 7*(6), 579.
35. Goyanes, A., Det-Amornrat, U., Wang, J., et al. (2016). 3D scanning and 3D printing as innovative technologies for fabricating personalized topical drug delivery systems. *Journal of Controlled Release, 234*(1), 41–48.
36. Goyanes, A., Wang, J., Buanz, A., et al. (2015). 3D printing of medicines: Engineering novel oral devices with unique design and drug release characteristics. *Molecular Pharmaceutics, 12*(11), 4077–4084.
37. Isreb, A., Baj, K., Wojsz, M., et al. (2019). 3D printed oral theophylline doses with innovative 'radiator-like' design: Impact of polyethyleneoxide (PEO) molecular weight. *International Journal of Pharmaceutics, 564*(1), 98–105.
38. Melocchi, A., Parietti, F., Loreti, G., et al. (2015). 3D printing by fused deposition modeling (FDM) of a swellable/erodible capsular device for oral pulsatile release of drugs. *Journal of Drug Delivery Science and Technology, 30*(2), 360–367.
39. Zhang, J., Feng, X., Patil, H., et al. (2017). Coupling 3D printing with hot-melt extrusion to produce controlled-release tablets. *International Journal of Pharmaceutics, 519*(1–2), 186–197.
40. Beck, R. C. R., Chaves, P. S., Goyanes, A., et al. (2017). 3D printed tablets loaded with polymeric nanocapsules: An innovative approach to produce customized drug delivery systems. *International Journal of Pharmaceutics, 528*(1–2), 268–279.

41. Melocchi, A., Parietti, F., Maroni, A., et al. (2016). Hot-melt extruded filaments based on pharmaceutical grade polymers for 3D printing by fused deposition modeling. *International Journal of Pharmaceutics, 509*(1–2), 255–263.
42. Gültekin, H. E., Tort, S., & Acartürk, F. (2019). An effective technology for the development of immediate release solid dosage forms containing low-dose drug: Fused deposition modeling 3D printing. *Pharmaceutical Research, 36*(9), 128.
43. Lee, K. J., Kang, A., Delfino, J. J., et al. (2003). Evaluation of critical formulation factors in the development of a rapidly dispersing captopril oral dosage form. *Drug Development and Industrial Pharmacy, 29*(9), 967–979.
44. Wang, C. C., Tejwani Motwani, M. R., Roach, W. J., et al. (2006). Development of near zero-order release dosage forms using three-dimensional printing (3-DP) technology. *Drug Development and Industrial Pharmacy, 32*(3), 367–376.
45. Hull, C. W. (1986). *Apparatus for production of three-dimensional objects by stereolithography*. UVP, Inc..
46. Melchels, F. P., Feijen, J., & Grijpma, D. W. (2010). A review on stereolithography and its applications in biomedical engineering. *Biomaterials, 31*(24), 6121–6130.
47. Wang, J., Goyanes, A., Gaisford, S., & Basit, A. W. (2016). Stereolithographic (SLA) 3D printing of oral modified-release dosage forms. *International Journal of Pharmaceutics, 503*(1–2), 207–212.
48. Tumbleston, J. R., Shirvanyants, D., Ermoshkin, N., et al. (2015). Continuous liquid interface production of 3D objects. *Science, 347*(6228), 1349–1352.
49. Cheah, C. M., Leong, K. F., Chua, C. K., et al. (2002). Characterization of microfeatures in selective laser sintered drug delivery devices. *Journal of Engineering in Medicine, 216*(6), 369–383.
50. Yu, L. X. (2008). Pharmaceutical quality by design: Product and process development understanding, and control. *Pharmaceutical Research, 25*(1), 781–791.
51. Olakanmi, E. O., Cochrane, R. F., & Dalgarno, K. W. (2015). A review on selective laser sintering/melting (SLS/SLM) of aluminium alloy powders: Processing, microstructure, and properties. *Progress in Materials Science, 74*(1), 401–477.
52. Wendel, B., Rietzel, D., Kühnlein, F., et al. (2008). Additive processing of polymers. *Macromolecular Materials and Engineering, 293*(10), 799–809.
53. Yu, D. G., Yang, X. L., Huang, W. D., et al. (2007). Tablets with material gradients fabricated by three-dimensional printing. *Journal of Pharmaceutical Sciences, 96*(9), 2446–2456.
54. Fina, F., Goyanes, A., Madla, C. M., et al. (2018). 3D printing of drug-loaded gyroid lattices using selective laser sintering. *International Journal of Pharmaceutics, 547*(1–2), 44–52.
55. Pietrzak, K., Isreb, A., & Alhnan, M. A. (2015). A flexible-dose dispenser for immediate and extended release 3D printed tablets. *European Journal of Pharmaceutics and Biopharmaceutics, 96*(1), 380–387.
56. Schiele, J. T., Quinzler, R., Klimm, H. D., et al. (2013). Difficulties swallowing solid dosage forms in a general practice population: Prevalence, causes, and relationship to dosage forms. *European Journal of Pharmacology, 69*(4), 937–948.
57. Zhang, J., Yang, W., Vo, A. Q., et al. (2017). Hydroxypropyl methylcellulose based controlled release dosage by melt extrusion and 3D printing Structure and drug release correlation. *Carbohydrate Polymers, 177*(1), 49–57.
58. Daly, R., Harrington, T. S., Martin, G. D., et al. (2015). Inkjet printing for pharmaceutics- A review of research and manufacturing. *International Journal of Pharmaceutics, 494*(2), 554–567.
59. Liu, C. Q., Wang, H. X., Zheng, L., et al. (2020). The research progress of 3D printing technology in the innovative development and application of traditional Chinese medicine. *Chinese Journal of Experimental Traditional Medical Formulae, 26*(3), 236–242.
60. Kuang, W. W., Wu, Z. F., Wan, N., et al. (2019). Discussion on research thought of dry granulation of traditional Chinese medicine: Research progress at home and abroad based on dry granulation technology. *China Journal of Chinese Materia Medica, 44*(15), 3195–3202.

61. Ma, W. (2018). Overview of 3D printing technology in pharmaceutical preparations research. *Pharmacy Today, 28*(3), 204–206.
62. Du, G., Sun, M. H., & Yin, X. Z. (2003). Treatment methods of volatile oil from traditional Chinese medicine in preparation. *Lishizhen Medicine and Materia Medica Research, 14*(3), 150–151.
63. Yi, Y. K., & Chen, Z. L. (2006). Evaluation of cyclodextrin inclusion of the volatile components in compound traditional Chinese medicine. *Journal of Southern Medical University, 26*(9), 1337–1340.
64. Thimma, R. T., & Tammishetti, S. (2013). Study of complex coacervation of gelatin with sodium carboxymethyl guar gum: Microencapsulation of clove oil and sulphamethoxazole. *Journal of Microencapsulation, 20*(2), 203–210.
65. Mule, S. T., Bhusnure, O. G., Waghmare, S. S., et al. (2020). Recent trends, opportunities and challenges in 3D printing technology for personalize medicine. *Journal of Drug Delivery and Therapeutics, 10*(4), 242–252.
66. Hang, L., Zhang, F., Zhang, D. K., et al. (2014). A preliminary study on the determination method of the content uniformity of traditional Chinese medicine preparation. *Chinese Herbal Medicines, 45*(15), 2125–2131.
67. Fan, L. L., Deng, J. W., & Hao, E. G. (2010). Research progress on correlation between dose and efficacy of traditional Chinese medicine. *Chinese Journal of Information on Traditional Chinese Medicine, 17*(10), 104–106.
68. Zhang, J. K., Zheng, H., & Feng, G. (2020). Professor ZHENG Qizhong's experience in treating pediatric diseases with modified Guizhi Tang. *Journal of Pediatrics of Traditional Chinese Medicine, 16*(5), 16–19.
69. Li, Y. Z., Tang, L., Yang, Y. D., et al. (2019). Preparation and preliminary evaluation of compound salvia miltiorrhiza orally disintegrating tablets by 3D printing. *Contemporary in Chinese Medicine, 26*(12), 48–51.
70. Yan, J. X., Wang, Y., Zhang, X., et al. (2019). Snakegourd root/Astragalus polysaccharide hydrogel preparation and application in 3D printing. *International Journal of Biological Macromolecules, 121*(1), 309–316.
71. Wu, S. T., Li, J. S., Mai, J., et al. (2018). 3D electrohydrodynamic printing and spinning of flexible composite structures for oral multi-drug forms. *ACS Applied Materials & Interfaces, 10*(29), 24876–24885.
72. Peng, C. J., Du, B., Sun, G. Q., et al. (2019). Three-dimensional printing beta-tricalcium phosphate scaffold loaded with icariin particles for repairing osteonecrosis of the femoral head in rabbits. *Chinese Journal of Tissue Engineering Research, 23*(14), 2162–2168.
73. Dankar, I., Haddarah, A., Omar, F. E. L., et al. (2018). 3D printing technology: The new era for food customization and elaboration. *Trends in Food Science and Technology, 75*(1), 231–242.
74. Zhu, S., Stieger, M. A., Goot, A. J., et al. (2019). Extrusion-based 3D printing of food pastes: Correlating rheological properties with printing behavior. *Innovative Food Science and Emerging Technologies, 58*(1), 102214.
75. Periard, D., Schaal, N., Schaal, M., et al. (2007). *Printing food: Report of Cornell University*. Cornell University.
76. Xiao, J. Y., Zhang, M. Q., Cong, R. H., et al. (2019). Study on 3D printing molding of chocolate containing functional factors of traditional Chinese medicine. *Science and Technology of Food Industry, 40*(5), 77–82.
77. Wang, J. L., Wang, Y., Cen, P. Q., et al. (2018). *A 3D printing material for gel marshmallows containing optional compound polysaccharides and its preparation method*. Hubei: CN108402264A.
78. Cao, S. W., An, B. C., Xiang, S. J., et al. (2019). Studies on the anti-acne effects and skin safety of 3D printing cryptotanshinone hydrogel mask. *The Chinese Journal of Dermatovenereology, 33*(3), 371–378.

79. Chen, W. W., Zhang, G. F., Chen, Y. H., et al. (2018). Clinical application of 3D printed decompression insole in prevention and treatment of diabetic foot. *Journal of Tongji University (Medical Science), 39*(6), 76–81.
80. Huang, B. Y., Liu, X. R., Wang, X. Q., et al. (2018). *A traditional Chinese medicine insole based on 3D printing*. China: CN207531979U.
81. Wang, Y. R., Li, H., Zhang, B. X., et al. (2010). Application of new excipients in Chinese medicine dispersible tablets. *Chinese Journal of Experimental Traditional Medical Formulae, 16*(10), 207–209.
82. Pham, D. T., & Gault, R. S. (1998). A comparison of rapid prototyping technologies. *International Journal of Machine Tools and Manufacture, 38*(10–11), 1257–1287.
83. Katstra, W. E., Palazzolo, R. D., Rowe, C. W., Giritlioglu, B., Teung, P., & Cima, M. J. (2000). Oral dosage forms fabricated by Three Dimensional Printing (TM). *Journal of Controlled Release, 66*(1), 1–9.
84. FDA. (2017). *Tablet friability general chapter guidance for industry annex 9.*
85. Matthew, D. P., James, C., David, H., et al. (2015). Additively manufactured medical products-The FDA perspective. *3D Printing in Medicine, 2*(1), 1–6.
86. FDA. (2017). *Technical considerations for additive manufactured medical devices.*
87. Liu, Q., Cao, S. W., An, B. C., et al. (2019). *A 3D printing orally disintegrating tablet of breviscapine and its preparation method.* Guangdong Province, CN106511285B.
88. Liu, Q., Cao, S. W., An, B. C., et al. (2017). *A 3D printed orally disintegrating tablet of Panax notoginseng saponins and its preparation method.* Guangdong Province, CN106511416A.
89. Zheng, Y. (2018). *A 3D printing doxofylline orally disintegrating tablet and its preparation method.* Shanghai, CN107669648A.

Chapter 14
Nanotechnology in Drug Delivery: How Compatible It Is for TCM Drug Delivery

Shijia Fu, Yi Lu, Rongrong Lai, Ziyi Liu, and Yuehong Xu

Abstract Traditional Chinese medicine (TCM) is a treasure of the traditional culture of the Chinese nation, although many Chinese medicine ingredients have strong pharmacological effects in vitro; they have many problems such as poor water solubility, poor stability, and low bioavailability, which severely limit their druggability and clinical application. Nanotechnology is possible to improve the water solubility, maintain stability, and increase the bioavailability of the active ingredients of Chinese medicines. The application of nanotechnology can greatly improve the clinical application value and practical significance of TCM.

Keywords Traditional Chinese medicine · Nanotechnology · Solubility · Stability · Bioavailability · Druggability · Therapeutic efficiency

Traditional Chinese medicine (TCM) is a treasure of the traditional culture of the Chinese nation and a unique form of human use of natural medicine and its artificial substitutes. For thousands of years, under the guidance of the TCM theory, Chinese medicines have played an important role in fighting diseases and safeguarding health for the Chinese nation. With the continuous in-depth research on the chemistry and pharmacology of Chinese medicine, more and more active ingredients of Chinese medicine with promising and attractive pharmacological effect have been discovered. Some of the active ingredients such as paclitaxel and artemisinin have also been recognized worldwide as first-line treatments for the diseases that are life-threatening or that dramatically affect the quality of life of the patients. Huperzine A and butylphthalide have also become characteristic therapeutic agents for related diseases. But at the same time, it was also found that although many Chinese medicine ingredients have strong pharmacological effects in vitro, they have many

---

Shijia Fu and Yi Lu contributed equally to this work.

S. Fu · Y. Lu · R. Lai · Z. Liu · Y. Xu (✉)
School of Pharmaceutical Sciences, Sun Yat-sen University, Guangzhou, China
e-mail: lssxyh@mail.sysu.edu.cn

N. Feng, Z. Yang (eds.), *Novel Drug Delivery Systems for Chinese Medicines*,
https://doi.org/10.1007/978-981-16-3444-4_14

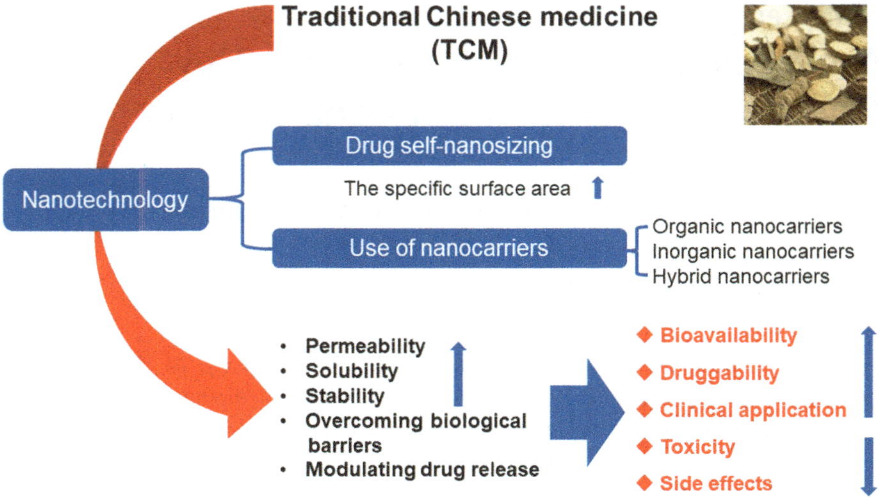

Fig. 14.1 Schematic diagram of applications of nanotechnology for TCM

problems such as poor water solubility, short half-life, poor stability, low and variable bioavailability, and large toxic and side effects, which severely limit their druggability and clinical application (Fig. 14.1).

Nanotechnology is considered to be one of the three core technologies supporting human civilization in the twenty-first century. Nanotechnology has carried out extensive research and application in the field of biomedicine as follows. (1) Nanosizing of the drug itself. The drug is made into nanometer size to increase the specific surface area and improve absorption. (2) Loading drugs into nanocarriers, such as liposomes, micelles, nanoparticles, and nanoemulsions, to improve their solubility and overcome various barriers.

Through the application of nanotechnology, it is possible to improve the water solubility of the active ingredients of Chinese medicine and increase the bioavailability of the medicine; the active ingredients of Chinese medicine are encapsulated into the nano-carriers to prevent damage from light, pH, and enzymes and maintain its stability. Besides, the small size of the nano-carrier and the modification of surface functional groups can be used to improve the targeting of the active ingredients of Chinese medicine while reducing its systemic side effects. Nanotechnology applied to TCM preparations can greatly improve the clinical application value and practical significance of TCM.

14.1 Advances in Nanotechnology

Through the application of nanotechnology, the water solubility of poorly soluble drugs can be improved, and the bioavailability, stability, targeting, and bioadhesion of the drugs can be improved, thereby obtaining an ideal drug delivery system and effectively treating diseases. However, due to the wide variety and complex composition of Chinese medicines, different effective ingredients need to be processed in combination with different nanotechnology. There are currently two main methods: one is to prepare active ingredient nanoparticles such as nanocrystals or nanosuspensions; the second is to combine nano-carrier systems such as nanoemulsions, liposomes, solid lipid nanoparticles, and phospholipid complexes to form a nano-TCM carrier system and improve its druggability. Nano-based drug delivery systems provide promise in overcoming the limitations of Chinese medicines including poor water solubility, insufficient absorption, and poor bioavailability (Table 14.1).

Based on Table 14.1, curcumin, an active ingredient of *Jianghuang* (*Curcumae Longae Rhizoma*), is the most widely developed in using nanotechnology to modify its properties such as poor solubility (1–10 μg/mL in water at room temperature and neutral pH) and poor stability for druggability [22, 23].

14.1.1 Nanometerization of Active Ingredients

14.1.1.1 Nanosuspension

Nanosuspensions are nano-colloidal dispersions formed by uniformly dispersing drug particles in the water phase with the help of the stability of surfactants or polymer materials. The preparation method can be divided into three types: emulsification, coagulation, and dispersion. Because the nanosuspension has a very small particle size, the drug has a larger specific surface area, and the dissolution rate of the drug reaches the maximum in a short time. Besides, it can extend the residence time of the drug in the gastrointestinal tract, thereby improving bioavailability. Therefore, nanosuspensions are widely used and have significant effects in solving the oral absorption of insoluble Chinese medicine active ingredients.

Curcumin is the main active component of Chinese medicine turmeric; it possesses good effects in regulating blood lipids and anti-inflammatory and anti-tumor growth. However, due to its extremely low water solubility, poor permeability, and poor stability, the oral bioavailability is low, which limits its clinical application. Gao et al. [24] prepared a curcumin nanosuspension with a particle size of 210 nm using a high-pressure homogenization method. After intragastric administration in rats, its oral bioavailability was 6.8 times that of curcumin suspension. Further studies have found that curcumin nanosuspension not only accelerates the fluidity of the intestinal mucosa but also changes the conformation of related intestinal

Table 14.1 Summary of typical nanotechnology applied to TCM

Nanotechnology		Effective monomers or components	Objective	Refs.
Nanoparticles	Solid lipid nanoparticles	Curcumin	Improve the stability of curcumin to light and oxygen	[1]
	PLGA Nanoparticles	Curcumin	Improve the stability of curcumin and bioavailability with sustained release	[2]
	Mesoporous carbon nanopowder	Baicalin	Improve solubility and drug loading	[3, 4]
	Chitosan Nanoparticles	Berberine	Improve adsorption and penetration of cell membranes to improve absorption in the small intestine	[5]
Nanosuspensions		Oleanolic acid	Improve saturated solubility, dissolution rate, and bioavailability	[6]
		Curcumin	Improve saturated solubility, dissolution rate, and bioavailability	[7]
		Puerarin	Improve saturated solubility, dissolution rate, and bioavailability	[8]
Microemulsion/ nanoemulsions		Baicalin	Surfactant and co-surfactant induced permeability enhancement, sustained release of yellow ical glycosides, and increased absorption of yellow ical glycosides by lymph	[3]
		Curcumin	Reduce skin irritation of curcumin, improve permeability and high drug loading	[7, 9, 10]
		Pseudolaric acid B	Improve skin permeability and vivo skin bioavailability	[11]
Self-microemulsifying drug delivery		Oleanolic acid Curcumin	Improve the solubility and dissolution rate; self-emulsifies into tiny droplets in the intestine so as to increase the surface area in contact with the small intestine and improve absorption; and can be transported through the lymph after absorption in the intestine to avoid the first pass effect	[12–14]
Liposomes		Baicalin	Improve solubility, drug stability, and bioavailability	[15]
		Camptothecin	Improve the stability to pH value, prolong blood circulation time, and improve accumulation in tumor tissue	[16]
Ethosomes		Curcumin	Improve adhesion and permeability to the gastrointestinal tract, thereby improving absorption and bioavailability in the gastrointestinal tract	[17]

(continued)

Table 14.1 (continued)

Nanotechnology	Effective monomers or components	Objective	Refs.
Nanocrystals	Puerarin	Improve the saturated solubility and bioavailability	[8, 18, 19]
	Myricetin	Significantly improve the solubility and dissolution rate of the drug	
Micelles	Curcumin	Improve stability and solubility in alkaline environment	[20]
Phospholipid complexes	Hydrocarbon camptothecin	Improve solubility and the permeability to intestinal mucosa, thereby improve the oral absorption	[21]

mucosal membrane proteins and improves the oral absorption of curcumin. With the advancement of nanotechnology, researchers increasingly pay attention to the surface modification of nanosuspensions, thereby changing the distribution of drugs in the body and the targeting effect of lesions and achieving applications in more fields. To increase tumor targeting of annona lactone, Hong et al. [25] prepared the nanosuspension and modified the nanosuspension with folic acid on its surface. The results show that compared with the non-modified nanosuspensions, folic acid-modified nanosuspensions can improve the accumulation of anti-tumor active ingredient annonaceous lactone at the tumor site and exert the improved anti-tumor effect on breast cancer mouse models. Therefore, nanosuspension is a very promising drug delivery system, but nanosuspension is a thermodynamically unstable system. Due to the increase in specific surface area, the nanosuspension is very easy to agglomerate. To date, many researchers have tried various strategies to address this problem. Using stabilizers such as surfactants and water-soluble cellulose derivatives is the main method to prevent the aggregation of high-energy nanosuspensions; they can provide both electrostatic and steric stabilizations. Moreover, optimization of nanosuspension preparation and solidification approaches are also performed to improve the stabilization of nanosuspensions [26]. Solidification of nanosuspension is re-dispersed into a nanosuspension prior to use [26].

14.1.1.2 Nano Co-crystal

Drug co-crystal refers to the combination of active pharmaceutical ingredient (API) and another or more neutral molecules (co-crystal former, CCF) in a fixed ratio under the action of hydrogen bonds or other non-covalent bonds. The pure state of API and CCF is both solid at room temperature. Its design relies on the supramolecular interactions between the effective functional groups of the eutectic components, which include hydrogen bonds, π-π stacking, van der Waals forces, and halogen bonds. Co-crystal technology is mainly used to improve or modify the physical and chemical properties of API in solid preparations, such as solubility, dissolution rate, melting point, stability, and bioavailability. At present, there are various preparation methods for drug co-crystals, among which the solution method and grinding method are the most commonly used preparation methods.

For example, myricetin, a typical flavonoid component, has good free radical scavenging ability and antioxidant activity and has many important biological activities, but its application has been limited by low solubility, poor stability, and low bioavailability. Nicotinamide was used to prepare myricetin-nicotinamide co-crystals by the solution method, which improved the solubility and dissolution rates of myricetin [19]. Further research on the use of the anti-solvent reprecipitation method to precipitate the co-crystal, combined with ultrasound to control the crystallization speed, successfully obtained myricetin nano-co-crystal. Compared with myricetin suspension, the nano-co-crystal significantly improved the solubility and dissolution rate under different pH conditions [27]. Compared with nano-carrier systems such as liposomes and nanoemulsions, nano-co-crystal, a technology aiming at the nanometerization of the drug itself, has a higher drug loading capacity and is suitable for large-dose administration while reducing the volume of administration. However, the selection of CCF is limited, that is, CCF is mostly selected from a structural point of view, commonly used such as nicotinamide, caffeine, etc. The safety of these CCFs in the human body is mostly unproven. This limits the development and application of nano-co-crystal.

14.1.2 Use of Nano-carriers

In the first place, the nano-drug delivery system (nano-carriers) can increase the chemical stability of drugs. The drug is encapsulated in the carrier to form a relatively closed environment, which can effectively prevent chemical changes such as oxidation, reduction, hydrolysis, and photolysis caused by external factors such as light, heat, moisture, and oxygen. Besides, the nano-drug delivery system can improve the physical stability of drugs, such as preventing drug aggregation. And it can increase the drug's biological stability in the digestive tract or blood, where the drug will be faced with various acid-base environment and enzyme damage. The nano-carriers are basically divided into organic nano-carriers, inorganic nano-carriers, and hybrid nano-carriers. However, considering the biocompatibility and safety, the organic nano-carriers especially prepared with the natural and biological original materials are more widely used.

14.1.2.1 Liposome

Liposomes are vesicle-like particles formed by self-assembly of amphiphilic phospholipid molecules. Its structure is similar to biomembrane, which can encapsulate hydrophilic and lipophilic drugs and improve the properties of drugs and has the characteristics of low toxicity and biodegradability. The particle size of liposomes is generally between tens of nanometers to tens of microns. Nano-scale liposomes have good stability and can passively target the lesion site and prolong the half-life of the drug in the blood circulation. Liposomes are mainly prepared by using phospholipids and cholesterol as membrane materials, using traditional methods such as thin-film dispersion, solvent injection, and ultrasonic dispersion.

Camptothecin (CPT) and its analogs have shown a broad spectrum of anti-tumor activity against many solid tumors in xenografts. However, the α-hydroxylactone ring, an essential group of CPTs, can be rapidly hydrolyzed into inactive forms under physiological conditions. Moreover, in the human body, the plasma protein preferentially combines with the inactive form of CPT, which shifts the balance and thus facilitates the conversion of CPT and its derivatives from the active form to the inactive form [28]. Masato Watanabe et al. [16] formulated CPT liposomes by the addition of 3,5-bis(dodecyloxy)benzoic acid to polyethylene glycol-containing liposomes and by coating the surface of the liposomes with human serum albumin (HSA, HSA-DB-L). The stability of CPT in vivo and the accumulation of CPT in the tumor site were significantly improved, and the anti-tumor effect was significantly improved. Yi et al. [28] prepared CPT liposomes by inserting the α-hydroxylactone ring into the liposomes' phospholipid bilayer, avoiding contact with the external pH environment and increasing its gastrointestinal stability.

The stability of anthocyanin is poor, and it is easy to degrade or oxidize under the influence of temperature, pH, light, metal ions, and other external factors [29]. Wang et al. [30] modified purple sweet potato anthocyanin liposome with three different concentrations of anionic polysaccharides to explore the stability of liposomes in the gastrointestinal environment under simulated conditions in vitro. It was found that the combination of polysaccharides and liposomes can increase the stability of the bilayer membrane of liposomes, which improves the stability of liposomes in gastric and intestinal fluids.

14.1.2.2 Solid Lipid Nanoparticles

Solid lipid nanoparticles (SLN) were nano-carriers developed in the early 1990s. They are made with natural or synthetic physiologically compatible high-melting lipids, emulsifiers, and water. The lipids construct the inner cores to encapsulate or adsorb drugs. This system has higher physical and chemical stability, can avoid the degradation of drugs, and has the characteristics of liposomes and emulsions with low toxicity and large-scale production. It is a new type of nano-drug system with great development prospects. The preparation methods mainly include high-pressure homogenization, emulsification ultrasound, and solvent emulsification evaporation methods. However, SLN show some disadvantages including an unpredictable gelation tendency, polymorphic transition, and low incorporation due to the crystalline structure of solid lipids. The new generation of lipid nanoparticles is nanostructured lipid carriers (NLC), which is prepared by the addition of liquid lipid into the solid lipid matrix leading to a special nanostructure to address the potential drawbacks of SLN. Compared with SLN, NLC can improve the drug loading and the inherent stability of nano-carrier and decrease the drug expulsion during storage.

Curcuminoids are antioxidants isolated from the rhizome of *Jianghuang* (*Curcumae longae rhizome*). Unfortunately, they are degraded by acidic and alkaline hydrolysis, oxidation, and photodegradation. Tiyaboonchai et al. [1] prepared curcuminoid-loaded SLN by micro-emulsification technology. The lyophilized curcuminoid SLN and non-encapsulated curcuminoid were prepared into the cream and stored in the absence of sunlight. After 6 months of storage in the absence of sunlight, the remaining curcumin in SLN cream was 91%; however, the non-encapsulated curcumin cream showed 80% curcuminoid loss. SLN significantly improved the stability of curcuminoid to light and oxidation during storage. Han et al. [31] prepared SLN of the volatile oil of *Jiangxiang* (*Dalbergiae odoriferae lignum*) by hot dispersion and sonication technique. The biocompatible lipid monostearate was used as a matrix of drug carrier, and soybean phospholipid and poloxamer F-68 were used as surfactants. The stability of volatile oil was increased. To improve the solubility and bioavailability of curcumin, Vijayakumar developed a ginsenoside-modified NLC for curcumin (G-NLC) against colon cancer; G-NLC was demonstrated to enhance the cellular uptake and cytotoxicity of curcumin as well as its oral bioavailability [32]. Rapalli et al. reported a NLC based on lipids of Precirol ATO 5 and Labrafac M 1944 for curcumin dermal delivery to enhance its skin retention and cellular uptake by keratinocytes [33].

14.1.2.3 Nanoemulsion

Nanoemulsion is a transparent or translucent dispersion composed of the water phase, oil phase, surfactant, and co-surfactant, with a particle size of 1–100 nm. Nanoemulsion mainly includes three types, water-in-oil, oil-in-water, and bicontinuous. Nanoemulsion has a simple preparation method and high safety. It is often used as a nano-carrier to improve the solubility and stability of poorly soluble drugs to increase bioavailability. The new type of nanoemulsion system can achieve the active target through surface modification or adjustment of the way the nanoemulsion is prepared.

Breviscapine is a cardiovascular drug extracted from *Dengzhanxixin* (*Erigerontis herba*), which can improve blood circulation and relieve blood stasis. However, it is stable only in acidic condition, but not in alkaline solution. Xiong et al. [34] prepared breviscapine nanoemulsion modified by monooleate-PEG-COOH, which enhanced the stability of breviscapine, prolonged the circulation time in vivo, and thus improved the bioavailability.

14.1.2.4 Cyclodextrin-Drug Inclusion Complex

Clathrate is a class of organic crystals. Its structure contains two structural units, that is, the inclusion compound is composed of two compounds: one is a compound that can trap other compounds in the cavities of its structural skeleton, called an inclusion agent or host molecule; the other is a compound trapped in the cavities or pores of the clathrate structure, called the clathrate or guest molecule. Clathrate is commonly used as nanotechnology to solve the solubilization technology of insoluble drugs. Currently, cyclodextrins used in delivering Chinese medicine include β-cyclodextrin and hydroxypropyl-β-cyclodextrin. *Yuxingcao* (*Houttuyniae Herba*) is known as TCM antibiotic. Volatile oil is its main effective component, mostly terpenoids. Zhang et al. [35] prepared hydroxypropyl β-cyclodextrin inclusion complex of volatile oil from *Yuxingcao*. The characteristics of hydroxypropyl β-cyclodextrin can make insoluble drug molecules enter into its cavity and form inclusion complex, avoiding the direct contact between drugs and the environment; reducing the influence of light, heat, oxygen, and hydrolysis; protecting the active components; and prolonging the efficacy and storage life, so as to improve the quality of the drug and to have high stability.

The volatile oil of *Aiye* (*Artemisia argyi folium*) is unstable, and it is easy to degrade when exposed to light, heat, and oxidation, thus affecting its curative effect. The stability of β-cyclodextrin inclusion complex of volatile oil from *Aiye* was studied by classical constant temperature method [36]. After inclusion with β-cyclodextrin, the $t_{0.9}$ of volatile oil from *Aiye* increased by 111.8%, and the validity period was prolonged. This is due to the special molecular structure of β-cyclodextrin inclusion of volatile oil, forming a "molecular capsule." Cordycepin, an active ingredient of *Dongchongxiacao* (*Cordyceps*), has poor water solubility and poor stability, so its application in pharmaceutical preparations is limited. Bao et al. [37] prepared cordycepin-cyclodextrin inclusion compound with dimethyl-β-cyclodextrin, which greatly improved the solubility and stability of cordycepin.

Inclusion technology has been more and more widely used in the research of TCM preparations. However, due to the limitations of the inclusion compound itself, this technology still has some drawbacks such as poor solubility improvement and low inclusion efficiency for some Chinese medicines. Moreover, the inclusion materials approved by regulation are limited.

14.1.2.5 Micelles

Micelles are nano-carriers based on polymers or lipids possessing both hydrophilic and hydrophobic groups; they can form micelles in water and encapsulate drugs. Screening its hydrophobic core helps to carry drugs of different properties. The hydrophilic shell can be chemically modified to make micelles have specific functions, such as targeting and temperature sensitivity.

Jiang et al. [21] prepared the phospholipid complex of CPT by solvent method. The phospholipid complex was dispersed into nano-micelles by ultrasonic probe method. The proportion of lactone type was significantly increased, the ring-opening phenomenon was reduced, and the stability of the drug was improved.

To improve the blood stability of curcumin, methoxy polyethylene glycol polycaprolactone block copolymer capped by tert-butoxycarbonylphenylalanine was synthesized, and curcumin copolymer micelles were prepared by solid dispersion process [38]. The results showed that the plasma elimination half-life of curcumin micelles was significantly longer than that of curcumin solution, and the clearance rate was significantly reduced by 8 times, which indicated that the micelles significantly reduced the clearance rate of curcumin in blood and improved the blood stability of curcumin.

14.2 Nanotechnology Improves the Bioavailability of Active Ingredients of Chinese Medicines

Oral administration is one of the most common ways of administration of TCM drug. However, due to poor water solubility, low membrane permeability, or unstabillity in the gastrointestinal tract, the active ingredients of many Chinese medicines are poorly absorbed after oral administration and have low bioavailability, which severely limits the effectiveness of Chinese medicine. Therefore, improving the bioavailability of the active ingredients of Chinese medicine is the main aim in the current research of TCM preparation. To solve this problem, a series of drug delivery systems have been developed, among which nanotechnology is of great significance for improving the bioavailability of TCM preparations. The improvement of bioavailability can be obtained through improving solubility and permeability, preventing degradation, and the combination of these. Table 14.2 summarizes the active ingredients from Chinese medicines, of which the bioavailability is improved by the application of nanotechnology.

14.2.1 Improve the Solubility of the Effective Ingredients of Chinese Medicines

With the gradual development of research on the modernization of TCM, more and more effective ingredients of Chinese medicines have been discovered and confirmed, such as paclitaxel, berberine, artemisinin, etc. The effective ingredients of Chinese medicine not only have strong pharmacological activity in vitro but also have good therapeutic effects on many diseases. However, the active ingredients in many Chinese medicines have low solubility and poor oral bioavailability, especially when the drugs are the Biopharmaceutics Classification System (BCS) Class II; their bioavailability correlates with their solubility. An increase in solubility should result in the increase of in vivo bioavailability. By loading these effective ingredients into nano-carriers or nanometerization, their solubility can be significantly improved, thereby further improving their bioavailability.

Table 14.2 Representative nanotechnologies to improve the bioavailability of Chinese medicines

Chinese medicine monomer/ component	Source	Nanotechnology	Advantages	Refs.
Puerarin	*Gegen* (*Puerariae Lobatae Radix*)	Microemulsion	Improve bioavailability	[39]
		Nanoparticles	Improve bioavailability	[40]
		Nanocrystals	Improve solubility and bioavailability	[18]
Baicalin	*Huangqin* (*Scutellariae Radix*)	Liposome	Improve bioavailability	[15]
		Nanoemulsion	Improve oral bioavailability	[9]
		HLA-based nanogel system	Improve transdermal flux and bioavailability	[41]
		Mesoporous carbon nanopowder	Improve solubility and bioavailability	[3]
Curcumin	*Jianghuang* (*Curcumae Longae Rhizoma*)	Solid lipid nanoparticles	Enhancing the drug solubility	[1]
		Nanoemulsion gel	Improve skin permeation	[10]
		PLGA Nanoparticles	Improve stability and bioavailability	[2]
		Self-microemulsifying drug delivery system	Improve solubility and bioavailability	[14]
		Ethosomes	Improve bioavailability	[17]
		Solid lipid nanoparticles	Improve stability and bioavailability	[42]
		Nano-micelles	Reduced skin irritation, improved permeation, and drug loading	[20]
Oleanolic acid	*Nvzhenzi* (*Ligustri Lucidi Fructus*)	Nanosuspensions	Improve solubility	[6]
		Self-microemulsifying drug delivery system	Improve bioavailability	[12, 13]
		Nanoparticles	Improve bioavailability	[4]
20 (S)-ginsenoside Rg3	*Hongshen* (*Ginseng Radix et Rhizoma Rubra*)	Nanospheres	Improve solubility and bioavailability	[43]
Pseudolaric acid B	Tujingpi (*Pseudolaricis Cortex*)	Microemulsion	Improve solubility and permeability	[11]
Camptothecin	*Xishu* (*Camptotheca acuminata*)	Liposomes	Increased stability, enhanced anti-tumor effect	[16]

(continued)

Table 14.2 (continued)

Chinese medicine monomer/ component	Source	Nanotechnology	Advantages	Refs.
Breviscapine	*Dengzhanxixin* (*Erigerontis Herba*)	Lipid emulsions	Enhance the pharmacological activity	[34]
Myricetin	Many fruits such as grapes, onions, berries, vine tea	Co-crystal	Enhancing the solubility	[19]

The nanometerization of the effective ingredients of Chinese medicines is an important means to improve the solubility of Chinese medicines. At present, the main methods for preparing Chinese medicine nanosuspensions include medium milling, high-pressure homogenization, emulsification, and nano-spray drying. Because the drug particles in the nanosuspension have a smaller particle size and a larger specific surface area, the solubility and dissolution rate of the drug are significantly improved, and the bioavailability of the oral drug is further improved [44]. Huang et al. [45] prepared a high drug loading triptorubin nanosuspension with poloxamer 188 as a stabilizer, and the drug loading amount was as high as 86.39%. Xie et al. [46] prepared luteolin nanosuspension by the medium milling method, which significantly improved the dissolution rate of luteolin in vitro.

In addition, loading the poorly soluble effective ingredients into nano-carriers is another important means to improve the solubility. For example, the hydrophobic part of the micelle has high solubility for poorly soluble drugs; loading the poorly soluble drugs into the hydrophobic core of the micelle can improve the solubility of the poorly soluble drugs. Curcumin has strong anti-tumor activity in vitro, but its poor water solubility and low bioavailability limit its clinical application. Abedanzadeh [20] successfully loaded curcumin into amphiphilic block copolymer micelles with variable hydrophobic length, which significantly increased the solubility of curcumin by 400 times. After the lipid components in the solid lipid nanoparticles are digested by the digestive enzymes in the gastrointestinal tract, they will work together with bile salts and other secretions to form mixed micelles, thereby improving the drug solubility in the gastrointestinal tract [47]. Artemisinin and its derivative artemether are specific drugs for a variety of drug-resistant malaria and are also considered promising anticancer drugs. However, artemisinin has poor water solubility and low oral bioavailability, which reduces the efficacy of oral administration of artemisinin. Dwivedi [48] developed a solid lipid nanoparticle loaded with artemether, which significantly increased the solubility and oral bioavailability of artemether. Compared with the suspension of artemether, the relative bioavailability was improved to 7461% in Sprague-Dawley rats.

14.2.2 Improve the Permeability of the Effective Ingredients of Chinese Medicines

Many active ingredients with poor membrane permeability also have limited oral bioavailability, which are the drugs of BCS III and IV. These drugs often require injection in clinical practice. The development of oral preparations of such drugs is difficult. Nano-preparations can effectively solve this problem. For example, liposomes have good compatibility with cell membranes and can fuse with gastrointestinal mucosal cells through pinocytosis and phagocytosis, thereby increasing the bioavailability of drugs. The lipid components in nanoemulsion can help open the tight junctions of the intestinal wall, thereby improving the permeability of low-permeability drugs.

It is reported that after the total saponins of *Sanqi* (*Panax notoginseng*) are made into liposomes and administered orally, the AUC is significantly higher than that of the marketed preparation *Xueshuantong* Capsules, and the absolute bioavailability is significantly improved [49]. Silymarin is hydrophobic and oleophobic. After oral administration, only 20–50% is absorbed by the gastrointestinal tract and rapidly metabolized and eliminated, so its bioavailability is extremely low. After preparing silymarin into proliposomes, the absolute bioavailability is increased by about 3 times compared with its suspension formulation, the average retention time (MRT) of the drug in the body is increased by about 2 times, and the peak concentration (Cmax) is increased by about 5 times [50].

In recent years, new types of nano-carriers have been developed to further improve the membrane permeability of the effective ingredients of Chinese medicines. For example, the positively charged chitosan nanoparticles can electrostatically adsorb with the negatively charged cell membrane, thereby promoting the endocytosis of the nanoparticles and improving the transport and permeability of berberine, an insoluble component of Chinese medicines, in the gastrointestinal cells [5, 51]. With the exception of enhancing the drug permeability, reducing the efflux by some transporters is also one strategy to improve drug permeability.

14.2.3 Improves the Bioavailability of the Effective Ingredients of Chinese Medicines

The development of nanotechnology has paved a new way for the clinical application of TCM. The combination of TCM components and nanotechnology can improve the problems of poor water solubility, poor permeability, and poor stability of Chinese medicine monomers, so as to overcome the shortcomings of short half-life and low bioavailability [52]. The rate of drug absorption is affected by the solubility and dissolution rate of the drug in the body fluids at the site of absorption. The results showed that the dissolution rate of the effective ingredients was closely related to the characteristics of the pulverized product particles [53]. The dissolution rate is proportional to the surface area of the drug. The smaller the size and the larger the surface area, the more favorable the dissolution and absorption of the drug. Therefore, the dissolution rate of drugs reaching the nanoscale increases greatly, thus improving bioavailability [53]. Moreover, the adhesion and small particle size on the surface of nanoscale drugs are conducive to the increase of retention during local drug administration, achieving the sustained release effect, increasing the contact area and contact time between drugs and the intestinal wall, and improving the bioavailability. In addition, nanoscale drugs can change the membrane transport mechanism and increase the permeability of drugs to biofilms, which is conducive to drug transdermal absorption, intracellular efficacy, and bioavailability.

In the following part, we introduce several examples of improving bioavailability of active ingredients of Chinese medicine through nanotechnology. Curcumin has been found to have a wide range of pharmacological effects, such as antioxidant, anti-inflammatory, anticancer, and antibacterial. Despite its safety, curcumin has not been used clinically because of its low bioavailability. Major reasons contributing to the low plasma and tissue levels of curcumin appear to be due to poor absorption, rapid metabolism, and rapid systemic elimination. The bioavailability of curcumin can be improved to a certain extent by using nano-technologies such as liposomes, micelles, and nanoparticles. The formulation of SMEDDS is composed of 20% ethanol, 60% Cremophor RH40®, and 20% isopropyl myristate, which improved the oral bioavailability of curcumin significantly, and the relative oral bioavailability of SMEDDS compared with curcumin suspension was 1213% [14]. Pueraria is a bioactive flavonoid in some Chinese medicines. In recent years, the research on improving the bioavailability of puerarin has developed rapidly. Various nanotechnology and preparation technologies, including microemulsions and SMEDDS, dendrimers, nanoparticles, and nanocrystals, have been used to improve the bioavailability of puerarin [8]. The preparation of amorphous butadienolactone nanomaterials by wet grinding can improve the solubility and stability of butadienolactone, an anti-tumor component of *Chansu* (*Bufonis Venenum*), and realize the rapid and synchronous dissolution of multicomponent preparations, which may increase the bioavailability of drugs with poor water solubility [54]. Baicalin is an active ingredient for the treatment of ischemic cerebrovascular diseases, but its clinical application is limited due to its poor water solubility, poor bioavailability, and short half-life. Compared to the baicalin suspension, the $AUC_{0\text{-}t}$ and C_{max} values of the baicalin nanoemulsion were increased by 10.5-fold and 3.12-fold, respectively, which mean that nanoemulsion increases the bioavailability of baicalin [9]. 20 (S)-ginsenoside Rg3 was extracted from red ginseng. However, its poor water solubility and low oral bioavailability limit its clinical application. A magnetic human serum albumin nanoparticle loading 20 (S)-ginsenoside Rg3 was prepared to improve its water solubility and bioavailability [55]. *Xionghuang* (*Realgar*) is widely used in TCM, but its poor water solubility, potential toxicity, and low bioavailability hinder its clinical application. Application of nanotechnology to realgar may overcome these problems. *Xionghuang* is insoluble in water. Several types of nanoparticles (NPs) have recently been developed, some of which also have the unique optical properties of quantum dots. Therefore, realgar nanoparticles have been developed to improve the shortcomings of realgar's poor water solubility and strong toxicity [56]. Oleanolic acid, a naturally derived triterpene, is clinically used in the treatment of hepatitis in China, but its poor solubility often leads to poor bioavailability. A novel oleanolic acid nanoparticle-loaded lactoferrin nanodelivery system can enhance in vitro oleanolic acid dissolution and improve oral absorption and bioavailability. An effective in vivo bioavailability (340.59%) was achieved compared to the free drug following oral administration to rats [4].

14.3 Improve the Transdermal and Mucosal Absorption of Active Ingredients of Chinese Medicines

Transdermal and transmucosal administration of Chinese medicines is a common way of administration. The effective components of TCM are absorbed into the systemic circulation through the skin and mucosa to produce systemic or local therapeutic effects. Since the penetration of Chinese medicine through the skin or mucosa is limited, it is particularly important to improve the transdermal or transmucosal efficiency of the effective ingredients of Chinese medicines for the development of transdermal and transmucosal administration of Chinese medicine.

14.3.1 Improve the Transdermal Absorption

Modern pharmacy can improve the absorption of the effective ingredients of Chinese medicine in the skin by preparing the effective ingredients of Chinese medicine into nano-preparations. Transdermal delivery system is considered to be a safe option given the higher patient compliance and controlled release compared to other delivery systems. Nanotechnology used in transdermal drug delivery system can effectively enhance the solubility of compounds, interact with the skin, and deliver the ingredient across the skin or along the hair follicular pathway, thus improving the transdermal efficiency. Figure 14.2 presents the improvement transdermal efficiency of nanotechnology on transdermal delivery.

Solid lipid nanoparticles do not use high-concentration surfactants in their preparation process; they can form a film on the skin surface, and promote the drug absorption through epidermal hydration after partial sealing, and increase the contact time and area of the drug with the stratum corneum. This facilitates the transdermal absorption of the drug. Mei et al. [57] screened the percutaneous penetration and anti-inflammatory activity of triptolide using solid lipid nanoparticles and found that triptolide solid lipid nanoparticles have a stronger effect on adjuvant arthritis caused by complete adjuvant and can reduce the toxicity of triptolide to the liver, kidney, and other tissues. Microneedles have recently emerged as a novel transdermal drug delivery system, which can transiently break through the barrier properties of the

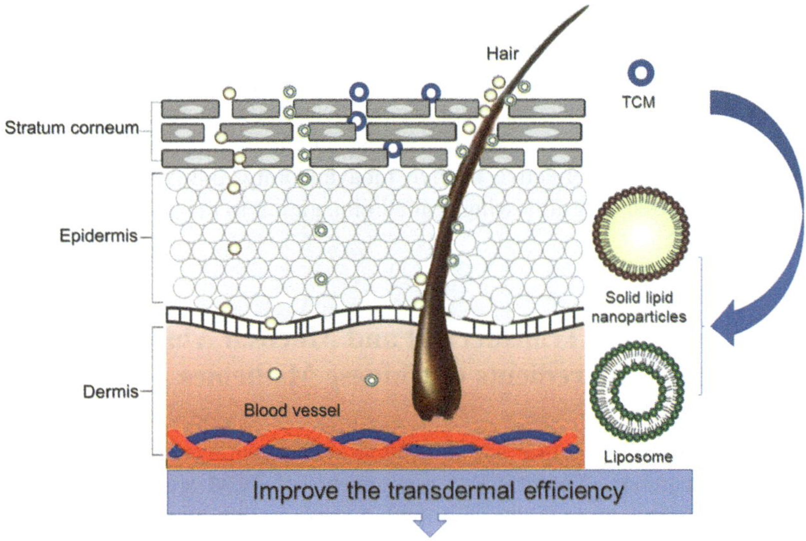

Fig. 14.2 Improve the transdermal efficiency of TCM with nanotechnology

skin and enhance the permeation of vaccines, macromolecules, and nanoparticles. Guo et al. [58] prepared aconitine-loaded solid lipid nanoparticles into dissolving microneedles, which significantly increased drug penetration in the skin and reduced the toxicity of aconitine. In addition, the area under the concentration-time curve of aconitine obtained with microneedles was 1.95-fold higher than those of solid lipid nanoparticles applied onto the skin.

Ethosomes are lipid vesicles containing phospholipids and relatively high concentrations of low molecular alcohols. Owing to their high deformability, they can transport active agents through the stratum corneum into deeper layers of the skin more effectively than traditional liposomes. Shen et al. [59] designed a novel delivery vehicle for apigenin that can enhance drug loading by increasing apigenin's solubility and transdermal absorption. Ethosomes showed the highest in vivo skin deposition at 2 h and the highest in vitro skin deposition at the end of the test period of 12 h compared with liposomes and deformable liposomes. In addition, Zhang et al. [60] developed a new phospholipid vesicle that is co-hybridized with hyaluronic acid (HA) and ethanol, as transdermal delivery vehicles for eugenol and cinnamaldehyde in order to increase drug loading, improve formulation stability, and enhance transdermal drug delivery. The HA-immobilized ethosomes significantly improved vesicle stability and reduced permeation of loaded lipid-soluble drugs out of the phospholipid membrane, thereby decreasing the leakage and release of the drug when they penetrated deep skin.

Microemulsion (ME), as a colloidal nanosize carrier system, has emerged as a promising vehicle for topical administration of drug with poor water solubility, and its potential for drug percutaneous delivery was mainly attributed to the properties of having excellent solubilizing capacity and being penetration enhancers. Although pseudolaric acid B (PAB) exhibited unique fungicidal activity, PAB tincture is a strong irritant to the skin owing to the high ethanol content of more than 70%. Wan et al. [11] developed microemulsion-based carbopol1940 hydrogel for PAB that improved the solubility and eventually the dermal permeability and bioavailability of PAB. In vitro sensitivity against *C. albicans* test indicated that 8 mg/g of PAB microemulsion-gel exhibited a higher efficacy than that of 20 mg/g miconazole nitrate cream after 7-day treatment.

14.3.2 Improve the Mucosal Absorption

Intranasal administration of Chinese medicines has a local effect on nasal cavity, or Chinese medicine delivered from nose to brain shows a central nervous treatment as well as works in curing systemic diseases [61].

The liposome can better encapsulate hydrophilic or lipophilic drugs, has obvious advantages in transmucosal penetration of poorly soluble drugs, and can be used to increase the concentration of local poorly soluble drugs. It can also be used as a drug reservoir to achieve a sustained release effect by increasing the retention time of the drug in the mucosa. Yan et al. [62] compared the nasal mucosal absorption of ligustrazine phosphate-loaded liposomes and ligustrazine phosphate solutions using a rat and in vivo nasal circulation perfusion method and found that the absorption of ligustrazine phosphate from liposome through the nasal mucosa was significantly higher than that of the solution. *Xinyi* (*Magnoliae flos*) has the functions of dispelling wind chill and clearing nose orifice, and its main effective component is volatile oil. The volatile oil nanoliposomes could significantly reduce the ear swelling caused by xylene in mice, significantly inhibit the capillary permeability caused by acetic acid in mice, and effectively fight against nasal itching, sneezing, and runny nose caused by allergic rhinitis in rats, with better therapeutic effect than the free volatile oil of *Xinyi* [63].

Phospholipid complex can effectively improve the oil-water partition coefficient of the active ingredients of Chinese medicine with poor solubility and improve its transmucosal absorption efficiency. Shi et al. [64] prepared the poorly soluble extract of *Huangqin* into a phospholipid complex, which can effectively improve its oil-water partition coefficient. The absorption rate of *Huangqin* extract and phospholipid complex in vivo through a rat nasal circulation absorption experiment showed that the phospholipid complex can promote the absorption of baicalin, and its absorption rate constant is 30% higher than that of the extract. Wu et al. determined that the baicalin phospholipid complex was obviously superior to the other two drug loading systems by evaluating the permeability of liposome, cyclodextrin inclusion compound, and phospholipid complex through the nasal mucosa of isolated animals [65].

Zhang et al. [66] prepared chitosan modified gardenin-loaded polylactic acid-hydroxyacetic acid nanoparticles (CS-PLGA-NPs) by compound emulsion and solvent evaporation method. It was stable in nasal lotion and had no nasal ciliary toxicity. CS-PLGA-NPs could promote the direct transport of drugs into the brain through nasal cavity, which is expected to be an ideal carrier for nasal administration.

Zhang et al. [67] used phase transfer technology to prepare high-dose tanshinone IIA nasal submicroemulsion, which is administered through the nasal cavity and aims to obtain the brain targeting effect. It is expected to be an effective preparation for treating ischemic brain injury. The preparation process is stable and feasible, and the drug load is higher than the traditional method, which can meet the needs of various drug use ways.

14.4 Conclusion

As an emerging novel technology with great market potential, nanotechnology will have a profound impact on the development of TCM. And TCM is a traditional cultural treasure with a long history. It has many and complex ingredients, but the research technology in the field of Chinese medicine is relatively backward, and there is an urgent need to apply new technologies to TCM. Applying modern nanotechnology to TCM can solve the problem of low solubility, poor stability, permeability, and low bioavailability of Chinese medicines. However, the application of nanotechnology to TCM should pay more attention to the following items. First, Chinese medicine includes material, complex prescription, bioactive ingredients, and bioactive parts; the application of different nanotechnology methods to these Chinese medicine is different. The mechanical crushing technology is the main approach for nanolization of TCM material and complex prescription, and nanoparticulate drug delivery system is the main approach for nanolization of bioactive ingredients or bioactive components in TCM. Choosing the suitable nanotechnology for different Chinese medicines is based on the compatibility. Second, the commercialization or scale-up of the nanotechnology for TCM is difficult. There are several anticancer nanomedicines including liposome, albumin nanoparticles, and polymeric nanoparticles approved for clinical use in cancer patients in the past few decades. However, the scale-up nanomaterial synthesis used in liposome or nanoparticles and formulation from the lab to industrial scale is difficult, and the complex technology and high cost of liposome and nanoparticles limit their scale-up. The future study includes choosing the suitable nanotechnology for TCM based on the compatibility of the technology with the properties of Chinese medicines and the requirements of druggability of Chinese medicines.

References

1. Tiyaboonchai, W., Tungpradit, W., & Plianbangchang, P. (2007). Formulation and characterization of curcuminoids loaded solid lipid nanoparticles. *International Journal of Pharmaceutics, 337*(1–2), 299–306.
2. Zheng, Y., Zheng, S. S., & Wang, Z. S. (2014). Curcumin-PLGA nanoparticles improve the bioavailability of oral administration. *The Chinese Journal of Modern Applied Pharmacy, 31* (06), 717–721.
3. Huang, T., Liu, Y., & Zhang, C. (2019). Pharmacokinetics and Bioavailability Enhancement of Baicalin: A Review. *European Journal of Drug Metabolism and Pharmacokinetics, 44*(2), 159–168.
4. Xia, X., Liu, H., Lv, H., Zhang, J., Zhou, J., & Zhao, Z. (2017). Preparation, characterization, and in vitro/vivo studies of oleanolic acid-loaded lactoferrin nanoparticles. *Drug Design, Development and Therapy, 11*, 1417–1427.
5. Yuan, X. Y., Xu, H. H., Shao, F. P., Yin, D. K., & Yang, Y. (2018). The effect of chitosan nanoparticles on the transport of berberine through Caco-2 cell monolayer membrane. *Chinese Journal of New Drugs, 27*(6), 708–713.
6. Chen, Y., Liu, J., Yang, X., Zhao, X., & Xu, H. (2005). Oleanolic acid nanosuspensions: Preparation, in-vitro characterization and enhanced hepatoprotective effect. *The Journal of Pharmacy and Pharmacology, 57*(2), 259–264.
7. Shome, S., Talukdar, A. D., Choudhury, M. D., Bhattacharya, M. K., & Upadhyaya, H. (2016). Curcumin as potential therapeutic natural product: A nanobiotechnological perspective. *The Journal of Pharmacy and Pharmacology, 68*(12), 1481–1500.
8. Zhang, L. (2019). Pharmacokinetics and drug delivery systems for puerarin, a bioactive flavone from traditional Chinese medicine. *Drug Delivery, 26*(1), 860–869.
9. Xu, Q., Zhou, A., Wu, H., & Bi, Y. (2019). Development and in vivo evaluation of baicalin-loaded W/O nanoemulsion for lymphatic absorption. *Pharmaceutical Development and Technology, 24*(9), 1155–1163.
10. Naz, Z., & Ahmad, F. J. (2015). Curcumin-loaded colloidal carrier system: Formulation optimization, mechanistic insight, ex vivo and in vivo evaluation. *International Journal of Nanomedicine, 10*, 4293.
11. Wan, T., Xu, T., Pan, J., Qin, M., Pan, W., Zhang, G., Wu, Z., Wu, C., & Xu, Y. (2015). Microemulsion based gel for topical dermal delivery of pseudolaric acid B: In vitro and in vivo evaluation. *International Journal of Pharmaceutics, 493*(1–2), 111–120.
12. Yang, R., Su, L. Q., Huang, X., & Zhai, G. X. (2010). Pharmacokinetics of oleanolic acid self-microemulsion in rats. *Chinese Journal of Hospital Pharmacy, 30*(11), 925–928.
13. Yang, R., Huang, X., Dou, J., Zhai, G., & Su, L. (2013). Self-microemulsifying drug delivery system for improved oral bioavailability of oleanolic acid: Design and evaluation. *International Journal of Nanomedicine, 8*, 2917–2926.
14. Hong, C., Xie, Y., Yao, Y., Li, G., Yuan, X., & Shen, H. (2011). Self-microemulsifying drug delivery system improves curcumin dissolution and bioavailability. *Drug Development and Industrial Pharmacy, 37*(1), 15–23.
15. Xiang, Y., Long, Y., Yang, Q., Zheng, C., Cui, M., Ci, Z., Lv, X., Li, N., & Zhang, R. (2020). Pharmacokinetics, pharmacodynamics and toxicity of Baicalin liposome on cerebral ischemia reperfusion injury rats via intranasal administration. *Brain Research, 1726*, 146503.
16. Watanabe, M., Kawano, K., Toma, K., Hattori, Y., & Maitani, Y. (2008). In vivo antitumor activity of camptothecin incorporated in liposomes formulated with an artificial lipid and human serum albumin. *Journal of Controlled Release, 127*(3), 231–238.
17. Zhao, J., Li, Y., Shi, M. X., Wang, X., & Zhang, J. B. (2017). The pharmacokinetics of curcumin liposomes in rats in vivo. *Journal of Sichuan University (Medical Edition), 48*(02), 290–294.

18. Xiong, S., Liu, W., Li, D., Chen, X., Liu, F., Yuan, D., Pan, H., Wang, Q., Fang, S., & Chen, T. (2019). Oral delivery of puerarin nanocrystals to improve brain accumulation and anti-Parkinsonian efficacy. *Molecular Pharmaceutics, 16*(4), 1444–1455.
19. Hong, C., Xie, Y., Yao, Y., Li, G., Yuan, X., & Shen, H. (2015). A novel strategy for pharmaceutical cocrystal generation without knowledge of stoichiometric ratio: Myricetin cocrystals and a ternary phase diagram. *Pharmaceutical Research, 32*(1), 47–60.
20. Abedanzadeh, M., Salmanpour, M., Farjadian, F., Mohammadi, S., & Tamaddon, A. M. (2020). Curcumin loaded polymeric micelles of variable hydrophobic lengths by RAFT polymerization: Preparation and in-vitro characterization. *Journal of Drug Delivery Science and Technology, 58*, 101793.
21. Jiang, H. B., Ding, C. N., Xu, S., & Cui, D. F. (2010). Preparation of hydroxycamptothecin phospholipid complex nanomicelles and improvement of the stability of its effective form. In *Biological Particle and Powder Preparation and Application Technology Seminar 2010: Shanghai, China.*
22. Nelson, K. M., Dahlin, J. L., Bisson, J., Graham, J., Pauli, G. F., & Walters, M. A. (2017). The essential medicinal chemistry of curcumin. *Journal of Medicinal Chemistry, 60*(5), 1620–1637.
23. Ma, Z., Wang, N., He, H., & Tang, X. (2019). Pharmaceutical strategies of improving oral systemic bioavailability of curcumin for clinical application. *Journal of Controlled Release, 316*, 359–380.
24. Gao, Y., Wang, C., Sun, M., Wang, X., Yu, A., Li, A., & Zhai, G. (2012). In vivo evaluation of curcumin loaded nanosuspensions by oral administration. *Journal of Biomedical Nanotechnology, 8*(4), 659–668.
25. Hong, J., Sun, Z., Li, Y., Guo, Y., Liao, Y., Liu, M., & Wang, X. (2017). Folate-modified Annonaceous acetogenins nanosuspensions and their improved antitumor efficacy. *International Journal of Nanomedicine, 12*, 5053–5067.
26. Wang, P., Cao, X., Chu, Y., & Wang, P. (2019). Ginkgolides-loaded soybean phospholipid-stabilized nanosuspension with improved storage stability and in vivo bioavailability. *Colloids and Surfaces. B, Biointerfaces, 181*, 910.
27. Liu, M., Hong, C., Li, G., Ma, P., & Xie, Y. (2016). The generation of myricetin-nicotinamide nanococrystals by top down and bottom up technologies. *Nanotechnology, 27*(39), 395601.
28. Yi, X. J., Wang, S. J., Gao, R. X., Cheng, F., & Liu, W. W. (2012). The effect of liposomes on the stability of 7-ethyl-10-hydroxycamptothecin. *Journal of Shenyang Pharmaceutical University, 29*(7), 491–496.
29. Niu, W. H., Feng, S. L., Zhou, Z. B., Zhang, W. N., Liu, Q., & Kong, L. Y. (2015). Preparation of black rice bran anthocyanin liposomes by reverse-phase evaporation combing with pH gradient. *Science and Technology of Food Industry, 36*(16), 238–242.
30. Wang, J. X., Lv, X. L., Li, J., & Zhu, L. (2018). Preparation and in vitro digestive stability of modified anthocyanin liposomes. *Food Science and Technology, 43*(01), 277–281.
31. Han, J., Tang, X., & Ba, D. C. (2004). Preparation of solid lipid nanoparticles containing volatile oil of Lignum dalbergia odorifera. *Chinese Patent Medicine, 06*, 6–9.
32. Vijayakumar, A., Baskaran, R., Baek, J. H., Sundaramoorthy, P., & Yoo, B. K. (2019). In vitro cytotoxicity and bioavailability of ginsenoside-modified nanostructured lipid carrier containing curcumin. *AAPS PharmSciTech, 20*, 88.
33. Rapalli, V. K., Kaul, V., Waghule, T., Gorantla, S., Sharma, S., Roy, A., et al. (2020). Curcumin loaded nanostructured lipid carriers for enhanced skin retained topical delivery: Optimization, scale-up, in-vitro characterization and assessment of ex-vivo skin deposition. *European Journal of Pharmaceutical Sciences, 152*, 105438.
34. Xiong, F., Xiong, C., Yao, J., Chen, X., & Gu, N. (2011). Preparation, characterization and evaluation of breviscapine lipid emulsions coated with monooleate–PEG–COOH. *International Journal of Pharmaceutics, 421*(2), 275–282.
35. Zhang, Z. L., Wang, Y. F., Rong, X. Z., Zhao, Z. H., Zhang, X. J., & Wang, G. F. (2017). Preparation of Houttuynia cordata volatile oil hydroxypropyl-β cyclodextrin inclusion compound. *Chinese Patent Medicine, 39*(05), 926–933.

36. Sun, Y., Zhou, Z. L., & Song, M. Y. (2007). Investigation on the stability of the volatile oil-β-cyclodextrin inclusion compound of mugwort. *Liaoning Journal of Traditional Chinese Medicine, 02*, 207–208.
37. Bao, Q. L., Xia, D. Z., Yang, J. L., Zhang, J. X., Dai, T., Li, G. D., & Yang, L. J. (2020). Study on inclusion behavior of cordycepin and dimethyl-β-cyclodextrin. *Journal of Yunnan University: Natural Sciences Edition, 42*(5), 958–965.
38. Li, C. C., Gong, F. R., Cheng, S. J., Han, X. X., & Zhang, L. L. (2014). Polymeric micelles for sustained release of curcumin: Preparation, characterization and in vivo evaluation of overcoming multidrug resistance for cytotoxic drug. *Journal of East China University of Science and Technology (Natural Science Edition), 40*(05), 18–23.
39. Tang, T., Hu, X., Liao, D., Liu, X., & Xiang, D. (2013). Mechanisms of microemulsion enhancing the oral bioavailability of puerarin: Comparison between oil-in-water and water-in-oil microemulsions using the single-pass intestinal perfusion method and a chylomicron flow blocking approach. *International Journal of Nanomedicine, 8*, 4415.
40. Luo, C., Yuan, M., Chen, M., Liu, S., Zhu, L., Huang, B., Liu, X., & Xiong, W. (2011). Pharmacokinetics, tissue distribution and relative bioavailability of puerarin solid lipid nanoparticles following oral administration. *International Journal of Pharmaceutics, 410* (1–2), 138–144.
41. Wei, S., Xie, J., Luo, Y., Ma, Y., Tang, S., Yue, P., & Yang, M. (2018). Hyaluronic acid based nanocrystals hydrogels for enhanced topical delivery of drug: A case study. *Carbohydrate Polymers, 202*, 64–71.
42. Ramalingam, P., Yoo, S. W., & Ko, Y. T. (2016). Nanodelivery systems based on mucoadhesive polymer coated solid lipid nanoparticles to improve the oral intake of food curcumin. *Food Research International, 84*, 113–119.
43. Yang, R., Chen, D., Li, M., Miao, F., Liu, P., & Tang, Q. (2014). 20(s)-ginsenoside Rg3-loaded magnetic human serum albumin nanospheres applied to HeLa cervical cancer cells in vitro. *Bio-Medical Materials and Engineering, 24*(6), 1991–1998.
44. Wang, L. L., Zu, M. H., Liu, Z. P., & Zhang, J. Q. (2017). Research progress of nanosuspension drug delivery system. *Chinese Pharmacy, 28*(10), 1415–1818.
45. Huang, T. T., Sheng, Y. P., Lu, L. K., Sun, X. Q., & Wang, X. T. (2020). High drug loading celastrol nanosuspensions: Preparation and in vitro evaluation. *Chinese Herbal Medicine, 51* (08), 2125–2133.
46. Xie, H., & He, J. Y. (2020). Preparation and quality evaluation of luteolin nanosuspension. *Tianjin Traditional Chinese Medicine, 37*(06), 711–716.
47. Liu, Y. D., & Xie, S. Y. (2020). Research progress on solid lipid nanocarriers promoting drug absorption. *Chinese Journal of Veterinary Medicine, 54*(3), 63–71.
48. Dwivedi, P., Khatik, R., Khandelwal, K., Taneja, I., Raju, K., Wahajuddin, S., Paliwal, S. K., Dwivedi, A. K., & Mishra, P. R. (2014). Pharmacokinetics study of arteether loaded solid lipid nanoparticles: An improved oral bioavailability in rats. *International Journal of Pharmaceutics, 466*(1–2), 321–327.
49. Lv, J. Y., & Liang, L. L. (2017). Preparation and pharmacokinetics of total panaxnotoginsen osides oral liposome in rats. *Zhongnan Pharmaceutical, 15*(07), 902–907.
50. Chu, C., Tong, S., Xu, Y., Wang, L., Fu, M., Ge, Y., Yu, J., & Xu, X. (2011). Proliposomes for oral delivery of dehydrosilymarin: Preparation and evaluation in vitro and in vivo. *Acta Pharmacologica Sinica, 32*(7), 973–980.
51. Chen, M., Mi, F., Liao, Z., Hsiao, C., Sonaje, K., Chung, M., Hsu, L., & Sung, H. (2013). Recent advances in chitosan-based nanoparticles for oral delivery of macromolecules. *Advanced Drug Delivery Reviews, 5*(6), 865–879.
52. Gao, C. F., Xia, J. X., Zhu, Y., Ren, H. W., Hong, C., Lu, W. G., & Wang, J. X. (2018). Application of nanotechnology in improving druggability of active ingredients of Chinese materia medica. *Chinese Herbal Medicine, 49*(12), 2754–2762.

53. Li, M. Y., Ni, J., & Yin, X. B. (2016). Research progress in preparation technology for improving oral bioavailability of traditional Chinese medicine. *Chinese Journal of Traditional Chinese Medicine, 34*(2), 307–311.
54. Zuo, W., Qu, W., Li, N., Yu, R., Hou, Y., Liu, Y., Gou, G., & Yang, J. (2018). Fabrication of multicomponent amorphous bufadienolides nanosuspension with wet milling improves dissolution and stability. *Artificial Cells, Nanomedicine, and Biotechnology, 46*(7), 1513–1522.
55. Yang, R., Chen, D., et al. (2014). 20 (s)-ginsenoside Rg3-loaded magnetic human serum albumin nanospheres applied to HeLa cervical cancer cells in vitro1. *Bio-medical Materials and Engineering, 24*, 1991–1998.
56. An, Y., Nie, F., Wang, Z., & Zhang, D. (2011). Preparation and characterization of realgar nanoparticles and their inhibitory effect on rat glioma cells. *International Journal of Nanomedicine, 6*, 3187–3194.
57. Mei, Z. N., Yang, X. L., & Yang, Y. J. (2003). Study on transdermal penetration and anti-inflammatory activity of triptolide solid lipid nanoparticles. *Chinese Pharmaceutical Journal, 38*(11), 854–857.
58. Guo, T., Cheng, N., Zhao, J., Hou, X., Zhang, Y., & Feng, N. (2019). Novel nanostructured lipid carriers-loaded dissolving microneedles for controlled local administration of aconitine. *International Journal of Pharmaceutics, 572*, 118741.
59. Shen, L., Zhang, Y., Wang, Q., Xu, L., & Feng, N. (2014). Enhanced in vitro and in vivo skin deposition of apigenin delivered using ethosomes. *International Journal of Pharmaceutics, 460* (1–2), 280–288.
60. Zhang, Y., Zhang, H., Zhang, K., Li, Z., Guo, T., Wu, T., Hou, X. F., & Feng, N. (2020). Co-hybridized composite nanovesicles for enhanced transdermal eugenol and cinnamaldehyde delivery and their potential efficacy in ulcerative colitis. *Nanomedicine: Nanotechnology, Biology and Medicine, 28*, 102212.
61. Wu, W., Zhang, H., Song, W., He, Y., Li, F., Zheng, Q., & Yang, M. (2011). Study on intranasal administration of traditional chinese medicine. *Chinese Journal of Experimental Traditional Medical Formulae, 17*(20), 288–292.
62. Yan, Y. L., Zhou, L. L., Ye, Y., & An, Q. (2007). Study on the absorption of ligustrazine phosphate liposome in rats in vivo nasal mucosa. *Chinese New Drugs and Clinical Pharmacology, 18*(5), 406–408.
63. Wu, M., Lu, X., & Zhang, X. (2007). Pharmacologic action of the Magnolia biondiiPamp volatile oil nanometer bangosome. *Journal of Shanghai Jiaotong University (Medical Science), 27*(4), 392–394.
64. Shi, Y. J., Shi, J. H., & Yang, M. (2015). Study on rat nasal mucosal absorption of Scutellaria baicalensis extract and its phospholipid complex and submicron emulsion preparation. *Chinese Materia Medica, 38*(10), 2172–2175.
65. Wu, P., Xu, R., Su, Z., Wei, P., Ling, Y., Yang, M., & Qin, Z. (2009). The nasal mucosa permeability and toxicity of baicalin carrier systems liposomes, β-cyclodextrin inclusion compound, and phospholipid complex. *Acta Pharmaceutica Sinica, 44*(04), 417–424.
66. Zhang, H., Chen, X., Wan, N., Yang, J., Wang, J., Zheng, Q., & Yang, M. (2010). Study on preparation of geniposide chitosan-coated poly lactic acid-glycolic acid nanoparticles and intranasal cavity delivery for brain targeting. *Chinese Journal of New Drugs and Clinical Remedies, 29*(06), 448–453.
67. Zhang, S., Guo, L., Shi, Y., Liang, Y., & Wang, Y. (2017). A study on preparation of high drug-loading Tanshinone II_A nasal submicron emulsion. *Shaanxi Traditional Chinese Medicine, 38* (09), 1298–1300.

The manufacturer's authorised representative in the EU is Springer Nature Customer Service Centre GmbH, Europaplatz 3, 69115 Heidelberg, Germany. If you have any concerns regarding our products, please contact ProductSafety@springernature.com

Printed and bound by CPI Group (UK) Ltd, Croydon, CR0 4YY

30/09/2026

02225245-0009